Clinical Nursing Practices

Commissioning Editor: Ninette Premdas
Development Editors: Mairi McCubbin, Fiona Conn
Project Manager: Elouise Ball
Design Direction: Erik Bigland
Illustration Manager: Merlyn Harvey
Illustrator: Cactus, Paul Bernson

Clinical Nursing Practices

Edited by

Elizabeth M. Jamieson BSc (Hons) MSC RN ONC RCT RNT
Senior Lecturer, School of Nursing, Midwifery and Community Health,
Glasgow Caledonian University, Glasgow, UK

Janice M. McCall BA RN
Former Lecturer, School of Nursing, Midwifery and Community Health,
Glasgow Caledonian University, Glasgow, UK

Lesley A. Whyte BA MPhil RN DN RNT
Lecturer, School of Nursing, Midwifery and Community Health,
Glasgow Caledonian University, Glasgow, UK

FIFTH EDITION

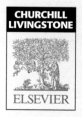

Edinburgh   London   New York   Oxford   Philadelphia   St Louis   Sydney   Toronto
2007

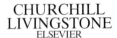

CHURCHILL
LIVINGSTONE
ELSEVIER

First edition 1988
Second edition 1992
Third edition 1997
Fourth edition 2002
Fifth edition 2007
  Reprinted 2007

ISBN 13: 978 0 443 10270 7
ISBN 10: 0 443 10270 8

British Library Cataloguing in Publication Data
A catalogue record for this book is available from the British Library

Library of Congress Cataloging in Publication Data
A catalog record for this book is available from the Library of Congress

Note
Knowledge and best practice in this field are constantly changing. As new research and experience
broaden our knowledge, changes in practice, treatment and drug therapy may become necessary or
appropriate. Readers are advised to check the most current information provided (i) on procedures
featured or (ii) by the manufacturer of each product to be administered, to verify the recommended dose
or formula, the method and duration of administration, and contraindications. It is the responsibility of
the practitioner, relying on their own experience and knowledge of the patient, to make diagnoses, to
determine dosages and the best treatment for each individual patient, and to take all appropriate safety
precautions. To the fullest extent of the law, neither the publisher nor the editors assume any liability
for any injury and/or damage to persons or property arising out or related to any use of the material
contained in this book.   *The Publisher*

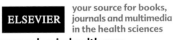

Working together to grow
libraries in developing countries

www.elsevier.com | www.bookaid.org | www.sabre.org

ELSEVIER   BOOK AID International   Sabre Foundation

ELSEVIER   your source for books,
journals and multimedia
in the health sciences

www.elsevierhealth.com

The
publisher's
policy is to use
**paper manufactured
from sustainable forests**

Printed in China

Contents

Contents

Contributors

Alison Brown MSc, BSc(Hons), RGN, RNT
Lecturer, School of Nursing and Midwifery,
  The Robert Gordon University, Aberdeen, UK
25 Moving and Handling

Mary Dowds BSc, RGN RCNT
Lecturer, School of Nursing, Midwifery and Community Health,
Glasgow Caledonian University, Glasgow, UK
13 Eardrops: Instillation of; 16 Exercises: Active and Passive;
17 Eye Care; 28 Nutrition; 37 Skin Care; 41 Toileting

Kate Goodhand BA(Hons), PGCE(FE), PGCE(TLT), NT, RGN
Lecturer, School of Nursing and Midwifery,
  The Robert Gordon University, Aberdeen, UK
2 Administration of Medicines

Pauline Hamilton MN, DipAsthma, RNT, RCNT, RGN, RMN
Lecturer, Adult Nursing, School of Nursing,
  Midwifery and Community Health, Glasgow Caledonian University,
  Glasgow, UK
12 Chest Drainage: Underwater Seal; 23 Lumbar Puncture;
26 Nebuliser Therapy

Dora C. Howes BSc, MN, PGCert, RGN, NDN
Lecturer, School of Nursing, Midwifery and Community Health,
  Glasgow Caledonian University, Glasgow, UK
1 Frameworks for Practice

Neil Johnson BA(Hons), MSc, PGCTLT, RGN
Lecturer, School of Nursing and Midwifery, The Robert Gordon University,
  Aberdeen, UK
6 Body Temperature; 34 Pulse/Radial Pulses; 42 Tracheostomy Care

Heather McAskill BA, RGN, DipDN, PGCert HELT
Lecturer, School of Nursing and Midwifery, The Robert Gordon University,
  Aberdeen, UK
2 Administration of Medicines

Evelyn McElhinney BSc, SPQ Anaesthetics, RGN
Lecturer,
  Glasgow Caledonian University
  Glasgow, UK
18 Gastric Aspiration; 32 Preoperative Nursing Care; 33 Postoperative Nursing Care

Alison McLennan BSc, MSc, RGN, RNMH, RNT
Senior Lecturer, School of Nursing and Midwifery, The Robert Gordon University,
  Aberdeen, UK
25 Moving and Handling

Sarah Murdoch BA, MPH, SRN, ENBCert329
Public Health Infection Control Nurse, Forth Valley NHS Board, Stirling, UK
19 Infection Prevention and Control: Principles of; 22 Isolation Nursing

Elizabeth S. Pirie BSc, MSc, RGN, PGCert, ILTM
Transfusion Nurse Specialist, Scottish National Blood Transfusion Service,
  Edinburgh, UK
5 Blood Transfusion; 7 Bone Marrow Aspiration

Theresa E. Price BSc (Hons), MSc, RN CertEdFE
Lecturer, School of Nursing, Midwifery and Community Health,
  Glasgow Caledonian University, Glasgow, UK
*4 Blood Pressure; 11 Central Venous Pressure; 21 Intravenous Therapy; 27 Neurological
Examination; 29 Oxygen Therapy; 36 Respiration; 44 Unconscious Patient*

Sarah Renton BSc, Specialist Nursing(Ortho), PGCE, RGN, DipN
Lecturer, School of Nursing, Midwifery and Community Health,
  Glasgow Caledonian University, Glasgow, UK
*9 Care of the Deceased Person; 24 Mouth Care; 43 Transfer of Patients Between
  Care Settings; 45 Urine Testing*

Fiona R.T. Rodgers MSc, RN,ALS, EPLS
District Nursing Sister, Clydebank Health Centre, Clydebank, UK
*3 Blood Glucose Monitoring; 10 Catheterisation: Urinary; 14 Ear Syringing; 15
  Enema; 35 Rectal Examination; 40 Suppositories; 48 Venepuncture; 49 Wound Care*

Elizabeth Simpson BSc., RN, ALS, EPLS
*Lecturer in Adult Nursing, Glasgow Caledonian University,
  Glasgow, UK.*
Formerly, Resuscitation offices, NHS Greater Glasgow and Clyde.
8 Cardiopulmonary Resuscitation

Mary Speirs RGN, BA(Hons)
Stoma Care/Colorectal Clinical Nurse Specialist, Monklands Hospital, Airdrie, UK
39 Stoma Care

Alison Ward RGN, SCMDipDiabetes
Practice Sister, Shaftesbury Medical Practice, Glasgow, UK
*3 Blood Glucose Monitoring; 38 Specimen Collection; 46 Vaginal Examination;
47 Vaginal Ring Pessary Insertion*

Preface

The first edition of this book was published in 1988. Subsequent editions have evolved in response to the many changes that have taken and are taking place in nurse education and practice; however, the core philosophy of this book is still to encourage readers to deliver the highest quality care to each individual patient.

As we are no longer in the front line of delivering nursing care, for this edition we have taken on the role of editors. A team of clinical and education experts has been commissioned to update the core practices, advise us of any obsolete ones and incorporate new ones.

Previous editions have linked each practice to the Roper–Logan–Tierney model for nursing. This link has been removed in this edition and a chapter giving a brief overview of a variety of frameworks for practice has been included. We hope that this will make the text more flexible and therefore more easily incorporated onto the framework used by the reader.

We have continued to emphasise the importance of current evidence-based practice by updating the references, including new ones and adding some useful website addresses. To encourage reflective practice, self-assessment questions have been developed. We have also added a section called Additional Information, which does not relate directly to the technical practice but should be considered as part of a holistic approach to care.

Some practices such as Moving and Handling, Cardiopulmonary Resuscitation and Blood Transfusion have been written with general descriptions rather than detailed guidelines and rationale. The editors acknowledge that these particular practices are likely to evolve within the lifetime of this edition.

We very much appreciate the enthusiasm, suggestions and material from our contributing team and hope this edition will continue to be useful to all our readers, whatever the setting.

Elizabeth M. Jamieson
Janice M. McCall
Lesley A. Whyte

Practice 1
Frameworks for Practice

Introduction

Nursing, as Jamieson et al (2002) suggest, is constantly evolving in an effort to meet the demands of health care in the 21st century. Central to that process is the need for nurses to deliver appropriate care in an educated and skilled manner (NHS Education for Scotland 2005). Given the increasing complexity in nursing roles and practice (Pearson et al 2005), the context within which the practice of nursing takes place is of paramount importance. This chapter will look at a variety of frameworks for practice that have been developed in order to assist that process. As it is recognised that this book will be used as a source of reference, rather than read from cover to cover, a broad overview of some commonly used traditional and contemporary frameworks are offered here. These are:

- Roper, Logan & Tierney model
- Orem's self-care framework
- Team nursing
- Primary nursing and the named-nurse concept
- Evidence-based practice
- Multi-disciplinary working and integrated-care pathways.

Roper, Logan & Tierney model

As a starting point it is useful to look at the Roper, Logan & Tierney model of nursing. This model was introduced in 1980 and represents the first British conceptual framework for practice. It is still widely used while becoming increasing well known internationally (Pearson et al 2005). The model was developed at a time when clinical practice during pre-registration education was seen as 'increasingly fragmented' (Tierney 1998:78). There was a need to design a framework which assisted learners to 'develop a way of thinking about nursing' (Tierney 1998:79), that enabled them to provide effective and compassionate patient care within a variety of healthcare settings and to different patient/client groups whilst recognising their age, need and background (Roper et al 1980). It was regarded as a concerted attempt to move away from the bio-medical model that had prevailed up until that point (Tierney 1998) and as a vehicle for distinctive professional recognition (Wimpenny 2002).

The framework itself is based on a 'model of living', which recognises an inextricable link between health, illness and lifestyle (Tierney 1998). The need for nursing intervention is normally considered to be on a short-term basis with an outcome emphasis on minimal disruption to people's established lifestyles (Tierney 1998). Prevention rather than cure is promoted (Aggleton & Chalmers 2000). Roper et al (2001) acknowledge that it is impossible to represent the complexities of living in a simplistic model so they attempt to identify only the main features of it. Roper et al (2001:13–14) describe five main conceptual components:

1. Activities of living (ALs).
2. Lifespan.

3. Dependence/independence continuum.
4. Factors influencing the ALs.
5. Individuality of living.

The focus is on the individual and their participation in the process of living throughout their lifespan. People move in a unidirectional mode from birth to death and this progression can involve moving from a state of dependence to independence depending on age, circumstances and the environment (Pearson et al 2005).

To clarify the process of living further, twelve specific 'activities of living' are identified (Roper et al 1980). It is not the intention of this overview to address each of the activities individually; rather a broad-based consideration is provided. If you are interested in exploring them in greater depth, there are a number of texts by authors such as Aggleton & Chalmers (2000), Pearson et al (2005) and Roper et al (2001) themselves, which may be of use. The activities identified by Roper et al (1980) range from those that are essential to human life to those that enhance its quality. Some have a biological basis whereas others are more socially and culturally determined (Aggleton & Chalmers 2000). However, common to them all is the possibility that they may be influenced by physical, physiological, sociocultural, environmental and politico-economic forces (Pearson et al 2005). Consequently, a person will be affected by a unique range of influencing factors that determine the way he/she lives and how he/she experiences illness.

Use of a concept such as 'activities of living' has the advantage of being familiar to a variety of allied health professionals and as such is important for reminding nurses that they are part of a wider multi-disciplinary team, capable of delivering optimum standards of care (Jamieson et al 2002). However, in order to gain an appreciation of how the model appears when all the contributing dimensions are placed together, it is easiest to view a diagrammatic representation of it (Fig. 1.1).

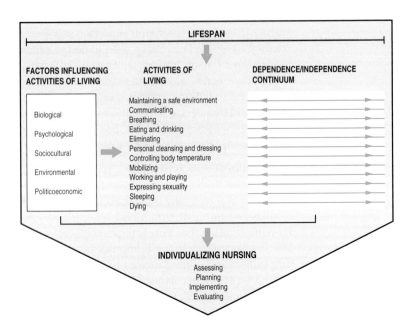

FIGURE 1.1
The model of nursing

Application of the model directs nursing intervention towards the process of 'helping people to prevent, alleviate, solve or cope with problems (actual or potential) related to the Activities of Living' (Roper et al 1990:37 cited in Tierney 1998:79). The framework makes explicit the relationship of the practice of nursing to the individual patient and the wider theoretical base of nursing (Jamieson et al 2002). While the model may not be considered to be highly original as it draws upon ideas contained within Henderson's classic definition of nursing (Tierney 1998), it is to be appreciated for its clarity, providing an enduring contribution for nurses to take forward (Pearson et al 2005).

Orem's self-care framework

In a similar, but slightly different context to that of Roper, Logan & Tierney's model, a framework for nursing emerged from the USA that also focused on individual independence. This framework is also widely used and is deemed to be popular with British and American nurses alike (Pearson et al 2005). The work of a well-known and respected nursing theorist, Dorothea Orem, the framework was also developed in a climate where external influences on nurse education programmes such as medicine prevailed (Phillips 1977 cited in Fawcett 2000), and where there was a need to identify nursing as a discrete art and science (Fawcett 2000).

The framework, which was first published in 1971, is similar to that of Roper, Logan & Tierney in so far as it draws upon the theory of human needs (Meleis 1991 cited in Pearson et al 2005), however it differs in the interpretation of 'independence'. For Orem (1995) the notion of independence may be regarded as 'self-care' focusing on the ability humans have to be self-determining. People endeavour to be self-caring either on their own merits or with the assistance of friends or family (Walsh 1998). An inability in any area preventing the achievement of this goal would result in a 'self-care deficit' requiring nursing intervention (Walsh 1998). Interestingly, it is not only the ability to self-care that is important for Orem, but also the ability to care for others. Her model considers the capacity to care for others as integral to human behaviour (Walsh 1998) and in this sense legitimises the role of the nurse.

People within Orem's framework are regarded as whole entities rather than the amalgamation of a number of subsystems (Aggleton & Chalmers 2000). They are capable of independent thought and action giving them the potential to acquire the knowledge, skills and motivation to care for themselves, their families and dependants. This capacity to self-regulate life, health and wellbeing is referred to as 'self-care agency' (Cox & Taylor 2005) and is dependent upon a number of factors including age, gender, developmental stage, socio-economic status, cultural orientation, environmental influences and adequacy of resources (Orem 1991 cited in Aggleton & Chalmers 2000). The acknowledgement of influences upon the individual in relation to health is similar to the Roper, Logan & Tierney model, but instead of the individual moving along a dependence/independence continuum, a balance is sought between needs and abilities. When a mid-point is reached, which is of equal weighting either side, a state of health is deemed to have been achieved (Fig. 1.2).

Like the Roper, Logan & Tierney model, Orem identifies a significant number of needs, which she entitles 'universal self-care needs'. She identifies eight in total

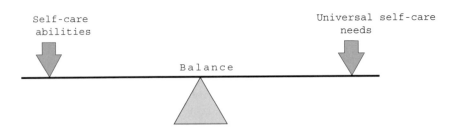

FIGURE 1.2
A healthy individual

encompassing physical, psychological and social dimensions. However, in contrast to Roper, Logan & Tierney, Orem does not specify any particular way of meeting these needs and accepts that individuals will vary in the extent to which they may wish to satisfy them (Aggleton & Chalmers 2000). Indeed, her theory of self-care deficit proposes that individuals need to undertake a number of actions in a timely and adequate manner each day to maintain their health, life and well-being (Cox & Taylor 2005).

In addition to universal self-care needs, health deviation and developmental self-care needs are identified within Orem's framework (Aggleton & Chalmers 2000). Health deviation self-care needs reflect the extra demands placed on the ability to self-care by illness, while developmental self-care needs acknowledge an individual's stage of growth and development (Aggleton & Chalmers 2000). The need for nursing intervention, therefore, arises when any of these needs (singly or in combination) shift the balance away from the healthy mid-point previously described.

The diversity of dependency acknowledged within the framework indicates that nurses not only have a caring role, but they may also be required to be a health educator (Walsh 1998). It is a framework, therefore, that finds appeal from healthcare professionals working in the areas of health promotion and disease prevention alike (Pearson et al 2005). This is an important consideration given contemporary thinking about nursing and its future direction (Royal College of Nursing 2004). Similarly, the framework places a focus on the family (Taylor 2001) and in that respect reflects the current World Health Organization (WHO) 'Health for all' policy framework (World Health Organization, 1998), which is receiving widespread interest and attention.

While what appears here may be viewed as simplistic, it is worth noting that, in reality, Orem's framework is a complex one and should not be underestimated. For a more detailed insight into the framework, authors such as Fawcett (2000) and Marriner Tomey & Alligood (2005) are advised. Equally, the frameworks discussed so far are not in themselves exclusive, there are others including Roy's adaptation model (1976), Neuman's systems model (1982), King's goal-attainment model (1981) and Peplau's developmental model (1952), to name but a few. While acknowledging their importance, these models tend not to be encountered as frequently as those mentioned above and as such are not discussed here.

Team nursing

The development, by theorists, of models and frameworks for practice in nursing are important as they offer clarity and identity (Tierney 1998), however they are not the only frames of reference used by nurses when practising (Fawcett 2003). Historically, nursing has been organised either by assigning patients or tasks (Tiedeman & Lookinland 2004). One approach that has utilised both is team nursing. Team nursing emerged in the 1950s as a model of care delivery that eased the shortage of nurses following World War II while utilising the available, differing levels of skilled healthcare workers (Tiedeman & Lookinland 2004). The model of care requires the formation of a team led by an experienced, qualified member of nursing staff (Brooker & Nicol 2003). The underlying philosophy is that a team of people working collaboratively together can deliver better quality care than the same group of individuals working independently (Tiedeman & Lookinland 2004).

The team is responsible for the care of a group of patients throughout their stay in hospital (Brooker & Nicol 2003) and, as such, has a collective responsibility for all aspects of the patients' care. The focus of the duties by team members, as indicated previously, may be task or patient orientated depending on the style of implementation adopted by the team leader (Tiedeman & Lookinland 2004). The team leader allocates care duties in accordance with the complexity of the patient needs and the level of ability of the caregiver (Tiedeman & Lookinland 2004). While being an attractive framework for practice, as it acknowledges and effectively utilises the skill mix within contemporary healthcare, it is also open to some criticism. A team's responsibility to its patients lasts only for the duration of its shift and a patient–team assignment may vary from shift to shift or adopt a permanent team allocation for the duration of the hospital stay (Tiedeman & Lookinland 2004). This disparity, along with the differing modes of deployment of staff, may lead to care of a variable standard and quality. Equally, the fact that the team, and not a named individual, has responsibility for all aspects of patient care can create a vagueness surrounding the line of accountability (Brooker & Nicol 2003). Not withstanding these weaknesses, it is a framework for practice that is still widely used and readily recognisable on entering clinical areas.

Primary nursing and the named-nurse concept

In recognition that the organisation of nursing staff and patient care can affect the quality and outcome of the care delivered (Ryan 1998), a framework for practice was developed that placed the individual at the centre of caring while emphasising the autonomy, accountability and authority of the nurse engaged in the process. Primary nursing may be described as an approach whereby a nurse provides comprehensive, continuous, co-ordinated and individualised care to a patient who is assigned to him/her for the duration of their hospital stay (Manthey 1992, Ryan 1998). In practice this means that the primary nurse has the 'responsibility and authority to assess, plan, organise, implement, co-ordinate and evaluate care in collaboration with the patient and his/her family' (Tiedeman & Lookinland 2004:295). Decisions are made at the bedside rather than centrally with the nurse having the opportunity to make independent clinical judgements while being accountable for the action(s) taken.

The primary nurse assumes 24-hour responsibility and accountability for the patient and when not available transfers these duties to an associate nurse who follows the set plan of care (Brooker & Nicol 2003, Tiedeman & Lookinland 2004). The advantage of the approach is the small numbers of patients under the care of a nurse at any one time. This facilitates 'hands on' patient involvement and holistic care addressing physical, psychological, emotional and spiritual needs while offering the potential to develop a good patient relationship with real knowledge and understanding (Brooker & Nicol 2003). Equally, primary nursing resolves many of the previously mentioned issues surrounding the team approach. The approach is also attractive in its flexibility. It is not simply confined to hospitalised patients but is equally applicable in the community where nurses have a caseload and small teams of nurses and healthcare assistants are available to care for patients (Brooker & Nicol 2003).

The individualised nature of the care given and the one-to-one nurse–patient relationship that is formed promotes the concept as a philosophy as well as a framework for practice (Reed 1988, Manthey 1988 cited in Ryan 1998) and, as such, may be viewed as appealing. Indeed, it could be regarded as the precursor to the concept of 'named nursing', introduced by the British Government in 1991 (Steven 1999). Against a background of consumerism, market forces and capitalism, the government introduced a 'Patient's Charter' in which it was stated that a patient should have a named, qualified nurse, midwife or health visitor who would be responsible for their nursing or midwifery care (Steven 1999). Implicit within the declaration is the notion of continuing responsibility and accountability causing the approach to closely resemble primary nursing. This may account for the synonymous and interchangeable use of the terms.

The named nurse, like the primary nurse, is normally a qualified registered nurse who focuses on assessing, planning and evaluating individualised care. Such are the similarities between the two approaches that named nursing has been considered to be a diluted version of primary nursing being implemented when resources are scarce (Steven 1999). However, there are distinct differences between the two. For example, named nursing is a framework for practice emanating from governmental policy imposed upon nurses whereas primary nursing was the result of enthusiastic practising nurses looking to develop the quality of their practice (Steven 1999). Similarly, primary nursing assumes holistic care giving whereas named nursing assumes accountability for care, but not necessarily the scope of that care. Indeed, there is the possibility that while a clinical area claims to employ primary nursing it may actually be named nursing that is in operation as Ryan (1998) suggests there is considerable variation in the extent to which primary nursing is practised.

As a framework for practice, the effectiveness of primary nursing is variable with evidence being inconclusive (Ryan 1998) and the resources demanded problematic where areas have high staff turnover (Brooker & Nicol 2003). Nevertheless, primary nursing is practised widely and as such you are likely to encounter it or its derivative at some stage of your professional career.

Evidence-based practice

Tiedeman & Lookinland (2004) describe the driving forces behind the implementation of the primary nursing care framework for practice as including the possibility of using an individualised problem-solving approach and the application of scientific methods. Given the changes within the NHS in the

1990s emphasising cost-effectiveness, value for money and quality (White 1997), problem solving and applying scientific methods have become skills of the utmost importance and evidence-based practice encourages the practitioner to use both. While not being directly associated with primary nursing, evidence-based practice provides nurses with an approach to care that is based on finding, appraising and applying scientific evidence to the treatment and management of patients (Hammer 1999 cited in Dale 2005). The underlying premise is that patients are given high-quality, clinically effective care within the resources available (Colyer & Kamath 1999).

Clinical problems are turned into questions and then systematically appraised using contemporary research findings (Rosenberg & Donald 1995). The outcome of the appraisal, along with individual clinical expertise and patient preference, is then used as the basis for care (Sackett et al 2000). While the approach is commonly referred to as evidence-based practice, it may also be presented as medicine- or evidence-informed nursing (Rosenberg & Donald 1995, Sackett et al 1996, McSherry et al 2002).

Implicit within the approach is the portrayal of the nurse as a 'knowledgeable doer'. He/she is expected to understand the importance of practice based on evidence, be familiar with the research process and have the skills and expertise to implement and manage care in such a way as to ensure that it is done in the right way for the right patient at the right time (Royal College of Nursing 1996, Muir Gray 1997, McSherry et al 2002). In effect, nurses must be able to justify their care interventions and no longer rely on ritual and/or tradition (McSherry et al 2002). By doing so, the path to the professional recognition of nursing as a distinct and unique discipline may be progressed.

In carrying out the process of evidence-based practice, nurses have a hierarchy of five levels of evidence to draw upon to appraise research (McSherry et al 2002). The hierarchy is determined by research design, whereby studies that incorporate measures to minimise the researcher from influencing the findings are ranked top (McSherry et al 2002). Thus, experimental approaches in the format of well-designed randomised controlled trials are placed at the top of the hierarchy with expert opinion, committee reports and descriptive studies at the bottom (Dale 2005). Such is the importance placed on the type of evidence accessed, that the highest level is accorded a gold standard, which then attaches a value system to the hierarchy.

The resultant emphasis towards randomised controlled trials is problematic for nursing as important evidence to guide practice comes from across the spectrum of research and not simply from experimental quantitative approaches. For example, understanding patients' experience of an illness episode is invaluable when providing care for other patients in similar circumstances (Dale 2005). This type of research is most likely to be qualitative in nature and so may be given a low value, if not excluded from the hierarchy altogether. This means that there is the potential for substantial areas of nursing knowledge and clinical expertise to be excluded in preference to purely experimental evidence (Dale 2005). This is concerning as nursing has a limited amount of quantitative studies with which to underpin practice (McSherry et al 2002). Nonetheless, the framework is an important one for nurses to be aware of because contemporary healthcare is being determined by evidence-based practice (Dale 2005) and nurses have a pivotal role within this arena (Pearson & Craig 2002).

Multi-disciplinary working and integrated-care pathways

A significant strength of evidence-based practice is that it can be applied across professional boundaries (White 1997). Multi-disciplinary working is very much the 'buzz word' for the 21st century emanating from key policy documents such as 'Partnership for Care' (Scottish Executive 2003), 'The NHS Plan: a plan for investment, a plan for reform' (Department of Health 2000), 'Our National Health: a plan for action, a plan for change' (Scottish Executive 2000) and 'The new NHS: modern and dependable' (Department of Health 1998). While there are many forms in which multi-disciplinary or inter-professional working may take place, one that involves evidence-based care and is most likely to be encountered in clinical practice, is that of an integrated-care pathway (ICP). An ICP is 'a tool which is locally agreed, multi-disciplinary, based on guidelines and evidence if available, for a specific patient/client group forming all or part of the clinical record documenting the care given while facilitating the evaluation of outcomes for continuous quality improvement' (National Association Pathways 1998:1 cited by Overill 1998:93). Also known as care maps, coordinated care pathways, anticipated recovery pathways, critical pathways, multi-disciplinary pathways of care, collaborative care pathways and care protocols (Kitchiner & Bundred 1996 cited in Nyatanga & Holliman 2005), ICPs offer a structured approach to developing and implementing local care protocols based on clinical evidence (Campbell et al 1998, Simmons 2002).

As a framework for practice an ICP provides a context in which care is specified and evaluated with the purpose of improving the quality of clinical practice (Nyatanga & Holliman 2005). The ICP documentation replaces part or all traditional records of care such as nursing care plans, while providing clear guidance on the roles and responsibilities of the multi-disciplinary team. However, it must meet the professional needs of all those involved in the delivery of care (Nyatanga & Holliman 2005). In this respect nurses will find themselves working alongside doctors and allied healthcare professionals such as physiotherapists and dieticians. Working together has the advantage of promoting communication, discussion and decision making between professions, which is regarded as essential in the current climate, but it can also lead to a perceived loss of individual professional judgement in particular circumstances (Campbell et al 1998). Therefore, all those involved in the development of an ICP must be clear about the identified need.

The purpose of an ICP is to outline the expected pathway of care of a patient with a specific clinical condition by describing the required tasks, sequence, timing and member of the multi-disciplinary healthcare team needed to carry them out (Campbell et al 1998). The ICP itself is either condition specific, which means that it may consider the management of a patient who has been diagnosed as having a condition such as a myocardial infarction or a stroke, or it can be symptom based, where the focus is on the investigation and treatment of a specific symptom such as pain (Nyatanga & Holliman 2005). Occasionally, specific procedures or therapeutic guidelines may be included (Nyatanga & Holliman 2005).

Given the particular nature of the focus, ICPs are not suitable for all types of patients although Campbell et al (1998) indicate that they exist for over 45 different conditions or procedures. They are easier to implement when the expected pathway that most people will follow is known and predictable. Where diseases are complex, for example, with multiple pathologies, or where clinical judgement varies, an ICP is much more difficult to create (Nyatanga & Holliman 2005). Nevertheless, when implemented appropriately, ICPs have the overall benefit of providing care that is patient focused, cost effective, based on evidence and multi-disciplinary.

Having described a number of frameworks for practice, which nurses may encounter in their professional careers, it is clear that irrespective of the framework utilised, the role of the nurse is pivotal in delivering patient-centred care. As Kitson (1999:46) states, 'Nursing is the "cement" in the structure that keeps the different parts of healthcare delivery together'. The framework may be the binding agent, but the practice skills carried out by nurses provide a significant proportion of the constituent ingredients.

This brief overview of frameworks for practice has given a flavour of current thinking on underlying philosophies for care delivery. The intention is that the reader will integrate the following clinical practices within an appropriate framework to help ensure the delivery of holistic care.

References

Aggleton P, Chalmers H 2000 Nursing models and nursing practice, 2nd edn. Palgrave, Houndsmills, Basingstoke, UK

Brooker C, Nicol M (eds) 2003 Nursing adults: the practice of caring. Mosby, Edinburgh, pp 10–15

Campbell H, Hotchkiss R, Bradshaw N et al 1998 Integrated care pathways. British Medical Journal 316: 133–137

Colyer H, Kamath P 1999 Evidence-based practice. A philosophical and political analysis: some matters for consideration by professional practitioners. Journal of Advanced Nursing 29(1): 188–193

Cox KR, Taylor SG 2005 Orem's self-care nursing theory: pediatric asthma as exemplar. Nursing Science Quarterly 18(3): 249–257

Dale AE 2005 Evidence-based practice: compatibility with nursing. Nursing Standard 19(40): 48–53

Department of Health 1998 The new NHS: modern and dependable. The Stationery Office, London

Department of Health 2000 The NHS Plan: a plan for investment, a plan for reform. The Stationery Office, London

Fawcett J 2000 Analysis and evaluation of conceptual models of nursing, 3rd edn. FA Davis Company, Philadelphiaea, PA

Fawcett J 2003 On bed baths and conceptual models of nursing. Journal of Advanced Nursing 44(3): 229–230

Hammer S 2005 Evidence-based practice. In: Hammer S, Collinson G (eds) Achieving evidence-based practice: a handbook for practitioners. Baillière Tindall, Edinburgh

Jamieson E, McCall J, Whyte LA 2002 Clinical nursing practices, 4th edn. Churchill Livingstone, Edinburgh

King I 1981 A theory for nursing: systems, concepts process. Wiley, New York

Kitchiner D, Bundred P 1996 Integrated care pathways. Archives of Disease in Childhood 75(2): 166–168

Kitson A 1999 The essence of nursing. Nursing Standard 13(23): 42–46

Manthey M 1988 Can primary nurses survive? American Journal of Nursing 8(5): 644–648

Manthey M 1992 The practice of primary nursing. Kings Fund, London

Marriner Tomey A, Alligood MR 2005 Nursing theorists and their work, 6th edn. Mosby, Missouri

McSherry R, Simmons M, Pearce P 2002 An introduction to evidence-informed nursing. In: McSherry R, Simmons M, Abbot P (eds) Evidence-informed nursing: a guide for clinical nurses. Routledge, London

Meleis AI 1991 Theoretical nursing: development and progress, 2nd edn. Lippincott, Philadelphiapa, PA

Muir Gray JA 1997 Evidence-based healthcare: how to make health policy and management decisions. Churchill Livingstone, New York

National Association Pathways (ed) Definitions of a pathway. National Association Pathways Newsletter, Spring:1. In: Overill S (ed) A practical guide to care pathways. Journal of Integrated Care in Practice 2: 93–98

Neuman B 1982 The Neuman systems model: application to nursing education and practice. Appleton-Century-Croft, New York

NHS Education for Scotland 2005 NHS Education for Scotland strategic work plan 2005–2008. NHS, Edinburgh

Nyatanga T, Holliman R 2005 Integrated care pathways (ICPs) and infection control. Clinical Governance: An International Journal 10(2): 106–117

Orem DE 1991 Nursing: concepts for practice, 4th edn. CV Mosby, St Louis, MO

Orem DE 1995 Nursing: concepts for practice, 5th edn. CV Mosby, St Louis, MO

Pearson A, Vaughan B, FitzGerald M 2005 Nursing models for practice, 3rd edn. Butterworth Heinemann, Edinburgh

Pearson M, Craig JV 2002 Evidence-based practice in nursing. In: Craig JV, Smyth RL (eds) The evidence-based practice manual for nurses. Churchill Livingstone, Edinburgh

Peplau HE 1952 Interpersonal relations in nursing. GR Putman, New York

Phillips JR 1977 Nursing systems and nursing models, Image 9: 4–7. In: Fawcett J (ed) Analysis and evaluation of conceptual models of nursing, 3rd edn. FA Davis Company, Philadelphia, PA

Reed S 1988 A comparison of nurse-related behaviour, philosophy of care and job satisfaction in team and primary nursing. Journal of Advanced Nursing 13(3): 383–395

Roper N, Logan W, Tierney AJ 1980 The elements of nursing. Churchill Livingstone, Edinburgh

Roper N, Logan W, Tierney AJ 1990 The elements of nursing: a model for nursing based on a model of living, 3rd edn. Churchill Livingstone, Edinburgh, p 37

Roper N, Logan W, Tierney AJ 2001 The Roper, Logan, Tierney model of nursing: based on activities of living. Churchill Livingstone, Edinburgh

Rosenberg WMC, Donald A 1995 Evidence based medicine: an approach to clinical problem-solving. British Medical Journal 310(6987): 1122–1126

Roy C 1976 Introduction to nursing: an adaptation model. Prentice Hall, Old Tappin, NJ

Royal College of Nursing 1996 Clinical effectiveness: the Royal College of Nursing guide. RCN, London

Royal College of Nursing 2004 The future nurse: the RCN vision. RCN, London

Ryan AA 1998 Developing an audit tool for primary nursing. Journal of Clinical Nursing 7(5): 417–423

Sackett DL, Rosenberg WMC, Muir Gray JA et al 1996 Evidence based medicine: what it is and what it isn't. British Medical Journal 312(7023): 71–72

Sackett DL, Strauss SE, Richardson WS et al 2000 Evidence-based medicine. How to practice and teach EBM, 2nd edn. Churchill Livingstone, London

Scottish Executive 2000 Our National Health: a plan for action, a plan for change. The Stationery Office, Edinburgh

Scottish Executive 2003 Partnership for care. The Stationery Office, Edinburgh

Simmons M 2002 Benefits of research to nursing practice. In: McSherry R, Simmons M, Abbot P (eds) Evidence-informed nursing: a guide for clinical nurses. Routledge, London

Steven A 1999 Named nursing: in whose best interest? Journal of Advanced Nursing 29(2): 341–347

Taylor SG 2001 Orem's general theory of nursing and families. Nursing Science Quarterly 14(1): 7–9

Tiedeman ME, Lookinland S 2004 traditional models of care: what have we learned? Journal of Nursing Administration 34(6): 291–297

Tierney AJ 1998 Nursing models: extant or extinct? Journal of Advanced Nursing 28(1): 77–85

Walsh M 1998 Models and critical pathways in clinical nursing, 2nd edn. Baillière Tindall, London

White SJ 1997 Evidence-based practice and nursing: the new panacea? British Journal of Nursing 6(3): 175–178

World Health Organization 1998 Health 21. WHO Regional Offices for Europe, Copenhagen, Denmark

Wimpenny P 2002 The meaning of models to practising nurses. Journal of Advanced Nursing 40(3): 346–354

Practice 2
Administration of Medicines

There are seven parts to this section:

1 **Principles of medicine administration**

2 **Routes of medicine administration**

3 **Immunisation**

4 **Anaphylaxis**

5 **Syringe driver pumps**

6 **Patient-controlled analgesic devices**

7 **Patient compliance devices**

Learning outcomes

By the end of this section, you should know how to:
- support and prepare the patient for this practice
- collect and prepare the equipment
- carry out the administration of medicines safely and accurately
- educate the patient on follow-up care.

Background knowledge required

A review of:
- the pharmacology of the medicine to be administered (Downie et al 2003, McGavock 2005)
- the metric system of volume and weight used in the dose calculation of a medication (Lapham & Agar 2003, Downie et al 2006)
- Medicines Act (1968) as amended
- the Misuse of Drugs Act (1971 reprinted 1985), including all its amendments
- the 'Guidelines for the administration of medicines' (Nursing and Midwifery Council 2004b)
- the Medicinal Products: Prescription by Nurses Act (1992)
- the document 'Immunisation against infectious disease' (Department of Health 1996)
- 'Guidelines for records and record keeping' (Nursing and Midwifery Council 2005)
- health authority policy regarding the patient's medicine prescription and recording documents, the administration of drugs, the disposal of equipment and the management of anaphylactic shock.

Indications and rationale for the administration of medicines

A medication can be administered by a variety of routes and for many different reasons:

- *to prevent disease*
- *to cure disease*
- *to alleviate pain or other symptoms caused by disease, injury or surgery*
- *to alleviate a manifestation of disease.*

Professional issues to consider prior to procedure

The role of the nurse involved in drug administration is multi-faceted, therefore prior to commencing any procedure it is important to be aware of the following issues:

1. The nurse in charge of the ward, department, and unit or treatment room at any time of the day or night is responsible for maintaining the safe and correct storage of all medicines, these storage requirements being enforced by law through the Medicines Act (1968) and the Misuse of Drugs Act (1971). Medicines kept in patients' own homes are their responsibility, but the community nurse has an important role in educating patients on all aspects of their regimen. The manufacturer's recommendations for the storage environment and expiry date should be adhered to or the composition of the medicine may be altered. Vaccines, in particular, need to be stored under very stringent conditions (recommendations being provided by both the manufacturer and the health authority).

2. A nurse can administer a medicine only on the written instruction of an authorised prescriber (Nursing and Midwifery Council 2004b). Changes to regulations in May 2006 enabled nurses who are trained as independent prescribers to prescribe any licensed medicine within their level of experience and competence. District nurses and health visitors will continue to be entitled to prescribe from a limited formulary known as the 'Nurse Prescribers' Formulary for Community Practitioners', which can be accessed in the British National Formulary (BNF; British Medical Association 2006). The Nursing and Midwifery Council (NMC) Standards for Nurse/Midwifery Prescribing (2006) and health authority policy should be followed with respect to this practice.

3. The medicine prescription should be written in black indelible ink, giving the date, the patient's full name and age, the name (preferably generic title) of the medication, the dosage to be given and the time of administration. The whole prescription should be legible (Nursing and Midwifery Council 2004b, 2005).

4. The nurse is responsible for the correct administration and documentation of a prescribed medication. Recording the administration may be performed only once the nurse is satisfied that the patient has received the prescribed medication.

5. A student nurse should be supervised by a member of staff who is registered with the NMC while administering medicines.

6. Should any error occur during administration, this must be reported using local policy so that the appropriate action can be implemented (Nursing and Midwifery Council 2004b, 2005).

7. The nurse should be familiar with the use, action, and common side-effects and therapeutic dose of the medicine being administered. This will help in the

education of patients and assists in identifying any adverse reaction that may develop. When an adverse effect is not life threatening, it may be necessary for the patient to adjust to a change in his or her activity of living. The nurse, therefore, has a role as an educator and facilitator during the adjustment. It is important to observe the effectiveness of a medicine, for example following the administration of an anti-emetic or analgesic. Any sign of the development of a side-effect, of non-effectiveness or of dependence should be reported to the medical practitioner or prescriber.

Reference books available to healthcare professionals include: the British National Formulary (British Medical Association 2006) the Monthly Index of Medical Specialities (http://www.mims) and the Data Sheet Compendium (ABPI 2000). The ward pharmacist or on-call pharmacist is another invaluable resource.

Outline of the procedure

The administration of medicine encompasses many different procedures depending on the needs of the patient. The NMC (2004b) lays great emphasis on issues of accountability for any nurse undertaking this practice. It is important that the following guidelines are used in conjunction with health authority policy as there may be policy or procedural differences, such as the grade and number of nurses required to undertake these practices (Crown 1999).

Equipment

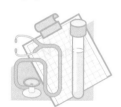

1. Means of identifying the patient
2. Patient's medicine prescription and recording documents
3. Trolley, tray or a suitable work surface for equipment
4. Medication to be administered
5. Equipment for use during medicine administration, e.g.
   — oral administration: medicine glass or spoon, glass of water
   — injection: appropriately sized sterile needles and syringe, disposable gloves, alcohol-impregnated cleansing swab, cotton wool, adhesive plaster
6. Sharps box
7. Receptacle for soiled material
8. Equipment/medication for the treatment of anaphylactic shock (as per health authority policy).

1. PRINCIPLES OF MEDICINE ADMINISTRATION

Guidelines and rationale for this nursing practice

All forms of medicine administration

▪ discuss the procedure with the patient, asking whether he or she has any known allergy to this drug or other drugs or substances such as eggs, which are used as a carrier substance in some medications, and obtain consent (this may not always be possible, for example when the patient is unconscious) *to inform the patient about the procedure, discuss any concerns or queries, identify any known allergies and ensure that the patient is aware of his or her rights as a patient*

▪ wash the hands to reduce the risk of cross-infection

- select a suitable clean surface and lay out the equipment **to provide a suitable protected work surface**
- observe the patient throughout this procedure **to identify any potential reactions to the medicine**
- identify the medicine to be administered on the prescription document. The prescription should be complete and legible **to ensure that all details about the medicine can be clearly identified on the prescription documentation**
- check that the medicine has not already been administered **to ensure that only one dose of the medicine is given**
- select the appropriate medicine against the prescription documentation **to ensure that the correct medicine is administered**
- check the medicine's name, dosage, timing and expiry date. If the medication has been dispensed to a specific patient, check that his or her name is on the container **to ensure that all the relevant details are listed on the medicine container**
- remove the prescribed dosage from the container to ensure that the correct amount of medicine is removed from the container
- check the prescription and dosage against the medicine container **to ensure that the medicine details match**
- identify the patient to whom the medicine is to be administered. In an institution, this will normally be achieved by checking the details on the patient's identification bracelet. In a community setting, verbal verification should be obtained from either the patient or the carer **to ensure that the medicine is administered to the correct patient**
- administer the medicine by the route prescribed
- ensure that the patient is comfortable following the administration of the medicine **to identify any reaction to the medication or to the chosen route of delivery**
- follow local policy regarding the time that a nurse must remain with a patient following the administration of certain medicines. This is particularly relevant when the medicine is being administered in the patient's own home or in a treatment room **to ensure prompt recognition and treatment of any reaction to the drug** (*see* 'Anaphylaxis', p. 24)
- record the medication details on the patient documentation, monitor any after-effects and report abnormal findings immediately **to ensure that there is a permanent record of the medicine administration and that any side-effects are reported to medical staff**
- dispose of contaminated equipment according to health authority policy **to prevent the transmission of infection or the poisoning of other persons/to allow for checking if the patient has an adverse reaction**
- if the patient has difficulty swallowing an oral preparation, the nurse may request that the medicine be supplied in another form. The pharmacist should be consulted before any tablet is crushed or halved (as this may affect the composition or absorption of the medicine). Pills, capsules and cachets should be supplied in the dosage stated on the prescription sheet
- in undertaking this practice, nurses are accountable for their actions, the quality of care delivered and record-keeping according to the Code of Professional Conduct (Nursing and Midwifery Council 2004a), Guidelines for Administration

of Medicines (Nursing and Midwifery Council 2004b) and Guidelines for Records and Record Keeping (Nursing and Midwifery Council 2005).

Controlled medicines   *Institutional setting*

The administration of a controlled medicine within an institutional setting must involve two nurses, or a nurse and another approved professional such as a medical practitioner or operating department practitioner. One nurse must be a registered nurse practitioner and may, according to local policy, need to be employed within that healthcare setting. A controlled drug register is kept on each ward or department, giving details of the stock and administration of controlled drugs.

- as for 'All forms of medicine administration' up to the guideline 'check that the medicine has not already been administered'
- remove the appropriate medicine from the controlled drug store, check the stock number with the number detailed in the register, along with the other nurse, *to ensure that the number of drugs in the container matches the number recorded in the register*
- check the date of the prescription *to ensure that the medicine is administered on the correct date*
- check the time of administration *to ensure that the medicine is given at the correct time*
- check the method of administration *to ensure the correct route of administration*
- remove the appropriate dose from the stock of controlled medicine, checking the name and dosage with the second nurse. Check and record the stock number of the remaining controlled medicine *to ensure that the correct dose is withdrawn from the container and the remaining balance recorded*
- enter into the controlled medicine record sheet the appropriate details *to ensure a permanent record of the administration details (date, time, patient's name, drug dosage and initials of staff)*
- continue as for 'All forms of medicine administration'.

Community setting

The administration of a controlled medicine within the patient's own home may be carried out by the patient or carer (this being the normal practice for medicines in tablet or liquid form). When medicines are given by injection, as a suppository or via a syringe driver, this is normally carried out by the community nurse(s). The number and grade of staff depend on health authority policy.

Controlled medicines belong to the patient and remain within his or her home. Advice should be given to the patient/carer on the safe storage of these medicines. A controlled medicine record sheet giving details of any medicine administered by the nurse and a balance of stock should be placed in the patient's house, along with a special prescription sheet for controlled medicines (completed and signed by the general practitioner or hospital consultant in charge of the patient's care). A guide to good practice in the management of controlled drugs in primary care (England) is available at the National Prescribing Centre (2006), available at http://www.npc.co.uk/index.htm.

- as for 'All forms of medicine administration' up to the guideline 'check that the medicine has not already been administered'
- check the stock number of medicines against the number detailed in the controlled drug record sheet **to ensure the number of medicines in the container matches the number recorded in the drug record**
- check the date of the prescription **to ensure that the medicine is administered on the correct date**
- check the time of administration **to ensure that the drug is given at the correct time**
- check the method of administration **to ensure the correct route of administration**
- remove the appropriate dose from the stock of controlled medicines, checking the name and dosage. Check and record the stock number of the remaining controlled medicines **to ensure that the correct dose is withdrawn from the container and the remaining balance recorded**
- enter into the controlled drug record sheet the appropriate details **to ensure a permanent record of the administration details (date, time, medicine dosage and signature of staff)**
- continue as for 'All forms of medicine administration'.

2. ROUTES OF MEDICINE ADMINISTRATION

Oral preparation

- as for 'All forms of medicine administration' up to the guideline that begins 'remove the prescribed dosage'
- remove the required number of tablets, pills or cachets from the medicine container without contaminating the preparation. Place into the medicine glass or medicine spoon **to ensure that the correct drug dosage is dispensed**

  or

- shake the liquid medicine preparation well. Pour into the appropriate container at eye level and on a solid flat surface, pouring away from label, to preserve label to allow future recognition of contents. **Wipe bottle (to prevent contamination)**. If the medicine is a powder that needs to be mixed with water, the instructions on the container should be followed **to ensure that the medicine moves efficiently down the oesophagus into the stomach**

  or

- draw up into a syringe **to ensure accurate drug dose measurement**
- check the medicine prescription and dosage against the container **to ensure that the correct medicine and dosage has been dispensed**
- identify the patient according to local policy **to ensure that the medicine is administered to the correct person**
- administer the medicine and offer the patient water (if allowed) **to aid the swallowing of an oral preparation**
- continue as for 'All forms of medicine administration'.

Injection preparations – intramuscular and subcutaneous routes

Equipment 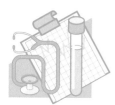	1. Appropriately sized needles (21G, 23G and 25G) and syringes 2. Alcohol-impregnated swab 3. Drug ampoule or vial 4. Ampoule breaker 5. Diluent if required 6. File 7. Disposable gloves 8. Gauze swab 9. Sterile adhesive plaster (if required).

Guidelines and rationale for injections

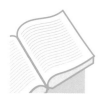

- as for 'All forms of medicine administration', follow the guideline that begins 'check the medicine's name, dosage, timing and expiry date'
- put on gloves *to prevent contamination by the medicine and to protect against blood-borne infection*.

Ampoule

- snap the neck of the ampoule using a gauze swab or an ampoule breaker *to protect the nurse from laceration by glass splinters should the medication be stored in a glass ampoule*
- if any glass enters the ampoule, discard the ampoule and start the process with a new one *as glass particles may have contaminated the medicine in some clinical areas, i.e. in children's wards filter needles can be used to draw up medication to prevent glass splinters*
- if the solution is already present in the ampoule, draw up the required amount of medicine into the syringe
- if the medicine is in powder form, draw up the required amount of diluent and inject it slowly into the powder within the ampoule *to enable the medicine to be dissolved in diluent*
- gently rotate the ampoule and inspect it for any visible particles of undissolved powder *to ensure that the powder is fully dissolved*
- withdraw the required amount of drug solution into the syringe *to ensure that the correct amount of medicine is dispensed*
- gently tap the side of the barrel with the finger to move any air bubbles to the neck of the syringe *to enable them to be expelled prior to injecting the solution*.

Vial

- remove the protective cap and cleanse the rubber top with an alcohol-impregnated swab *to cleanse the entry point*
- insert the first needle, ensuring that the tip is above the fluid level *to release the vacuum within the vial*
- draw air into the syringe attached to the second needle to equal the amount of solution to be withdrawn from the vial *to enable the easier withdrawal of solution from the vial*

- insert the second needle attached to the syringe, and expel the air into the vial. Draw up the required amount of drug, expelling any air bubbles prior to removing the needle from the vial **to prevent spray of the drug solution into the atmosphere on withdrawal of the needle**
- if the medicine is in powder form, draw up the required amount of diluent and inject it slowly into the powder within the vial **to enable the medicine to be dissolved in diluent**
- gently rotate the vial and inspect for any visible particles of undissolved powder **to ensure that the powder is fully dissolved**
- change the needle to the required size for the route of administration; **if an intramuscular injection is to be given, a clean needle prevents irritation of the subcutaneous tissue as the needle is being inserted into the muscle** (Workman 1999)
- place the prepared syringe and the empty ampoule or vial on a foil tray **to retain the original drug container so that a final check can be made prior to administering the medicine**
- identify the patient to whom the medicine is to be administered and recheck the prescription details with the medicine, container and dosage drawn up in the syringe **to ensure that the correct medicine is administered to the correct patient**
- ensure the patient's privacy
- cleanse the skin surface (if required); the policy on skin cleansing prior to injection varies according to the health authority concerned (Rodger & King 2000). Patients receiving insulin injections should not have the area cleansed with an alcohol-impregnated swab as this will toughen the skin over time
- expose the chosen site and inject the drug.

Intramuscular injection

Sites for intramuscular injection are shown in Figure 2.1. Rodger & King (2000) suggest five injection sites, including the ventrogluteal site; however despite its advantages its use is still very limited. The use of the Z track technique (Fig. 2.2) is essential with certain medications that can stain the skin or are particularly irritant; indeed its use for all intramuscular injections is now recommended (Workman 1999, Rodger & King 2000).

- using the non-dominant hand, stretch the skin over the site; with the dominant hand, insert the needle two-thirds in, at an angle of 90°, **to ensure that the needle is inserted into the muscle**
- withdraw the piston of the syringe. If blood is drawn up into the syringe, withdraw the needle and syringe from the patient's tissue. Replace the needle, and start the procedure again **to prevent the drug being injected into a blood vessel**
- if no blood is withdrawn into the syringe, inject the solution slowly at a rate of 1 ml per 10 seconds (Workman 1999) **to reduce patient discomfort and/or tissue damage**.

Subcutaneous injection

Sites for subcutaneous injection are shown in Figure 2.3.

- using a pinch skin technique (King 2003), as shown in Figure 2.4, introduce the needle at a 90° **to ensure that the drug is delivered into the subcutaneous tissue**.

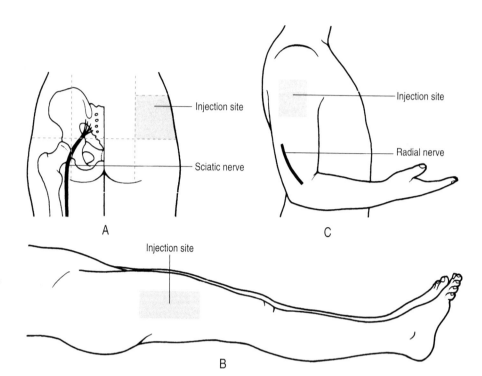

FIGURE 2.1
**Administration of medicines: sites used for intramuscular injection
A Upper outer quadrant of the buttock
B Anterior lateral aspect of the thigh
C Deltoid region of the arm**

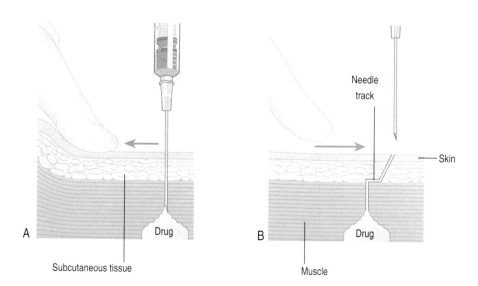

FIGURE 2.2
Z track technique

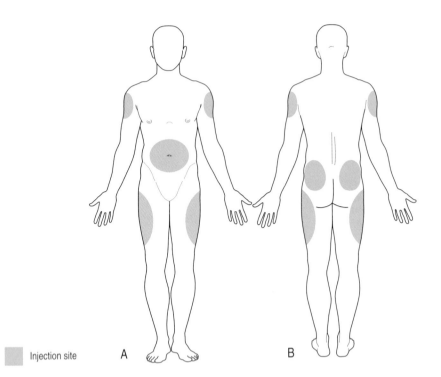

FIGURE 2.3
**Administration of
medicines: sites used for
subcutaneous injection
A Anterior aspect
B Posterior aspect**

Injection site

A

B

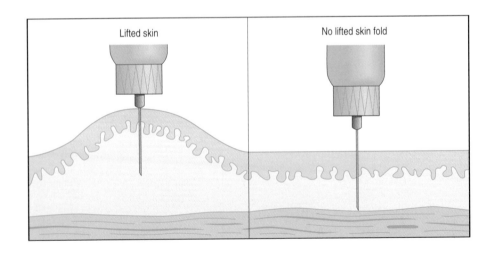

FIGURE 2.4
Pinch skin technique
From Becton Dickinson
UK Ltd, with permission

For subcutaneous injections there is no need to draw back as the needle size and the pinch skin technique will ensure that a blood vessel is not hit.
- if a patient is receiving subcutaneous injections over a period of time, the site of injection should be rotated **to reduce subcutaneous tissue irritation and maintain the medicine's absorption rate**.

For more information on insulin therapy, *see* 'Administration of insulin', below.

All injections

- hold the needle in situ for 10 seconds **to allow the diffusion of the drug into the tissues**
- withdraw the needle smoothly. **To prevent the occurrence of a needle-stick injury**, do not resheath the needle
- apply pressure to the site of the injection using a cotton wool ball or swab. If bleeding occurs, apply a small adhesive plaster **to prevent blood leakage**
- continue as for 'All forms of medicine administration'.

Specialised administration instructions provided by the manufacturer should always be followed.

The nurse should always be aware of the possibility of anaphylaxis following the administration of medicines. Health authority policy should be followed regarding the length of time for which the patient should be monitored following the administration of the medicine. This is particularly important for patients receiving medicines in the community. For further information, *see* 'Anaphylaxis', p. 24.

Administration of insulin

Insulin may be given via special insulin syringes or by an insulin pen device and is delivered subcutaneously. For patients who are self-administering insulin, the pen system is often more practical as the vial in the pen holds enough insulin for several doses. Some pen systems have a needle that is of a shorter length than the standard one used for subcutaneous injections. Various manufacturers advise that their pen be introduced at a 90° angle, but there has been some debate over whether this technique causes insulin to be injected into the muscle rather than the subcutaneous tissue (in patients who have less than 10 mm of subcutaneous tissue), thus increasing the absorption rate (King 2003). Patients injecting insulin should be taught the technique advised by the diabetic specialist within the health authority.

Some diabetics find injecting insulin through one layer of clothing more convenient when out socialising, for example, than the conventional technique requiring skin exposure (Strauss et al 2002) More details can be found by accessing the Royal College of Nursing web site available at: http://www.rcn.org.uk/publications/.

Intradermal route

According to Prausnitz et al (2004) transdermal drug delivery has been one of the most important innovations offering a number of advantages over the oral route. When used for immunisation such as BCG the nurse must meet the criteria for immunisation prior to administering this or any other vaccine via this route. The injection of a medicine into the dermis is a skilled injection technique. The sites where the injections can be given may vary according to the type of vaccination being administered; local health authority policy should therefore be followed. More detailed information on this technique is provided by the Department of Health (1996), the website can be accessed at http://www.dh.gov.uk.

Topical application

There is a growing trend for certain medicines to be administered via the topical route (http://bnf.org/bnf/), usually in the form of a 'skin patch'. Some drugs that can be given by this method include hormone replacement therapy and certain analgesics.

The patches should normally be applied to clean dry skin. The length of time they should be worn depends on the drug involved, so the manufacturer's instructions should be followed. The site of the patch should be rotated to reduce risk of a skin reaction, and care should be taken to ensure that only one patch is in place at a time, thus ensuring that the correct dose of medication is administered. Further information on drugs delivered via this route is available from individual manufacturers.

3. IMMUNISATION

Nurses working in both community and institutional settings are increasingly undertaking immunisation. This may include child immunisation regimens, vaccinations for travel abroad, the administration of influenza vaccines and the giving of anti-tetanus or hepatitis B vaccinations within accident and emergency units or treatment rooms. The Royal College of Nursing (2001a) examines some of the legal and professional aspects of immunisation by nursing staff and discusses the use of Patient Group Directions for this practice. Nurses participating in any immunisation programme must meet the following criteria (this is set out in the Immunisation Against Infectious Diseases 'Green book' Department of Health 1996). The most comprehensive, up-to-date and accurate information on vaccines, disease and immunisation in the UK is available at http://www.immunisation.nhs.uk/ (National Health Service 2006). The Royal College of Nursing also has a number of publications on vaccinations and injection technique available at http://www.rcn.org.uk. A knowledge of Patient Group Directions is also essential and these are set out by the NHS National Prescribing Centre (2004), available at http://www.npc.co.uk/index.htm

They must:
- undertake additional training on immunisation
- undertake training in the management of anaphylaxis
- be competent in the practice of immunisation and be able to recognise contraindications for vaccination
- be accountable for their practice.

4. ANAPHYLAXIS

Outline of the procedure

Anaphylaxis can result from an anaphylactic reaction (a reaction to a substance to which the body has previously been exposed and sensitised) or an anaphylactoid response (in which there has been no previous exposure). An anaphylactic reaction can lead to respiratory distress, shock, cardiac arrest or death and can occur at any time. It is essential that all nurses involved in the administration of medicines are familiar with the symptoms of an anaphylactic reaction. It is particularly important that nurses working in a community setting have the competence to both recognise and treat anaphylaxis (Chamberlain 1999); additional training being given to staff in order that they can undertake this procedure.

A reaction to a medicine may occur at any time following administration: it is not possible to give a time limit (Department of Health 1996). Ewan (1998) reports that a reaction frequently occurs within minutes of the patient receiving the injection (although it can also occur following the oral ingestion of medicines or certain foods, or through skin contact) but that it may also be delayed for up to several hours following administration.

The information provided in this section is based on the guidelines given by the Department of Health (1996); Royal College of Nursing (2001b) and the Resuscitation Council (UK), at http://www.resus.org.uk/pages/reaction.htm, but individual health authorities may provide additional guidance for staff.

Presenting characteristics	<ul><li>airway obstruction presenting as wheezing from bronchospasm and laryngeal oedema, dyspnoea and stridor</li><li>skin itching, flushing, urticaria and angio-oedema</li><li>change of skin colour, i.e. flushed/pale</li><li>extreme anxiety and a feeling of 'impending doom'</li><li>hypotension</li><li>tachycardia followed by bradycardia (secondary to profound hypotension).</li></ul>If untreated, the patient may eventually suffer respiratory and cardiac arrest.
Management of anaphylaxis	<ul><li>if the patient still has an adequate cardiac output, place him or her in the recovery position and insert an artificial airway **to maintain an airway** if the gag reflex has been lost</li><li>in an institutional setting: remain with the patient but get help urgently from other medical and nursing staff (in most units, it will be necessary to call the cardiac arrest team). When help arrives, inform the senior staff of the medication that the patient received prior to collapse **to initiate treatment and sustain life**</li><li>in a community setting: first summon help by dialling 999 and asking for an ambulance; then return to the patient and start treatment as soon as possible. When possible, send someone for medical help.</li></ul>Follow the Resuscitation Council UK Guidelines, see treatment algorithms (Fig. 2.5).<ul><li>commence the resuscitation procedure if the patient has suffered a respiratory and/or cardiac arrest (*see* 'Cardiopulmonary resuscitation', p. 71), **to initiate treatment as quickly as possible and sustain the patient's life**</li><li>any patient suffering an anaphylactic reaction should be admitted to hospital as soon as possible **in order that his or her condition may be monitored**. Fisher (1995) advises that a secondary reaction may occur up to 72 hours following the initial anaphylactic incident.</li></ul>

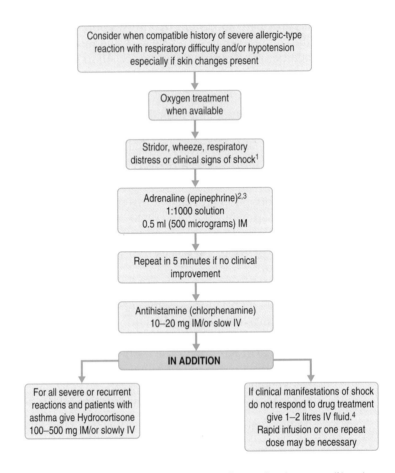

Consider when compatible history of severe allergic-type reaction with respiratory difficulty and/or hypotension especially if skin changes present

Oxygen treatment when available

Stridor, wheeze, respiratory distress or clinical signs of shock[1]

Adrenaline (epinephrine)[2,3]
1:1000 solution
0.5 ml (500 micrograms) IM

Repeat in 5 minutes if no clinical improvement

Antihistamine (chlorphenamine)
10–20 mg IM/or slow IV

IN ADDITION

For all severe or recurrent reactions and patients with asthma give Hydrocortisone 100–500 mg IM/or slowly IV

If clinical manifestations of shock do not respond to drug treatment give 1–2 litres IV fluid.[4] Rapid infusion or one repeat dose may be necessary

1. An inhaled beta$_2$-agonist such as salbutamol may be used as an adjunctive measure if bronchospasm is severe and does not respond rapidly to other treatment.
2. If profound shock judged **immediately** life threatening give CPR/ALS if necessary. Consider **slow** IV adrenaline (epinephrine) 1:10 000 solution. This is **hazardous** and is recommended only for an experienced practitioner who can also obtain IV access without delay.
   Note the different strength of adrenaline (epinephrine) that may be required for IV use.
3. If adults are treated with an adrenaline (epinephrine) auto-injector, the 300 micrograms will usuallly be sufficient. A second dose may be required. Half doses of adrenaline (epinephrine) may be safer for patients on amitriptyline, imipramine, or beta blocker.
4. A crystalloid may be safer than a colloid.

FIGURE 2.5
Resuscitation Council (UK) anaphylaxis algorithms
From Resuscitation Council (UK) 2005, with permission

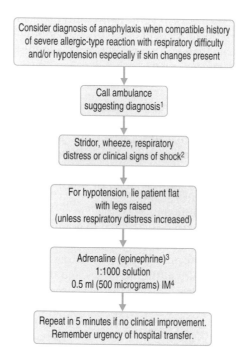

Consider diagnosis of anaphylaxis when compatible history of severe allergic-type reaction with respiratory difficulty and/or hypotension especially if skin changes present

Call ambulance suggesting diagnosis[1]

Stridor, wheeze, respiratory distress or clinical signs of shock[2]

For hypotension, lie patient flat with legs raised (unless respiratory distress increased)

Adrenaline (epinephrine)[3] 1:1000 solution 0.5 ml (500 micrograms) IM[4]

Repeat in 5 minutes if no clinical improvement. Remember urgency of hospital transfer.

**FIGURE 2.5   CONT'D
Resuscitation Council (UK) anaphylaxis algorithms**
From Resuscitation Council (UK) 2005, with permission

1. Ambulance will be equipped with oxygen, salbutamol and fluids which may be used as adjunctive therapy.
2. If profound shock judged to be **immediately** life threatening give CPR/ALS if necessary.
3. Half doses of adrenaline (epinephrine) may be safer for patients on amitriptyline, imipramine, or beta blocker.
4. If adults are treated with an adrenaline auto-injector, the 300 micrograms will usuallly be sufficient.
   A second dose may be required, but this should be considered ONLY if the patient's condition continues to deteriorate 5 minutes after the first dose.
   N.B. Remember the urgency of hospital transfer.

5.   SYRINGE DRIVER PUMPS

Indications and rationale for use of syringe driver

A patient who requires a continuous dose of medicine may be given it via a syringe driver pump, this facilitates good control of symptoms with little inconvenience or discomfort to the patient. More information can be obtained by accessing the British National Formulary available at http://www.bnf.org.

A pump may be used:

- *when the patient is unable to tolerate oral medication* (for example, because of a pathological lesion, unresolved nausea or vomiting, or a reduced level of consciousness)
- *when adequate pain control cannot be achieved by oral medication*
- *when a medicine needs to be administered via the subcutaneous route over a period of time*.

Outline of the procedure

The syringe driver administers a continuous amount of a prescribed medicine via the subcutaneous route over a set period of time (for example, 24 hours). It may be used when a continuous infusion of a medicine is required, such as to manage postoperative pain or to control symptoms during the terminal stage of an illness. More than one medicine may be administered at a time via this route. It is especially beneficial for patients being nursed in the community as it enables a more accurate titration of drug doses and therefore more effective symptom control.

In many settings, this practice has to be undertaken by two people, although policy may vary in the community setting. Within an institutional setting, the medicine may already be made up in the syringe by the pharmacist or doctor. In a community setting, the medicine is likely to be made up by the district nurse in the patient's own home. Health authorities may have different policies, which should be followed (Quinn 2000).

Different models of syringe driver with differing operating instructions are available, so it is essential that any nurse working with them is fully familiar with the particular manufacturer's instructions (Wilson 2000). Therefore it is possible to provide only general guidelines here, which should be followed in conjunction with health authority policy and the manufacturer's instructions. The Medicines and Healthcare Products Regulatory Agency website (available at http://www.mhra.gov.uk) may also be a useful resource.

Equipment 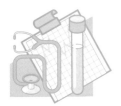	1. Syringe driver and battery (if required) 2. Manufacturer's instructions for the syringe driver 3. Patient's medicine prescription and recording documents 4. Trolley, tray or suitable work surface for equipment 5. Medication to be administered (including diluents) 6. 22G butterfly canola and giving set 7. Syringes (type and size as instructed by the manufacturer of the syringe driver) 8. Sterile needles 9. Disposable gloves 10. Cotton wool 11. Semi-permeable adhesive film dressing 12. Sharps box 13. Receptacle for soiled material 14. Adhesive label.

Guidelines and rationale for this practice

The following steps should be undertaken in conjunction with local policy and the instructions of the manufacturer of the syringe driver.

- as for 'All forms of medicine administration' (*see* p. 15), up to the guideline 'check that the medicine has not already been administered'. If a controlled drug is to be administered, the guidelines given under 'Controlled medicines' (*see* p. 17) should be followed
- ensure that the syringe driver is functioning by following the checking procedure advised by the manufacturer and health authority. This normally involves inserting the battery or attaching the pump to the mains supply and ensuring that the indicator light is lit. When applicable, a check on the inbuilt alarm system should also be carried out **to perform any recommended safety checks**
- in an institutional setting: collect the pre-prepared syringe containing the prescribed medicine and check the details on the syringe (patient's name and hospital number, date, medicine name(s) and diluent, dosage, total

volume of fluid in the syringe, starting time of administration, expiry date). This information should be checked with the details given on the patient's prescription sheet *to ensure that the medicine details on the syringe match those on the prescription sheet*

- in a community setting: prepare the medicine for administration as per the patient's prescription sheet (although the medicine dosage will be the same irrespective of the pump, the amount of diluent may differ). A label should be attached to the barrel of the syringe giving information on the contents of the syringe (date, name and dosage of the medicine, volume of drug and diluent, starting time of administration, signature of nurse) *in order that the contents are clearly identified*
- attach the giving set to the syringe and prime the tubing *so that all air is expelled from the tubing*
- elicit the duration of administration *as this will affect the rate of administration*
- set the prescribed rate according to the manufacturer's instructions *to ensure the correct infusion rate*
- select the site for infusion (the same as for 'Subcutaneous injection'), however insert the needle of the infusion set at a 45° angle (p. 22)
- secure the needle with the semi-permanent adhesive dressing *to prevent its becoming dislodged and to enable the entry site to be clearly visible*
- secure the syringe into the driver, ensuring that the plunger mechanism is correctly positioned and that any securing straps are in place to enable the administration of the medicine and *to ensure that the syringe does not become dislodged from the pump*
- start the syringe driver and observe it for the time specified by the health authority *to ensure that the driver is functioning*
- place the driver in a safe position (a carrying case is normally available for patients who are mobile) and ensure that it is kept away from water *to prevent the infusion set being dislodged from the syringe driver and to avoid damage to the machine*
- the syringe driver should be checked regularly and recordings such as fluid volume length (the length of fluid in the syringe barrel, measured normally in millimetres) documented (remembering that the checks to be carried out and their frequency may vary according to health authority policy) *to ensure that it is continuing to function correctly*
- check the infusion site regularly and report any signs of localised pain, inflammation or swelling; in the community, the patient or carer may be taught how to check the site. If any problems then resite the infusion set *to identify and rectify at an early stage any localised skin reaction*
- observe the patient's symptoms *to monitor the effectiveness of the drug therapy*
- in undertaking this practice, nurses are accountable for their actions, the quality of care delivered and record-keeping according to the *Code of Professional Conduct* (Nursing and Midwifery Council 2004a), *Guidelines for Administration of Medicines* (Nursing and Midwifery Council 2004b) and *Guidelines for Records and Record Keeping* (Nursing and Midwifery Council 2005).

The regular maintenance and calibration of the pump by the health authority or manufacturer is essential.

6. PATIENT-CONTROLLED ANALGESIC DEVICES

Devices that enable the patient to self-administer analgesia are becoming increasingly popular. These work via a pump system, which enables the patient to administer small doses of the prescribed analgesic, with an inbuilt safety mechanism preventing overdosage of the drug. The main administration routes are intravenous, subcutaneous and epidural. The benefits of this system are that the patient is more empowered and less anxious about effective pain control. Chumbley et al (2002) outline what information a patient requires about patient-controlled analgesia (PCA). The devices may be used by patients in both institutional and community settings. Reiff & Niziolek (2001) suggest troubleshooting tips for using PCA.

Patient-controlled analgesia may be prescribed for patients:
- following surgical procedures such as hysterectomy and hip replacement. *It allows the patient to administer frequent small boluses of analgesia for pain relief without becoming over-sedated. Good pain control enables the patient to mobilise earlier and enhances postoperative recovery*
- for pain relief as part of palliative care in terminal illness. This may be at home or in an institutional or hospice setting *and allows the patient to be alert and aware of the surroundings with adequate pain control*.

Equipment

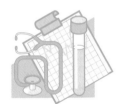

1. Venous or subcutaneous access
2. Specialised patient-controlled analgesia infusor (referring to the manufacturer's instructions).

The infusor consists of a reservoir balloon or a reservoir syringe that is prepared with the prescribed analgesic medication by the nursing staff. The fluid from the reservoir flows through a filter and a control nozzle on the demand button via its associated tubing (Fig. 2.6). Many devices are available, and the individual manufacturer's instructions must always be followed.

Patients administer their own dose of analgesia by pressing the demand button, which may take the form of a wrist button or a small hand-held demand set. When further analgesic is required, the demand button is again pressed, and a small amount of medication, usually 0.5–1 ml, is delivered. The equipment has an inbuilt safety mechanism that allows only a certain amount of fluid to be infused during 1 hour, so there is no possibility of a medication overdose. The strength of the individual bolus will be prescribed by the medical practitioner after assessing the patient's pain. The amount transfused each hour should be recorded, monitored and documented for evaluation of the patient's pain control.

7. PATIENT COMPLIANCE DEVICES

There are many types of device on the market to assist the patient to administer his or her medicines. All patients should be fully assessed before a medicine device is given, and checks made that the medicines can be stored in it. Interactions between medicines should also be checked, so it is essential that a pharmacist be

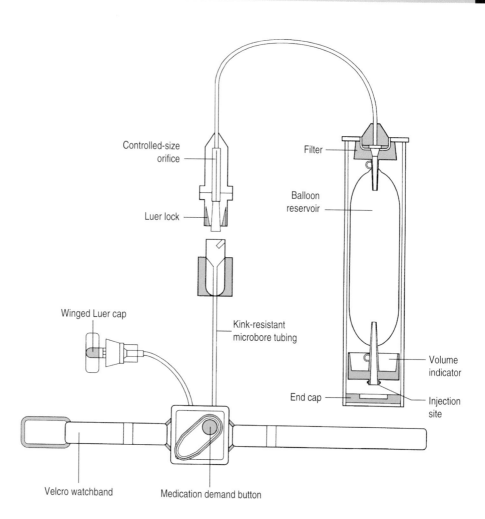

Controlled-size orifice

Filter

Balloon reservoir

Luer lock

Winged Luer cap

Kink-resistant microbore tubing

Volume indicator

End cap

Injection site

Velcro watchband

Medication demand button

FIGURE 2.6
Patient-controlled analgesia infusor

involved at all stages. The medicine device may comprise of individual trays for each day of the week, each with different compartments for the different times of day when the patient must take the medication. The trays are usually filled (by the patient or carer) with all the patient's medicines up to 1 week in advance. If the patient/carer is unable to perform this task then the pharmacist should be responsible for dispensing, labelling and sealing these compliance aids (Coleman 2005). Only in exceptional circumstances, when a community pharmacist is unavailable, should a nurse be required to fill these devices in which case the Guidelines for the Administration of Medicines (Nursing and Midwifery Council 2004b) as well as health authority policy, should be followed.

References

ABPI 2005 Compendium of data sheets and summaries of product characteristics: with the code of practice for the pharmaceutical industry. Association of British Pharmaceutical Industry.

British Medical Association 2006 British national formulary. British Medical Association and the Royal Pharmaceutical Society of Great Britain, London

Chamberlain D 1999 Emergency medical treatment of anaphylactic reactions. Project Team of the Resuscitation Council (UK) Emergency Medical Journal 16: 243–247

Chumbley GM, Hall GM, Salmon P 2002 Patient controlled analgesia: what information does the patient want? Journal of Advanced Nursing 39(5): 459–471

Coleman DJ 2005 Medication compliance in the elderly. Journal of Community Nurses 19: 8

Crown J 1999 Review of prescribing, supply and administration of medicines – final report. Department of Health, London

Department of Health 1996 Immunisation against infectious diseases. Stationery Office, London (available at http://www.dh.gov.uk/policyandguidance/HealthAndSocialCareTopics/GreenBook)

Downie G, MacKenzie J, Williams A 2003 Pharmacology and medicines management for nurses, 3rd edn. Churchill Livingstone, Edinburgh

Downie G, Mackenzie J, Williams A 2006 Calculating drug doses safely. Churchill Livingstone, Edinburgh

Ewan P 1998 ABC of allergies – anaphylaxis. British Medical Journal 316: 1442–1445

Fisher M 1995 Treatment of acute anaphylaxis. British Medical Journal 311: 731–733

King L 2003 Subcutaneous insulin injection technique. Nursing Standard 17(34): 45–52, 54–55

Lapham R, Agar H 2003 Drug calculations for Nurses, 2nd edn. Arnold, London

Medicinal Products: Prescription by Nurses Act 1992. HMSO, London

Medicines Act 1968. HMSO, London

McGavock H 2005 How drugs work, basic pharmacology for healthcare professionals, 2nd edn. Radcliffe Medical Press, Abingdon, Oxford

Misuse of Drugs Act 1971. HMSO, London

National Health Service 2006 Immunisations. NHS (available at http://www.immunisation.nhs.uk/)

National Prescribing Centre 2004 Patient group directions. National Prescribing Centre (available at http://www.npc.co.uk/index/htm)

National Prescribing Centre 2006 A Guide to good practice in the management of controlled drugs in primary care (England). National Prescribing Centre (available at http://www.npc.co.uk)

Nursing and Midwifery Council 2004a Code of professional conduct. NMC, London

Nursing and Midwifery Council 2004b Guidelines for the administration of medicines. NMC, London

Nursing and Midwifery Council 2005 Guidelines for records and record keeping. NMC, London

Nursing and Midwifery Council 2006 Standards of proficiency for nurse and midwifery prescribers. NMC, London

Prausnitz MR, Mitragotri S, Langer R 2004 Current status and future potential of transdermal drug delivery. Nature Reviews. Drug Discovery 3(2): 115–124

Quinn C 2000 Infusion devices: risks, function and management. Nursing Standard 14(26): 35–41

Reiff PA, Niziolek MM 2001 Troubleshooting tips for PCA. RN 64(4): 33–37

Rodger M, King L 2000 Drawing up and administering intramuscular injections: a review of the literature. Journal of Advanced Nursing 31(3): 574–582

Royal College of Nursing 2001a Immunisation. RCN, London

Royal College of Nursing 2001b UK guidance and best practice in vaccine administration. Shire Hall Communications, London

Strauss K, De Gols H, Letondeur C et al 2002 The second injection event (SITE) May 2000, Barcelona, Spain. Practical Diabetes International 19(1): 17–21

Wilson V 2000 Guidelines for use of the MS26 daily rate syringe driver in the community. British Journal of Community Health Nursing 5(4): 162–168

Workman B 1999 Safe injection techniques. Nursing Standard 13(39): 47–53

Websites

British National Formulary: http://www.bnf.org

Department of Health: http://www.dh.gov.uk/policyandguidance/

Journal of Community Nurses: http://www.jcn.co.uk/journal
Medicines and Healthcare Products Regulatory Agency: http://www.mhra.gov.uk
Monthly Index of Medical Specialities: http://www.mims
National Health Service: http://www.immunisation.nhs.uk/
National Prescribing Centre: http://www.npc.co.uk/
Resuscitation Council (UK): http://www.resus.org.uk/pages/reaction.htm

Self assessment

1. Make a note of all the acceptable methods a registered nurse may use to identify patients prior to administering any prescribed medication in your work area.
2. What advice would you give a patient who was self-administering insulin?
3. List the sites for intramuscular injections and state the advantages and disadvantages of each.
4. List the legislation that governs the administration of medicines and state what each act covers.
5. What are the signs and symptoms of anaphylaxis?
6. What is your hospital's policy on the use of alcohol swabs prior to injections?
7. What is the nurse's role in relation to patient education with regard to drug administration?
8. In what situation would a Patient Compliance Device be used in the community?
9. What documentation would be used in the community and institutional setting for controlled drug administration?
10. In what situation would a Patient Group Directive be used?

Practice 3
Blood Glucose Monitoring

Learning outcomes	**By the end of this section, you should know how to:** ▪ collect and prepare the equipment ▪ prepare the patient for this nursing practice ▪ carry out blood glucose measurement.
Background knowledge required	Anatomy and physiology of the endocrine system, with special reference to the regulation of blood glucose Clinical knowledge of insulin-dependent and non-insulin-dependent diabetes Target range of individual patient blood glucose level Knowledge of the normal range of blood glucose concentration Manufacturer's information on the selected test strip Knowledge of different blood glucose meters and devices used to obtain the blood sample and to measure blood glucose level Revision of local policy on blood glucose monitoring Principles of infection control with respect to blood-borne infection.
Indications and rationale for blood glucose estimation	Blood glucose estimation is the measurement of the level of blood glucose using a chemical test strip. This investigation may be carried out to: ▪ assist in the preliminary diagnosis of diabetes mellitus caused by pancreatic disease or other hormonal disorders *through the measurement of the level of glucose in the blood* ▪ monitor the blood glucose level in patients with established diabetes *in order to facilitate an acceptable blood glucose level and to detect abnormal levels (Watkins 2003)* ▪ monitor patients receiving parenteral nutrition (see p. 237) *to ensure that the blood glucose level is kept within an acceptable range*.
Outline of procedure	The nurse must be aware of the theory underpinning glucose monitoring practice and have a knowledge of the normal range of blood glucose level in order that any abnormal readings may be immediately recognised and treatment initiated according to local policy. Blood glucose levels are measured in mmol L^{-1}. Diabetes UK (http://www.diabetes.org.uk/home.htm) currently recommends that people with diabetes should aim to keep their blood levels between 4–6 mmol L^{-1} before meals (pre-prandial) and at no higher than 10 mmol L^{-1} two hours after meals (post-prandial). The acceptable range for each individual patient (particularly with long-standing diabetes) may vary slightly but should be identified by the medical practitioner and recorded in all patient documentation. Health promotion may be carried out in relation to an underlying disease, for example in a diabetic

patient attending for blood glucose monitoring. Aldridge (2005) advises that any education programme should take account of achievable patient goals, and individual preference for finger-pricking devices and glucose meters.

Equipment

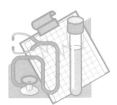

1. Finger-pricking device
2. Cotton-wool balls
3. Blood glucose testing strip
4. Disposable gloves
5. Tray for equipment
6. Sharps box
7. Receptacle for soiled material
8. Patient documentation and personal diabetic diary (if appropriate)
9. Blood glucose meter.

Guidelines and nursing practice

There are several different blood glucose pricking devices and meters available in the UK (Fig. 3.1), so the manufacturer's instructions for use must always be followed. Diabetes UK (http://www.diabetes.org.uk/home.htm) provides up-to-date information on a wide range of devices and meters.

- familiarise yourself with the instructions for the device you are using **to ensure a correct safe practice**
- check the expiry date of the test strip **to ensure that the strips are within the 'use by' date**
- confirm that the device is calibrated to the test strip **to reduce the risk of an error with the result**
- discuss the practice with the patient **to inform the patient about the practice and to discuss any concerns or queries**
- obtain consent from the patient to undertake the practice **to ensure that the patient is aware of his or her rights**
- select a suitable clean surface and lay out the equipment to provide an appropriate work surface
- cleanse the hands using an appropriate product **to reduce the risk of cross-infection**
- ask or assist the patient to wash his or her hands with soap and warm water, ensuring that all traces of soap have been rinsed off and that the hands are

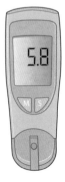
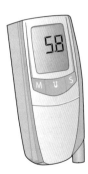
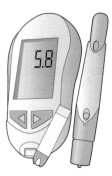

FIGURE 3.1
Blood glucose monitoring devices

dried thoroughly *to ensure that the skin surface is clean and that there is no residual soap, which may affect the accuracy of the reading. Heat will also help to dilate the small blood vessels in the fingertips*

- the patient's finger should not be cleansed with an alcohol-saturated wipe *as the alcohol acts as a contaminant and causes the skin to harden with constant use*
- any test strip accidentally contaminated by the nurse or patient must be discarded *as contamination of the test pad or the patient's blood could lead to inaccurate results*
- help the patient into a comfortable position (either sitting or lying supine) *to ensure patient comfort and prevent injury if the patient feels faint during the practice*
- select an appropriate puncture site (normally the soft flesh at either side of the top of the finger). If blood glucose monitoring is a regular practice, the site should be rotated *to avoid overuse of any one site and thus reduce discomfort for the patient*
- put on gloves *to protect the patient and nurse from potential blood-borne infection*
- using the pricking device prick the patient's finger *to pierce the skin with minimal discomfort*
- gently massage the finger to obtain an adequate drop of blood. *Obtain a suitable amount of blood to cover the test strip*
- allow the drop of blood to come into contact with the test strip as per the manufacturer's instructions without smearing and spreading the blood, *to ensure even coverage of the strip*
- continue as per the manufacturer's instructions for the specific device in use
- apply a clean cotton-wool ball with firm pressure to the skin site for approximately 30–60 seconds or until bleeding has stopped (the patient may be able to undertake this activity) *to prevent any further bleeding after the sample has been obtained and prevent haematoma formation*
- read the result on the glucose meter device *to obtain the blood glucose level*
- note and document the results in both the nursing/medical notes and the patient's personal diabetic diary (where applicable). Some meters can store results in the memory. Informing the patient of the result should normally be carried out in consultation with the medical practitioner who authorised the investigation *to ensure that the results are communicated to other healthcare professionals and the patient. It may not be appropriate for the nurse to give the result to the patient at this point if further investigations are required before an accurate diagnosis can be made*
- report any abnormal results to a medical practitioner as soon as possible. If the practice is being carried out in the patient's own home, the nurse may be required to remain with the patient until the glucose level has stabilised *to ensure that prompt and appropriate treatment can be initiated. There may be a local protocol to be followed when abnormal glucose readings are detected by nursing staff*
- dispose of any contaminated equipment according to local policy *to prevent the transmission of infection*
- remove the gloves and dispose of as above. Wash the hands *to prevent cross-infection*

- ensure that the patient is not feeling unwell after the practice (especially if the practice has been carried out in the patient's own home), *to ensure that any potential complications of the procedure are addressed promptly*
- discuss the points raised under 'Patient/carer education: key points', below. If the patient is unable to participate in follow-up self-care, this should be undertaken by the nurse or an appropriate adult carer *to ensure that the patient, carer and/or nurse are aware of, and understand, follow-up self-care*
- in undertaking this practice, nurses are accountable for their actions, the quality of care delivered and record-keeping according to the Code of Professional Conduct (Nursing and Midwifery Council 2004a), Guidelines for Records and Record Keeping (Nursing and Midwifery Council 2005), and Guidelines for the Administration of Medicines (Nursing and Midwifery Council 2004b).

The frequency of blood glucose monitoring will usually be advised by the medical practitioner.

Additional information

All test strips should be stored in a locked cupboard or drawer when not in use, in order to comply with health and safety at work regulations. The nurse in the community should encourage patients to keep all equipment in a safe place away from children. The manufacturer's recommendations for the conditions of storage and blood glucose monitoring technique must be observed, otherwise, inaccurate results may be obtained from the test strips.

It is advisable to record the date when the strips have been opened as they may need to be used within a certain time. Regular checking of the glucose meter device with the control solution provided by the manufacturer is recommended (Hall 1999).

The nurse should assess the blood glucose level at the specific time requested by the medical practitioner. There is evidence to suggest the value of testing at different points during the day to build up a profile over time (Watkins 2003).

Patient/carer education
Key points

In partnership with the patient and/or carer, ensure that they are competent to carry out any practices required. Information should be given on an appropriate point of contact for any concerns that may arise.

Diabetes UK has a wide range of education materials. Including 'Diabetes lifestyle', a newsletter providing invaluable information and advice specifically for black and minority ethnic (BME) communities (see website link).
- if the blood glucose results are not given immediately after undertaking the practice, the patient should be informed of when they will be available and of the process for obtaining them
- for newly diagnosed diabetic patients, the teaching of blood glucose estimation should be part of an individual education package on disease and symptom management. Teaching the patient about blood glucose estimation should incorporate the following main stages:

— education on the practice (including the rationale and the treatment of any abnormal readings) using verbal and written information
— demonstration of the blood glucose monitoring technique
— supervision of the patient carrying out blood glucose estimation
— regular monitoring of the technique as part of the ongoing management programme of care for the patient with diabetes

▪ patient education is likely to be shared between institutional and community staff
▪ patient education material is available from many of the manufacturers who produce test strips and devices and from the Diabetes UK website
▪ hospitalised insulin-dependent diabetics who are self-caring in this practice should be encouraged to continue with their monitoring as this provides an opportunity to assess their technique and reinforce good practice
▪ opportunity should be given for the patient and/or carer to discuss anxieties or issues concerning any newly diagnosed disease.

References

Aldridge V 2005 Facilitating self-management for diabetes patients. Practice Nurse 29(11): 33–34, 36, 38

Hall G 1999 Blood glucose monitoring. Practice Nurse 18(7): 469–471

Nursing and Midwifery Council (2004a) The NMC code of professional conduct: standards for conduct, performance and ethics. NMC, London

Nursing and Midwifery Council (2004b) Guidelines for the administration of medicines. NMC, London

Nursing and Midwifery Council 2005 Guidelines for records and record keeping. NMC, London

Watkins PJ 2003 ABC of diabetes, 5th edn. BMJ Books, London

Website
Diabetes UK Website: http://www.diabetes.org.uk/home.htm

Self assessment

1. What are the recommended ranges for normal blood glucose in healthy adults?
2. What part of the finger should you use for obtaining a sample of blood?
3. What action should you take if an abnormal blood glucose result is returned?
4. What patient education should you give a diabetic patient when teaching them to monitor their blood-glucose level independently?

Practice 4
Blood Pressure

Learning outcomes	**By the end of this section, you should know how to:** • prepare the patient for this nursing practice • collect and prepare the equipment • assess, measure, and record blood pressure.
Background knowledge required	Revision of the anatomy and physiology of the cardiovascular system.
Indications and rationale for regarding blood pressure	Blood pressure is the force exerted by the blood as it flows through the blood vessels. It is the arterial blood pressure that is normally recorded, and this may be indicated: • **to aid the diagnosis of disease** • **to aid in the assessment of the cardiovascular system during and after disease** • **to assess the efficacy of antihypertensive medication** • **preoperatively to assess the patient's usual range of blood pressure** • **to aid in the assessment of the cardiovascular system following surgery or trauma**.
Equipment 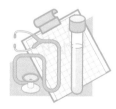	1. Sphygmomanometer: aneroid (Fig. 4.1A), electronic (Fig. 4.1B) or mercury (Fig. 4.1C) 2. Blood pressure cuff: different-sized cuffs are available for use on a baby, a child or an obese person (Williams et al 2004) 3. Stethoscope (for use with only an aneroid or mercury sphygmomanometer) 4. Swabs to clean stethoscope ear pieces and diaphragm.
Sphygmomanometers	Because of the health and environmental hazards associated with the use of mercury, mercury sphygmomanometers are increasingly being phased out and replaced with aneroid or electronic sphygmomanometers to monitor patients' blood pressure (Fig. 4.2). All sphygmomanometers should be calibrated at 6-monthly intervals by trained personnel to maintain the accuracy of the equipment (Williams et al 2004). Should nurses encounter any sphygmomanometers that they have not previously used, competency in the use of the equipment must be assured before assessing any patient's blood pressure.

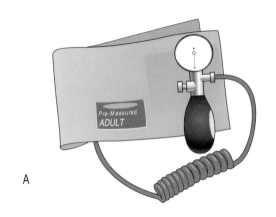

A

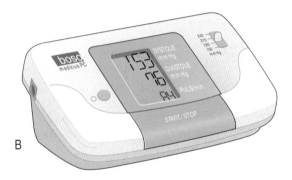

B

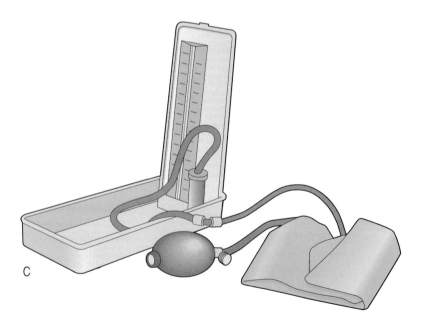

C

FIGURE 4.1
**Sphygmomanometers
used for blood pressure
measurement
A Aneroid
B Electronic
C Mercury**

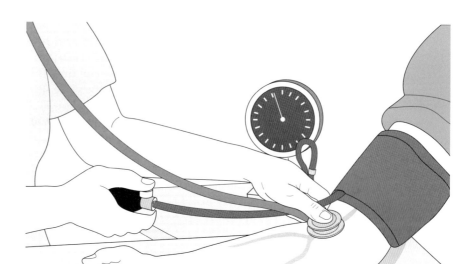

FIGURE 4.2
Stethoscope over the brachial artery

Guidelines and rationale for this nursing practice 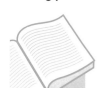	■ explain the nursing practice to the patient **to gain consent and co-operation** ■ wash the hands **to reduce the risk of cross-infection** ■ ensure the patient's privacy **to reduce anxiety and/or embarrassment** ■ collect the equipment **to assist in the planning and implementation of the practice** ■ observe the patient throughout this activity **to note any signs of distress** ■ help the patient into a suitable position, either sitting or lying, and remove any restrictive clothing from the arm. Avoid tightly rolled-up sleeves **as these prevent constriction of the vessels of the limb immediately before the practice and may lead to an inaccurate recording**.
Electronic sphygmomanometer	■ follow the manufacturer's instructions to achieving a recording, **thus ensuring an accurate measurement** ■ continue the practice as for 'All sphygmomanometers', below.
Aneroid sphygmomanometer	■ apply the cuff 3–5 cm above the point at which the brachial artery can be palpated. The cuff should be applied smoothly and firmly, covering 80% of the arm circumference (Williams et al 2004), the middle of the rubber bladder lying directly over the brachial artery **to permit access to the brachial artery by the stethoscope and ensure even pressure around the circumference of the limb. A bladder that is too large or too small will result in a respective under- or overestimation of the blood pressure** (Williams et al 2004) ■ if the patient is to have blood pressure measured both in a sitting and standing position then ask the patient to sit for 5 minutes or stand for 2 minutes before the blood pressure is recorded (Williams et al 2004)

- ask the patient to rest the straight arm, with forearm at heart level, on a suitable firm surface *to ensure patient comfort and prevent movement of the limb, which may lead to inaccurate results*
- palpate the radial pulse and inflate the cuff until the pulse has been obliterated. Inflate for a further 20 mmHg. Release the valve slowly, taking note of the reading on the dial when the radial pulse returns. Allow all the air to escape from the cuff. *This will provide an initial assessment of the systolic pressure*
- palpate the brachial pulse, place the stethoscope over the site (Fig. 4.3), and inflate the cuff to 20 mmHg above the previous reading. Release the valve of the inflation ball at a rate of 2 mmHg per second. When the first pulse is heard, the reading on the gauge should be noted – this is the systolic pressure (Williams et al 2004). *This provides an accurate assessment of the systolic pressure without excessive discomfort to the patient*
- continue to deflate the cuff, the pulse sounds changing to muffled sounds until they finally disappear. The reading at which the sound changes should be noted – this is the diastolic pressure (Williams et al 2004). *This provides an accurate assessment of the diastolic pressure*
- continue controlled deflation until a value 20 mmHg below the diastolic pressure has been reached *as this will eradicate the chance of a 'silent interval' leading to a false recording* (National Institute for Clinical Excellence 2004).

Mercury sphygmomanometer	<ul><li>position the sphygmomanometer at approximately heart height, ensuring that the mercury level is at zero and that the mercury column can be easily read. *This will reduce the incidence of over- or underestimation of the blood pressure* (Williams et al 2004)</li><li>if the patient is to have blood pressure measured both in a sitting and standing position then ask the patient to sit for 5 minutes or stand for 2 minutes before the blood pressure is recorded (Williams et al 2004)</li><li>apply the cuff 3–5 cm above the point at which the brachial artery can be palpated. The cuff should be applied smoothly and firmly, covering 80% of the arm circumference (Williams et al 2004), the middle of the rubber bladder being placed directly over the brachial artery *to permit access to the brachial artery by the stethoscope and even pressure around the circumference of the limb. A bladder that is too large or too small will result in under- and overestimation of the blood pressure respectively* (Williams et al 2004)</li><li>ask the patient to rest the arm on a suitable firm surface *to ensure patient comfort and prevent movement of the limb, which may lead to inaccurate results*</li><li>connect the cuff tubing to the manometer tubing and close the valve of the inflation ball, *creating a sealed unit within the equipment*</li><li>palpate the radial pulse and inflate the cuff until the pulse is obliterated. Inflate for a further 20 mmHg. Release the valve slowly, taking note of the reading on the mercury column when the radial pulse returns; the mercury level is read at the top of the meniscus. Allow all the air to escape from the cuff. *This will provide an initial assessment of the systolic pressure*</li><li>palpate the brachial pulse, place the stethoscope over the site (Fig. 4.3), and inflate the cuff to 20 mmHg above the previous reading. Release the valve of</li></ul>

the inflation ball at a rate of 2 mmHg per second. When the first pulse is heard, the mercury level should be noted – this is the systolic pressure (Williams et al 2004). ***This provides an accurate assessment of the systolic pressure without excessive discomfort to the patient***

- continue to deflate the cuff; the pulse sounds will become muffled until they finally disappear. The mercury level should now be noted – this is the diastolic pressure (Williams et al 2004). ***This provides an accurate assessment of the diastolic pressure***
- continue controlled deflation until a value 20 mmHg below the diastolic pressure has been reached ***as this will eradicate the chance of a 'silent interval' leading to a false recording***.

All sphygmomanometers	- completely deflate the cuff, disconnect the tubing and remove the cuff from the patient's arm ***to prevent further compression of the limb*** - ensure that the patient is left feeling as comfortable as possible ***to ensure the quality of this nursing practice*** - if a communal stethoscope has been used, clean the ear pieces with an alcohol-saturated swab ***to reduce cross-infection between staff*** - dispose of the equipment safely ***to comply with health and safety criteria and prolong the use of the equipment*** - document the nursing practice appropriately, comparing with past recordings: note any differences, detect trends, monitor the after-effects and report abnormal findings immediately. Blood pressure measurements can be recorded on a graded chart or abbreviated by placing the systolic pressure reading over the diastolic: 130/80 mmHg. ***This provides a written record and assists in the implementation of any action should an abnormality or adverse reaction to the practice be noted*** - in undertaking this practice, nurses are accountable for their actions, the quality of care delivered and record-keeping according to the Code of Professional Conduct: Standards for Conduct, Performance and Ethics (Nursing and Midwifery Council 2004) and Guidelines for Records and Record Keeping (Nursing and Midwifery Council 2005).
Additional information	Stressful situations such as admission to hospital or a visit to a healthcare professional are known to have an effect on people's blood pressure and can cause it to rise.
Patient/carer education Key points 	In partnership with the patient and/or carer, ensure that they are competent to carry out any practices required. Information should be given on an appropriate point of contact for any concerns that may arise. Inform the patient of the results and any action required should an abnormality be detected. Information regarding the common lifestyle factors that are known to affect blood pressure should be discussed with the patient. This may allow the patient to make an informed choice about whether or not to continue such practices.

References

National Institute for Clinical Excellence 2004 Clinical guideline 18 August 2004 Hypertension – management of hypertension in adults. In: Primary Care Online (available at http://nice.org.uk [accessed 28 November 2005])

Nursing Midwifery Council 2004 Code of professional conduct: standards for conduct, performance and ethics. NMC, London

Nursing Midwifery Council 2005 Guidelines for records and record keeping. NMC, London

Williams B, Poulter NR, Brown MJ et al 2004 Guidelines for management of hypertension: report of the fourth working party of the British Hypertension Society, 2004-BHS1V. Journal of Human Hypertension 18: 139–185

Website

Blood Pressure Association: http://www.bpassoc.org.uk

Self assessment

1. What are the main indications for measuring and recording a patient's blood pressure?
2. What considerations should be given to the machine, the cuff and bladder together with the inflation bulb and control valve (aneroid and mercury sphymomanometers) before using them to measure blood pressure?
3. How do you establish the point at which to cease inflation of the cuff/bladder when measuring the systolic pressure?
4. At which point is the diastolic blood pressure recorded?

Practice 5
Blood Transfusion

Learning outcomes	**By the end of this section, you should know how to:** ▪ prepare and support the patient receiving a blood component ▪ collect a blood component ▪ undertake the final patient identity check before administering a blood component ▪ monitor the patient, and take appropriate initial action in response to a possible transfusion reaction.
Background knowledge required	Revision of the anatomy and physiology of the blood, with a special emphasis on blood groups (*see* http://www.learnbloodtransfusion.org.uk) Review the adverse effects of blood transfusion, with special emphasis on the incorrect blood component reporting category (*see* http://www.shotuk.org.uk) Revision of 'Intravenous therapy' (*see* p. 169) Revision of 'Aseptic technique' (*see* p. 381) Review current national and European legislation and guidelines on blood transfusion (*see* http://www.transfusionguidelines.org.uk) Revision of local policy on blood transfusion.
Indications and rationale for a blood transfusion	The term 'blood transfusion' is used to describe the transfusion of red cells. Whole blood is rarely transfused nowadays. Red cells are supplemented with other blood components such as fresh frozen plasma or platelet concentrates if required, as this is considered more effective treatment (McClelland 2006). This practice will refer to the transfusion of red cells, however the same safety issues relate to the administration of all blood components. A 'blood transfusion' is the introduction of compatible donor red cells into the circulation of a recipient, and may be indicated for the following reasons: ▪ ***to support the patient who has lost a large volume of blood*** ▪ ***to enable a patient to have surgery that may involve the loss of a large volume of blood*** ▪ ***to support a patient receiving treatment for leukaemia or cancer*** ▪ ***to maintain or improve the lives of patients with some chronic conditions*** (Murphy 2005). Several countries have established a haemovigilance programme to collect data on the serious adverse effects of transfusion. The United Kingdom Serious Hazards of Transfusion (SHOT) scheme was launched in 1996. It is a voluntary scheme covering both NHS and independent hospitals, and aims to use the information gathered to improve safety standards for blood transfusion. The scheme has consistently reported that human error contributes significantly to the morbidity and mortality

of patients receiving blood transfusion (SHOT 1998–2005). The majority of these occurred because of an error in patient identification, either at the time of blood component collection from the storage site, or at the patient bedside. Correct identification of the patient is, therefore, the main focus of transfusion safety.

Outline of the procedure

The decision to transfuse a patient is made by a medical practitioner. Wherever possible the medical practitioner should discuss the risks and benefits of the proposed treatment with the patient. The USA and Canada have introduced written patient consent for blood transfusion, however there is no legal requirement in the UK to gain specific consent from the patient, for the transfusion of blood products. All patients, however, have a basic legal and ethical right to determine their treatment, and the patient should receive sufficient information to make an informed decision (Department of Health 2001). If the patient cannot communicate because, for instance, he or she is unconscious, it is essential that the proposed transfusion is explained to the patient's relative or carer.

When the decision to transfuse the patient is made, a venous blood sample will be taken and sent to the hospital transfusion laboratory along with a request for the blood component required. Tests will be undertaken on the sample to identify the patient's ABO, RhD group, and if there are any specific antibodies, before selecting a compatible donor unit for issue.

Each of the blood components have specific storage requirements (Table 5.1), and it is the responsibility of the hospital transfusion laboratory to ensure that blood components are stored appropriately (Guidelines for the Blood Transfusion Services in the UK 2005).

The final patient identification check is normally undertaken by two people, one of whom should be a registered medical practitioner or a 1st or 2nd level registered nurse. This practice has, however, been questioned as it may lead to a diffusion of responsibility and it has been suggested that it may be more appropriate for one registered practitioner to take full responsibility (British Committee for Standards in Haematology Transfusion Task Force 1999). It is therefore important to check current policy regarding the checking of patient identification.

Transfusion reactions

A reaction can occur with all blood components, therefore ensuring the patient's safety is the most important aspect of caring for a patient during the transfusion

---

TABLE 5.1
Blood components storage conditions

Component	Shelf-life	Storage conditions
Red blood cells; whole blood	35 days	4°C (± 2°C) in an authorised blood fridge
Platelets	5 days	+ 22°C (± 2°C) on an agitation rack in the hospital transfusion laboratory
Fresh frozen plasma	2 years	–30°C in the hospital transfusion laboratory
Cryoprecipitate	2 years	–30°C in the hospital transfusion laboratory

(Table 5.2). Any adverse event experienced by a patient should be considered as a possible transfusion reaction. Immediate recognition, and prompt nursing and medical action is required to prevent further complications, and possible death. This is particularly important if the patient is unconscious or cannot report symptoms.

If any transfusion reaction is suspected the transfusion must be ***stopped***, and urgent medical attention sought. Acute reactions can occur during, or within the first 24 hours of transfusion. Delayed transfusion reactions can occur days, weeks, months or even years later. These include delayed haemolytic reaction, and signs and symptoms of infectious disease such as hepatitis C or human immunodeficiency virus (HIV).

Treatment will depend on the cause and severity of the reaction, and is dictated by the patient's clinical condition. Close observation and monitoring of the patient should be maintained and this should include temperature, pulse, respiratory rate, blood pressure, blood loss and urinary output. All serious transfusion reactions must be reported to the hospital transfusion laboratory and duty haematologist, to ensure that the appropriate investigation, further management and reporting of the reaction occurs (Blood Safety and Quality Regulations 2005). There will be local policy for the method of reporting. The adverse event should also be documented in the patient's medical and nursing notes.

Equipment

As for intravenous infusion (*see* p. 169).

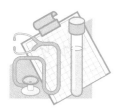

TABLE 5.2		
Acute transfusion reactions		
Type	*Cause*	*Symptoms*
Volume overload	Too much fluid is transfused or component transfused too rapidly	Dyspnoea, hypertension and tachycardia
Febrile	An immune response of the recipient to white cell antigens or white cell fragments in the blood component	Headache, mild fever (temperature rise of up to 1.5°C), and a moderate tachycardia without hypotension
Allergic, urticarial or anaphylactic	An immune response of the recipient to plasma proteins in the blood component	*Urticarial*: headache, rash and purititis without hypotension
		Anaphylaxis: nausea, vomiting, facial swelling, wheezing and laryngeal oedema
Haemolytic	The majority are the transfusion of an ABO incompatible component	Rigors, loin pain, muscle aches, tachycardia, hypotension and haemoglobinuria
Septic shock	A bacterially contaminated component	Chills, high fever, vomiting, abdominal cramps, diarrhoea and signs of shock

Additional equipment	1. Sterile blood administration set
	2. Infusion device
	3. Non-sterile gloves and apron (Gammon & Gould 2005).

In emergency situations	1. Intravenous fluid pressure infusion bag (Fenwal bag)
	2. Blood-warming equipment.

Guidelines and rationale for this nursing practice

In undertaking this practice, nurses are accountable for their actions, the quality of care delivered and record keeping according of the Code of Professional Conduct: Standards for Conduct, Performance and Ethics (Nursing and Midwifery Council 2004a), Guidelines for the Administration of Medicines (Nursing and Midwifery Council 2004b), and Guidelines for Records and Record Keeping (Nursing and Midwifery Council 2005). You should refer to your local transfusion policy, as there may be some variations in practice.

Practical aspects of transfusion

- blood components should be transfused via an intravenous route separate from all other infusions, *to prevent clotting of the transfused component in the infusion tubing*
- blood components must be administered through a blood administration set with an integral filter, *to filter macroaggregates (white cells, platelets and coagulum), which collect in stored blood*
- no drugs should be added to any blood component, *as they may contain additives such as calcium which can cause the citrated blood to clot*
- infusion devices, which are certified as suitable for use for blood components can be used to assist with regulation of flow rate.

Preparing the patient for transfusion

Gloves and apron should be worn to prevent contamination with body fluids.
- ensure that the blood component has been prescribed, and check the prescription for the following information:
  — the name and date of birth of the patient
  — the patient identification number
  — the date and time of the transfusion
  — the type of blood component prescribed, e.g., red cells or platelets
  — the number of units prescribed
  — the rate of transfusion ordered
  — the signature of the medical practitioner
- help to explain the nursing practice to the patient, *to gain consent and co-operation and encourage participation in care*
- collect and prepare the equipment, *making an efficient use of time and resources*
- ensure that the patient is in a setting where they can be directly observed, *to ensure visual observation of the patient*
- assist the patient into a comfortable position and ensure the patient's privacy, *to respect and maintain self-esteem and promote acceptance to the transfusion*

- prime the administration set with normal saline, **dextrose 5% or ringer lactate solution SHOULD NOT BE USED, as this may lead to clotting of the blood component**
- assist the medical practitioner with the insertion of an intravenous cannula if required.

Collecting blood components from the hospital transfusion laboratory or satellite fridge

- collect the blood component immediately before it is required, **so that the blood component is stored at the correct temperature until administered**
- in a non-emergency situation, collect one blood component at a time, **to reduce the risk of a patient identification error**
- take written patient identification information when collecting blood components, **as failure of correct patient identification is a major source of incorrect blood component incidents**
- check the written patient identification details against the information on the blood component label, **to ensure the patient identification details match**
- record the collection of the blood component on the blood fridge register, **to ensure traceability of the blood component** (Blood Safety and Quality Regulations 2005)
- deliver the blood component promptly to the clinical area, **to ensure that the transfusion is commenced without delay**.

Pre-administration checking procedure

- check the prescription for the blood component, **to identify if the patient has any special requirements, e.g. irradiated blood, or a concomitant drug, e.g. a diuretic**
- take a reading of the patient's temperature, pulse, respiration and blood pressure, **to provide a set of baseline observations before the start of the blood transfusion** (Gray et al 2005)
- check the expiry date of the component, and undertake a visual inspection of the component, **to ensure the component is safe to use** (Fig. 5.1)
- if there are any discrepancies do not proceed, **contact the hospital transfusion laboratory for advice and inform the nurse in charge and medical staff**.

Final patient identification checking procedure

- establish the patient's identity, wherever possible ask the patient to tell you their first name, surname and date of birth
  — check this information against the patient's wristband for accuracy
  — check that the patient's identification details on the wristband match the patient details on the compatibility/traceability label attached to the blood component
  — check that the blood group and donation number on the compatibility/traceability label are identical to the information on the blood component label (Fig. 5.2)
- if there are any discrepancies do not proceed, **contact the hospital transfusion laboratory for advice and inform the nurse in charge and medical staff**

Red Blood Cells

Compatibility/Traceability Label

The compatibility/traceability label is generated in the hospital transfusion laboratory. It is attached to the blood component and contains the following patient information *Surname, Forename(s), Date of birth, Gender, Hospital Number/ CHI Number, Hospital and Ward*

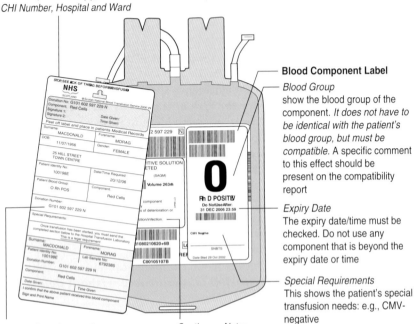

Blood Component Label

Blood Group
show the blood group of the component. *It does not have to be identical with the patient's blood group, but must be compatible.* A specific comment to this effect should be present on the compatibility report

Expiry Date
The expiry date/time must be checked. Do not use any component that is beyond the expiry date or time

Special Requirements
This shows the patient's special transfusion needs: e.g., CMV-negative

FIGURE 5.1
Blood component label and compatibility/ traceability label.
From Scottish Blood Transfusion Service, with permission

Unique Donation number
This is the unique number assigned to each blood donation by the Transfusion Service and allows traceability from donor to patient

Cautionary Notes
This gives instructions on storage conditions and the checking procedures for adminstering a blood component. It also includes information on the component type and volume

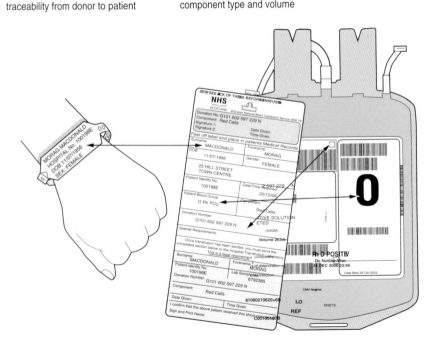

FIGURE 5.2
Checking the information on the patient's wristband and the compatibility/ traceability label attached to the blood component.
From Scottish Blood Transfusion Service, with permission

- transfer the donation number to the patient's transfusion record/chart and complete all documentation, *to ensure there is traceability of the transfused component and a record of professional responsibility*
- connect the blood component to the administration set, and commence the transfusion at the prescribed rate
- current recommendations advise that each unit of red cells should be transfused within 4 hours of removal from controlled storage.

Monitoring the patient during blood transfusion

- ensure the patient has access to the nurse call bell system, *to enable the patient to gain assistance immediately*
- observe the patient throughout the transfusion, with particular attention to the first 15 minutes, *as the majority of major transfusion reactions occur within this time period*
- monitor the patient's temperature and pulse every 15 minutes for the first hour of the transfusion (Gray & Illingworth 2004). Thereafter, continue to assess the temperature, pulse, respiration and blood pressure hourly, *to ensure early detection in the event of an adverse reaction*
- if a transfusion reaction is suspected, the transfusion must be stopped immediately and urgent medical advice sought, *to ensure prompt action in the event of an adverse reaction*.

On completion of the transfusion

- record the volume of the blood component transfused, *to ensure accurate monitoring of the patient's fluid balance status*. There are approximately 250–300 ml in a unit of red cells
- if other intravenous fluids are to be administered, change the blood administration set when the transfusion is completed, *as there may be residue of the blood component in the infusing tubing*
- dispose of the equipment safely, *to prevent the risk of sharp injuries and the transmission of infection*
- file all transfusion documentation in the patient's case notes, *to ensure compliance with traceability legislation* (Blood Safety and Quality Regulations 2005).

Patient/carer education

Key points

In partnership with the patient and/or carer, ensure that they are competent to carry out any required practices. Information should be given on an appropriate point of contact for any concerns that may arise.

- explain the reason for the transfusion, and state the time expected for the completion of each unit. This makes it easier for the patient to tolerate the practice
- advise the patient to notify you immediately if they become aware of any symptoms such as shivering, flushing, pain or shortness of breath or begin to feel anxious. This will enable early identification of any adverse effects of transfusion
- explain the importance of maintaining the cannula, by keeping the cannulated limb as still as possible. Emphasise the dangers of disconnection of the infusion lines

- explain the importance of immediately reporting any soreness or redness at the site of the transfusion, which may be a sign of local infection, even after completion of the transfusion
- if the patient has had a specific antibody identified on pre-transfusion testing, this will be documented by the hospital transfusion laboratory for future reference. The patient should also be given written information on the details of the particular antibody. They should be advised to give this to the doctor or nurse the next time they require to be transfused.

References

Blood Safety and Quality Regulations 2005 No. 50. The Stationery Office, London

British Committee for Standards in Haematology Blood Transfusion Task Force (Chairman: Kelsey P) 1999 [under revision 2006] Guidelines on the administration of blood components and the management of transfused patients. Transfusion Medicine 9: 227–238

Department of Health 2001 Good practice in consent. Implementation guideline: consent to examination or treatment. Department of Health, London

Gammon J, Gould D 2005 Universal precautions, a review of compliance and strategies to improve practice. Journal of Research in Nursing 10(5): 529–547

Gray A, Illingworth J 2004 Right blood, right patient, right time. RCN guidance for improving transfusion practice. Royal College of Nursing, London

Gray A, Howell C, Pirie E 2005 Improving blood transfusion: a patient-centred approach. Nursing Standard 19(26): 38–42

Guidelines for the Blood Transfusion Services in the UK 2005 (7th edn). The Stationery Office, London

McClelland DBL (ed) 2006 The handbook of transfusion medicine (4th edn in press). The Stationery Office, London

Murphy MF (ed) 2005 Practical transfusion medicine. Blackwell Science, Oxford

Nursing and Midwifery Council 2004a Code of professional conduct: standards for conduct, performance and ethics. NMC, London

Nursing and Midwifery Council 2004b Guidelines for the administration of medicines. NMC, London

Nursing and Midwifery Council 2005 Guidelines for records and record keeping. NMC, London

The United Kingdom Serious Hazards of Transfusion. Annual Report 1998–2005. SHOT, London

Websites

Department of Health: http://www.dh.gov.uk

Scottish National Blood Transfusion Service: http://www.learnbloodtransfusion. org.uk

Serious Hazards of Transfusion (SHOT): http://www.shotuk.org.uk

UK Blood Transfusion & Tissue Transplantation Service: http://www. transfusionguidelines.org.uk

Self assessment

1. What is the most common cause of an incompatible transfusion?
2. What checks should be completed when collecting a red cell unit from the hospital blood bank or satellite fridge?
3. What vital signs should be recorded on a patient receiving a red cell transfusion?
4. What is the first step you should take if you suspect a transfusion reaction?

Practice 6
Body Temperature

Learning outcomes	**By the end of this section, you should be able to:** ▪ demonstrate an understanding of the rationale for this practice ▪ prepare the patient for this nursing practice ▪ collect and prepare the equipment ▪ measure and record the body temperature at the axilla, in the oral cavity, ear canal or in the rectum, in both a community and a hospital setting.
Background knowledge required	Revision of the anatomy and physiology of the skin in relation to the control of body temperature and the temperature-regulating centre, and of the related body mechanisms associated with heat production and heat loss. Revision of the anatomy of the area where the temperature is to be measured.
Indications and rationale	Body temperature can be considered as the balance of heat lost from the body and heat gained by the body. Both behavioural and physiological mechanisms maintain *core* body temperature at 37°C ± 1°C. Abnormal body temperature recordings may be an indication that your patient has an infection, is becoming unwell or is experiencing an abnormal reaction to transfused blood products. The normal *range* of body temperature is 36–37.5°C, but this may vary, by as much as 0.6°C, according to the site used for measurement and from individual to individual. Factors naturally influencing the patient's body temperature include the ingestion of fluids and food, hormonal changes, smoking and a number of conditions that interfere with thermoregulation (Neno 2005). It is also important, where possible, to establish your patient's normal temperature at rest. The following terms are used to describe abnormal temperature ranges: ▪ Mild hypothermia (32–35°C) ▪ Moderate hypothermia (28–32°C) ▪ Severe hypothermia (below 28°C) ▪ Mild pyrexia (depending on your patient's normal baseline temperature, 37.2–38.9°C) ▪ Hyperthermia (above 40.6°C). The upper and lower limits of survival are not precisely known but are thought to be a body temperature of 44°C and 27°C respectively. The recording of body temperature may be required: ▪ **to establish a baseline temperature**, for example when patients are admitted to the hospital or clinic ▪ **to monitor fluctuations in temperature**, as may occur during the postoperative period, **as temperature fluctuations can indicate developing infection or the presence of a deep venous thrombosis**

- **to monitor signs of incompatibility when patients are receiving a blood transfusion**
- **to monitor the temperature of patients being treated for an infection**
- **to monitor the temperature of patients recovering from hypothermia**
- **to monitor temperature during and following invasive diagnostic procedures.**

The frequency of measurement will be dependent upon your patient's condition and recorded temperature.

Equipment

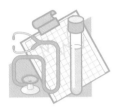

1. Tray
2. Appropriate thermometer, e.g.
   — disposable thermometer
   — electronic thermometer plus probe and disposable cover
   — tympanic thermometer and disposable cover
3. Alcohol-impregnated swabs
4. Watch with a second hand
5. Black pen
6. Observation chart
7. Tissues
8. Receptacle for disposable items.

The nature of this practice means that there is a risk of cross infection if the nurse does not adequately clean the thermometers between different patients. Digital electronic probes as well as tympanic thermometers with sheaths/covers still require cleaning with a swab containing 70% isopropyl after patient use to prevent the spread of infection (Carroll 2000).

Disposable thermometers

A variety of disposable thermometers are available for purchase, two of the more common ones being the chemical dot thermometer and the liquid crystal heat-sensitive synthetic strip (Fig. 6.1). These are for single use only, and the manufacturer's instructions for use must be followed to ensure an accurate recording. These thermometers tend to be used in a community or domestic setting.

Electronic thermometers

Electronic thermometers (Fig. 6.2) have replaced traditional mercury glass thermometers as one of the most popular methods of measuring body temperature in hospitals. The electronic thermometer can be used both orally and axillary and some may have a separate probe for rectal use. In addition to this, the electronic thermometer may require that the correct mode of use, e.g. oral or rectal is selected prior to use. Regardless of which site is selected, research indicates that the accuracy of the recording is dependent upon correct probe placement and the cleanliness of the equipment itself (Carroll 2000). The thermometer will automatically give out an audible signal when the temperature has been recorded. As an accountable nurse it is your personal responsibility that you know how to operate equipment and referral to the manufacturer's instructions is essential.

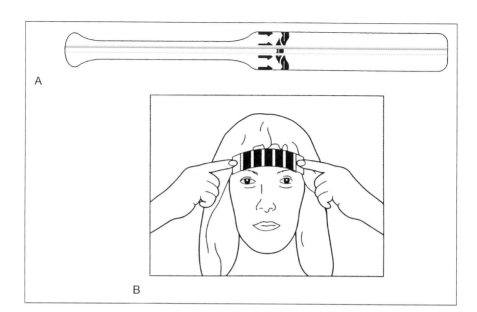

FIGURE 6.1
A Disposable chemical dot thermometer
B Liquid crystal disposable thermometer

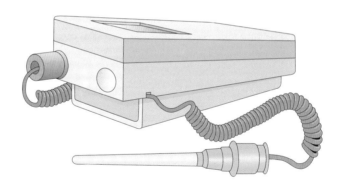

FIGURE 6.2
Example of an electronic thermometer
From Torrance & Semple 1998. Copyright Emap Public Sector Ltd 1998. Reproduced by permission of Nursing Times

Tympanic thermometers

Now in widespread use, tympanic thermometers (Figs 6.3 & 6.4) have a probe with a disposable cover that is inserted into the ear canal. They detect infrared energy that is emitted from the tympanic membrane at the end of the ear canal and surrounding tissue, this then being displayed digitally as a temperature reading. Literature suggests that tympanic thermometers represent a more accurate picture of actual body temperature due to the fact that the tympanic membrane shares the same arterial blood supply as the hypothalamus (the temperature regulating centre within the brain; Gallimore 2004).

The thermometer must be covered by a disposable cover in order to function, and the detection window must be kept clean in order to obtain an accurate result. False readings may arise from incorrect technique, a damaged lens or an inaccurate timing between measurements (Jevon & Jevon 2001).

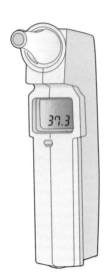
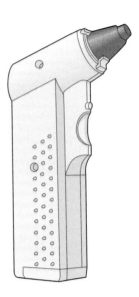

FIGURE 6.3
Example of a tympanic thermometer
From Torrance & Semple 1998. Copyright Emap Public Sector Ltd 1998. Reproduced by permission of Nursing Times

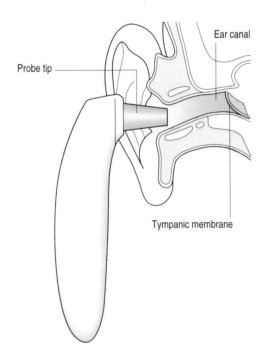

Ear canal

Probe tip

Tympanic membrane

FIGURE 6.4
Tympanic membrane thermometer; insertion of probe into ear canal
From Gallimore 2004. Copyright Emap Public Sector Ltd 2004. Reproduced by permission of Nursing Times

Guidelines and rationale for this nursing practice

The patient should be assessed carefully to identify the most appropriate site for temperature measurement, which will ensure an accurate and safe result. Once chosen, the same site should be used for consistent measurement.

Axilla

The axillary site is inappropriate in patients where peripheral circulation is shut down, such as patients with hypothermia (Stevenson 2004). In addition to this the axillary site is the least accurate site in reflecting core body temperature. In elderly patient groups there may be insufficient lean body mass to ensure that the probe is surrounded by skin tissue. The presence of surgical wounds around the site should indicate the avoidance of the site as a means of temperature measurement.

- wash the hands and clean thermometer *to prevent cross-infection* (Carroll 2000)
- explain the nursing practice *to gain consent and co-operation, and encourage participation in care*. Ensure that the patient has not recently had a hot bath, ingested fluid or food or been engaged in strenuous exercise *as these will cause a temporary rise in body temperature*
- ensure the patient's privacy *to respect individuality and maintain self-esteem*
- help the patient into a comfortable position, either sitting or lying, with the back and shoulders well supported *so that the position can be maintained for a few minutes*
- help the patient to remove or adjust the clothing *to expose one axilla*
- observe the patient throughout this activity *to monitor any adverse effects*
- dry the skin of the axilla by wiping with a tissue, *a film of moisture between the skin and the thermometer probe can cause an inaccurate reading*
- place the probe of the thermometer in the axilla where the skin surfaces will surround it *to gain an accurate temperature reading*
- help the patient to hold the arm across the chest *to retain the thermometer in the correct position*
- leave the thermometer in position as per the manufacturer's instructions *to ensure an accurate technique*
- remain with the patient if required *to reassure the patient and ensure that the thermometer remains in the correct position*
- remove the thermometer *when the optimum time for accurate recording has been reached*
- read the temperature measured by the thermometer *for an accurate recording to be monitored and documented*
- ensure that the patient is left feeling as comfortable as possible *to reassure the patient and reduce anxiety*
- clean/dispose of equipment safely *to prevent cross-infection*
- document the temperature reading in the patient's records, compare the reading with previous recordings, and report any abnormal findings

immediately. ***This will ensure safe practice and enable prompt, appropriate medical and nursing intervention to be initiated***
- in undertaking this practice, nurses are accountable for their actions, the quality of care delivered and record-keeping according to the Code of Professional Conduct (Nursing and Midwifery Council 2004), and Guidelines for Records and Record Keeping (Nursing and Midwifery Council 2005).

Oral cavity

Accuracy in measuring body temperature utilising this site is often determined by thermometer placement. Accuracy of the reading will also be affected by mouth breathing, oxygen therapy, fluid/food ingestion and smoking. The oral cavity should be avoided in patients who are at risk of seizure, patients who are confused and perhaps non-compliant and patients who have undergone oral surgery. These factors should be considered prior to proceeding to use this site.
- wash the hands and clean the thermometer ***to prevent cross-infection*** (Carroll 2000)
- explain the nursing practice ***to gain consent and co-operation***. Ensure that the patient has not recently had a hot or cold drink, or a hot bath, or been engaged in strenuous exercise ***as this may temporarily raise the body temperature***
- help the patient into a comfortable position ***so that he or she will more readily tolerate the thermometer probe***
- prepare the thermometer as per the manufacturer's instructions
- apply a disposable sleeve if required ***to prevent the transmission of infection***
- place the thermometer probe under the patient's tongue so that the probe lies adjacent to the frenulum at the junction of the floor of the mouth and the base of the tongue, on either the right or left side. ***A maximum temperature recording will be obtained from one of these two 'heat pockets' in the mouth*** (Fig. 6.5). This is also the position for disposable oral thermometers
- explain to the patient the importance of closing only the lips round the thermometer, and not biting it, ***so that the oral temperature is maintained and not distorted by the inspiration of air through the mouth***
- leave the thermometer in position for the required time ***for accurate recording to occur***
- remove the thermometer probe and proceed as for an axillary temperature recording.

Rectum

The rectal site should not be used in patients with rectal trauma, e.g. haemorrhoids, rectal surgery or patients who have difficulty in lying on their left side. In addition to this you should be aware that the presence of soft stool within the rectum can lead to an inaccurate result being obtained.
- wash hands, apply gloves, clean thermometer ***to prevent cross-infection*** (Carroll 2000)
- explain the nursing practice to the patient ***to gain consent and co-operation***
- ensure the patient's privacy ***to respect individuality and maintain self-esteem***

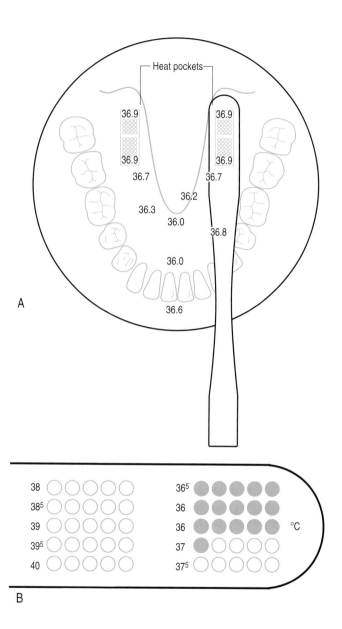

FIGURE 6.5
A Heat pockets in the oral cavity
B Recording area of a disposable thermometer

- help the patient into a comfortable position lying on his or her side with the knees bent *so that access is easier and the patient is least distressed*
- prepare the thermometer probe as per the manufacturer's instructions
- if suggested by the manufacturer, lubricate the end of the thermometer probe *to make insertion easier and prevent any damage to the mucosa*
- gently insert the thermometer probe into the patient's anus for 2–4 cm and hold it in position for the required time *for an accurate recording of the temperature to occur*
- remove the thermometer probe, dispose of the probe and soiled glove, and proceed as for an axillary temperature recording.

Ear canal – tympanic thermometer only

A number of factors must be considered prior to using the tympanic route. The comfort of your patient and accuracy of your recording could be affected by a range of factors. These are summarised in Box 6.1.

Once these have been considered you can then, if safe and appropriate, continue with tympanic measurement.

- wash the hands and clean the thermometer *to prevent cross-infection* (Carroll 2000)
- explain the nursing practice *to gain consent and co-operation*. Ensure that the patient has not recently had a hot or cold drink, or a hot bath, or been engaged in strenuous exercise *as this may temporarily raise the body temperature*
- help the patient into a comfortable position *in order to gain safe access to the ear canal and so that the patient will tolerate the practice more readily*
- prepare the thermometer as per the manufacturer's instructions *to ensure an accurate measurement*
- apply a disposable sleeve *to prevent the transmission of infection and allow the device to function*
- switch the device on *to ensure that it is calibrated and ready to take an accurate measurement*
- stabilise the patient's head *to ensure the safe introduction of the thermometer probe*
- gently pull the ear lobe upwards and position the probe so that it occludes the canal, *this will straighten the ear canal and permit the probe a view of the tympanic membrane without interference from ambient air temperature* (Fig. 6.6)
- hold the thermometer steady and take the recording as per the manufacturer's instructions *for accurate recording to occur*
- remove the thermometer probe, dispose of the cover, and return equipment to its storage case *to prevent breakage and prolong usage*
- proceed as for an axillary temperature recording.

Additional information

The measurement of body temperature is an invaluable observation regarding your patient's condition and one that can inform decisions made about your patient's treatment and care. It is vital that you utilise the correct equipment,

---

BOX 6.1
Factors affecting readings

Wax in the ear
Incorrect placement of the probe tip in the ear canal
Inner ear infection
Lying on the side of the head that will be measured before a temperature recording
Hair in the ear
The removal of a hearing aid up to 20 minutes before a reading is taken
Most studies acknowledge some of the above factors, but none consider them all

---

From Gallimore 2004. Copyright Emap Public Sector Ltd 2004. Reproduced by permission of Nursing Times

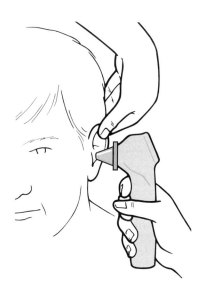

FIGURE 6.6
Using a tympanic thermometer

select the correct site and record your patient's temperature accurately, recognising abnormalities and irregularities and reporting these promptly. Body-temperature measurement can be obtained via either the oral, rectal, axillary or tympanic route. It should be noted that the core temperature can be more than 0.4°C higher than the oral temperature and more than 0.2°C lower than the rectal temperature. Oral, rectal and axillary temperature can be taken using a digital electronic probe and tympanically using a special hand-held device with a probe that is inserted into the patient's ear canal. For each patient, the preferred site should be used consistently so that any change in temperature can be accurately monitored. This should be based on an assessment of the most appropriate site for measurement to be recorded.

Traditionally, mercury glass thermometers have been used in recording body temperature. However, there are risks associated with their use, which means that they should no longer be used in recording body temperature, i.e. the safety hazard in relation to broken glass and exposure to mercury (Dean & Shobbrook 2003).

It is important to note that the measurement of body temperature does not rely solely on the thermometer alone, but should include a general observation of the patient: does the patient look flushed, is the skin hot or cold, is the patient sweating and clammy to touch, is the patient shivering or showing signs of confusion and disorientation?

Patient/carer education

Key points

In partnership with the patient and/or carer, ensure that they are competent to carry out any required practices. Information should be given on an appropriate point of contact for any concerns that may arise:

- explain the importance of monitoring the body temperature for evaluating the progress and treatment of the patient's condition
- the patient should understand the importance of the thermometer remaining in position for the correct period of time
- explain the importance of reporting headaches, excess sweating, shivering or general feelings of distress, which may indicate a change in body temperature

- patients with pyrexia should understand the importance of drinking an adequate amount of fluid in order to prevent dehydration
- elderly patients should be given advice on how to prevent heat loss at home and told of the dangers of hypothermia. This should be reinforced with written advice and specific information about the resources available, and should involve family and carers as applicable
- the procedure should be explained to the patient and instruction given as to their role in achieving accurate measurement, e.g. the need to restrain from speaking during oral recording.

References

Carroll M 2000 An evaluation of temperature measurement. Nursing Standard 14(44): 39–43.

Dean J, Shobbrook P 2003 Insights into adult nursing. In: Grandis S, Long G, Glasper A et al (eds) Foundation studies for nursing. Palgrave Macmillan, London, pp 138–173

Gallimore D 2004 Reviewing the effectiveness of tympanic thermometers. Nursing Times 100(32): 32–34

Jevon P, Jevon M 2001 Using a tympanic thermometer. Nursing Times 97(9): 43–44

Neno R 2005 Hypothermia: assessment, treatment and prevention. Nursing Standard 19(20): 47–52

Nursing and Midwifery Council 2004 Code of professional conduct: standards for conduct, performance and ethics. NMC, London

Nursing and Midwifery Council 2005 Guidelines for records and record keeping. NMC, London

Stevenson T 2004 Achieving best practice in routine observation of hospital patients. Nursing Times 100(30): 34–36

Torrance C, Semple M 1998 Practical procedures for nurses No 6.1. Recording temperature 1. Nursing Times 94(2): insert 2 pp

Self assessment

1. What is the normal temperature range in a healthy adult?
2. What observations could you use to assess your patient's temperature apart from the use of a thermometer?
3. Write down the numerical values of the following temperature ranges:
   —hyperthermia
   —mild hypothermia
   —borderline pyrexia
   —moderate hypothermia.
4. Identify the contraindications for the use of the following sites for recording temperature:
   —tympanic
   —oral
   —axillary
   —rectal.
5. Ray Martin is a 75-year-old gentleman who lives alone in sheltered accommodation. What advice would you give to Ray to prevent hypothermia?

Practice 7
Bone Marrow Aspiration

Learning outcomes

By the end of this section, you should know how to:
- prepare the patient for this procedure
- collect and prepare the equipment
- assist the medical practitioner during bone marrow aspiration
- monitor the patient for the adverse effects of bone marrow aspiration.

Background knowledge required

Revision of the anatomy and physiology of the blood, with special reference to the source and development of the red blood corpuscles
Revision of 'Wound care' technique (*see* p. 381)
Revision of local policy on bone marrow aspiration.

Indications and rationale for bone marrow aspiration

Soft tissue found in the inner cavities of the bones, which is responsible for the formation of blood cells, is known as 'red marrow'. Bone marrow aspiration is the removal of a sample of this fluid, and may be indicated for the following:
- to confirm the diagnosis of some anaemias, leukaemias and lymphomas
- to evaluate the effectiveness of treatment during the course of a disease
- to identify the source of a pyrexia of unknown origin
- to assess a person's ability to store iron.

Outline of the procedure

Bone marrow aspiration is carried out by a medical practitioner or a specially trained nurse. The procedure may take place as a day patient in an outpatient setting, or as an inpatient in hospital. It is considered best practice to obtain written consent, as bone marrow aspiration is an invasive procedure. The medical practitioner should ensure that the patient has received sufficient information about the procedure to make an informed decision (Department of Health 2001).

Positioning the patient

The position of the patient for the procedure is dependent on the site chosen for aspiration:

Posterior superior iliac crest

This is the preferred site, the patient is positioned in a right or left lateral position with knees flexed.

Anterior superior iliac crest

The patient can be positioned prone or on their side.

Sternum

The patient is required to lie supine with one pillow under the head.

Sternal aspiration should only be attempted in adults, since there is a higher incidence of complications in infants and children. Care is required to prevent cardiac injury, therefore the iliac crest should be considered as first choice as there are no vital organs near the puncture site.

Tibia

Aspiration of the anteromedial surface of the tibia is performed only in children under 18 months of age. The patient is positioned on their back.

Bone marrow aspiration is an aseptic procedure and takes approximately 20–30 minutes. The patient may be given a sedative prior to the procedure, to help them relax. Following correct hand-washing procedures the medical practitioner will administer a local anaesthetic into the chosen site and then apply sterile gloves. The skin over the aspiration site is cleansed using an antiseptic, a small stab incision is made, and the aspiration needle inserted through the skin and rotated until it penetrates the cortex, or outer covering of the bone, into the red bone marrow cavity.

The needle is specially designed and fitted with an adjustable protective guard to control its level of penetration (Fig. 7.1), thus preventing injury to the underlying vital organs. The stilette of the needle is removed and the syringe attached to the hub of the marrow needle.

Approximately 2.5 ml of bone marrow is aspirated, if additional marrow is needed the needle is repositioned, and a new syringe attached. The specimen of marrow is transferred from the syringe to the microscopic slides. Following the aspiration, the syringe is disconnected, the stilette replaced and the needle withdrawn. The slides are smeared with a preservative, allowed to dry, and sent to the laboratory for testing.

As the microscope slides are prepared, pressure should be applied to the puncture site until bleeding ceases. The puncture site should be covered with a sterile adhesive dressing.

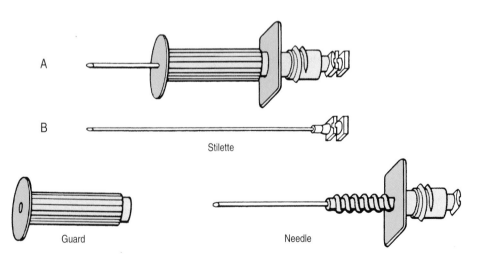

FIGURE 7.1
Bone marrow aspiration needle (disposable) showing the adjustable guard
A Complete needle
B Needle taken apart

If the patient has received sedation prior to the procedure, it is important to ensure that they have fully recovered from its effects before they mobilise.

Serious problems from a bone marrow aspiration are not common, however problems may include:

- excessive bleeding from the biopsy site. People with clotting problems may have a higher chance of this occurring
- infection of the bone at the biopsy site
- injury to the heart, lung or major blood vessel if the sample is taken from the sternum. A cardiac tamponade can develop when bleeding from a ruptured blood vessel in the myocardium causes pressure on the pericardial sac (Lewis et al 2004).

Equipment

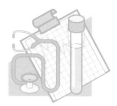

1. Trolley for equipment
2. Sterile gloves
3. Disposable plastic aprons
4. Sterile dressings pack
5. Alcohol-based antiseptic for cleansing the skin
6. Local anaesthetic and equipment for its administration
7. Sterile disposable scalpel or similar equipment
8. Sterile marrow aspiration needles
9. Sterile 20 ml syringe for aspiration of the marrow
10. Plastic spray dressing
11. Sterile adhesive dressing
12. Receptacle for soiled disposable items
13. Microscope slides, appropriately labelled, coverslips and slide fixative if the haematology technician service is not available
14. Sterile specimen containers appropriately labelled with a completed laboratory form and plastic specimen bag for transportation.

Guidelines and rationale for this nursing practice

- In undertaking this practice, nurses are accountable for their actions, the quality of care delivered and record-keeping according to the Code of Professional Conduct: Standards for Conduct, Performance and Ethics (Nursing and Midwifery Council 2004), and Guidelines for Records and Record Keeping (Nursing and Midwifery Council 2005). You should refer to your local policy, as there may be some variations in practice.

Preparing for the procedure

- identify the patient, **to ensure correct patient identification** (National Patient Safety Agency 2005)
- assist the medical practitioner to explain the procedure to the patient, **to gain consent and co-operation**

The medical practitioner should identify the following:
— medical history, **to identify medical problems that may complicate the procedure**

— current medication, including herbal supplements, **to identify potential complications with clotting**

— previous adverse reactions to medications or anaesthetics, **to identify if the patient has any allergies**

- prepare the equipment and trolley, **to ensure that all the equipment is available and ready for use**
- the patient's temperature, pulse, respiration and blood pressure should be recorded, **to provide a baseline reading, which will assist with monitoring the patient**

The procedure

- follow correct hand-washing procedures, **to reduce the risk of cross-infection** (Gammon & Gould 2005)
- if sedation is required, assist the medical practitioner with administration. **Sedation will help to reduce patient anxiety**
- help the patient into the correct position, depending on the chosen site, as this will permit easy access to the site and make satisfactory specimens easier to obtain
- remain throughout the procedure and assist the medical practitioner as necessary, **to ensure safe completion of the procedure**
- the patient may experience some discomfort such as a sharp sting, when the needle is inserted or when the marrow is aspirated, **encourage deep breathing and relaxation techniques**
- observe the patient throughout the procedure, **to note any signs of distress**
- on completion of the procedure apply pressure to the puncture site, and cover with a sterile dressing, **to ensure bleeding has stopped and the puncture site is protected**
- ensure that the patient is left feeling as comfortable as possible, **to maintain the patient's dignity and assist with their recovery**
- dispose of the equipment safely, **to prevent the risk of sharp injuries and the transmission of infection**
- dispatch the labelled specimens to the laboratory immediately with the completed laboratory forms, **to allow the microscopic examination of fresh body cells**
- take the patient's temperature, pulse, respiration and blood pressure, **to monitor the patient's condition**
- monitor the biopsy site, and report any abnormal findings immediately, **to ensure early detection and prompt action in the event of any adverse effects**
- document the nursing practice appropriately, **to provide a written record of the procedure**
- the patient should rest for at least 30 minutes following the procedure **to facilitate recovery**
- the puncture site should be monitored for signs of bleeding or haematoma. If bleeding occurs pressure should be applied to the site for a minimum of 10 minutes **to minimise discomfort and aid healing.**

Patient/carer education

Key points

In partnership with the patient and/or carer, ensure that they are competent to carry out any practices required. Information should be given on an appropriate point of contact for any concerns that may arise.

The medical practitioner and the nurse should explain why a bone marrow aspiration is necessary. An explanation of the procedure should be provided, including the rationale behind the position the patient needs to adopt for the aspiration. The patient and carer should be given time to ask questions and discuss any concerns they have about the planned procedure. If the patient is being discharged following the procedure, they should be collected and driven home by a relative or carer.

The patient should be advised:
- to rest for at least 30 minutes following the procedure
- to monitor the puncture site for signs of bleeding or haematoma. If bleeding occurs pressure should be applied to the site for a minimum of 10 minutes
- normal activities may be resumed when the patient feels ready
- some pain or soreness may be expected from the puncture site
- prescribed pain medication can be used to alleviate discomfort
- the area should be kept dry for 24 hours
- the adhesive dressing can be removed 2–3 days following the procedure.

The patient should be informed when the results will be available and, if applicable, the date and time of the next outpatient appointment should be provided (Grundy 2006).

References

Department of Health 2001 Good practice in consent. Implementation guideline: consent to examination or treatment. Department of Health, London

Gammon J, Gould D 2005 Universal precautions, a review of compliance and strategies to improve practice. Journal of Research in Nursing 10(5): 529–547

Grundy M 2006 Nursing in haematological oncology. Baillière Tindall, London

Lewis SM, Heitkemper MM, Dirksen SR 2004 Medical surgical nursing: assessment and management of clinical problems, 6th edn. Mosby, St Louis, MI

National Patient Safety Agency 2005 Safer patient identification alert. Notice 22 November (available at http://www.npsa.nhs.uk)

Nursing and Midwifery Council 2004 Code of professional conduct: standards for conduct, performance and ethics. NMC, London

Nursing and Midwifery Council 2005 Guidelines for records and record keeping. NMC, London

Websites

British Committee for Standards in Haematology: http://www.bcshguidelines.com

Department of Health: http//:www.dh.gov.uk

eMedicine specialties – Bone Marrow Aspiration and Biopsy: http://www.emedicine.com/med/topic2971.htm

National Patient Safety Agency: http://www.npsa.nhs.uk

Self assessment

1. What is the preferred site for bone marrow aspiration?
2. What after-effects may occur following bone marrow aspiration?
3. How long should the patient rest following bone marrow aspiration?

Practice 8
Cardiopulmonary Resuscitation: Adult Resuscitation

This section consists of five parts:

1 Identifying patients at risk of cardiac arrest in hospital

2 Using the ABCDE approach

3 Confirming cardiac arrest

4 Initiating in-hospital adult cardiopulmonary resuscitation

5 Initiating adult cardiopulmonary resuscitation in a community care environment

(Please note that some publishers and/or organizations use cardiorespiratory in place of cardiopulmonary.)

Within the context of the in-hospital environment, adult resuscitation involves management of the critically ill patient, with acute altered physiology in addition to cardiopulmonary resuscitation (CPR). This chapter will discuss a systematic approach to recognition and management of the 'at risk' patient; in-hospital CPR and out-of-hospital CPR for the healthcare provider. The procedures involved in advanced life support (ALS) are outside the remit of this chapter, therefore the focus will be on first responder CPR and use of automated external defibrillators (AED).

Learning outcomes	**By the end of this section, you should know how to:** ▪ identify patients at risk of cardiac arrest ▪ manage these patients using the ABCDE approach ▪ confirm cardiac arrest ▪ initiate in-hospital cardiopulmonary resuscitation ▪ initiate cardiopulmonary resuscitation in a community setting ▪ identify essential equipment required in a clinical emergency.
Background knowledge required	Revision of the anatomy and physiology of the cardiovascular and respiratory systems Review of the health authority and trust policy pertaining to the procedure of cardiopulmonary resuscitation.

Clinical Nursing Practices

1. IDENTIFYING PATIENTS AT RISK OF CARDIAC ARREST IN HOSPITAL

Indications and rationale for this practice

To maintain function of the vital organs, we require an airway that is open; the ability to breath in oxygen and to obtain adequate gaseous exchange in the lungs; and a pump that can circulate this oxygen to those organs to keep them perfused and alive. Failure at any point in this process will result in reduced oxygen delivery, organ failure and, ultimately, death.

The majority of in-hospital cardiac arrests are not sudden (Jevon 2006), unexpected events and as many as 80% of patients will demonstrate warning signs of altering physiology prior to the event. Close monitoring of the patient may allow early recognition of deteriorating physiology (Table 8.1), provide an opportunity for appropriate treatment and in some cases may prevent cardiac arrest (Resuscitation Council (UK) 2006a).

In hospital the most common cause of cardiac arrest is hypoxaemia due to deteriorating respiratory, circulatory and neurological systems (International Liaison Committee On Resuscitation 2005a). There are common clinical signs evident in the critically ill patient. These are:
- tachypnoea in an attempt to breath in more oxygen
- tachycardia as the body attempts to circulate oxygen to the vital organs
- hypotension as the cardiac output drops, the blood pressure will fall
- reduced conscious level as the perfusion of the brain is diminished (Resuscitation Council (UK) 2006a).

Equipment

1. Local health authority Early Warning Scoring system (EWSs) chart.

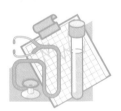

TABLE 8.1

Example of an early warning scoring system

Score	3	2	1	0	1	2	3
Respiration rate	—	< 8	9–10	11–20	21–25	26–30	> 31
Pulse	—	< 4	41–50	51–100	101–110	110–130	> 130
Systolic BP	< 84	85–89	90–100	101–199	—	> 200	—
GCS/AVPU*	< 8	9–13	14	15	—	—	—
	—	—	New agitation/ confusion	Alert	Voice	Pain	Unresponsive
Urine	< 10 ml h^{-1}	< 30 ml h^{-1}	—	—	—	—	—
Temp. (°C)	—	< 35	35–35.9	36–37.4	37.5–38.5	> 38.6	—
Spo$_2$%	< 87	88 –91	92–94	95–100	—	—	—

*See paragraph titled Disability in Section 2

Guidelines and rationale for this nursing practice

- the assessments associated with EWSs must be undertaken as quickly and efficiently as possible *to enable the required assistance to be summoned quickly*
- assess the patient's respiratory rate (*see* p. 293) *to identify an 'at risk' rate*
- assess the patient's pulse rate (*see* p. 279) *to identify an 'at risk' rate*
- assess the patient's blood pressure (*see* p. 41) *to identify an 'at risk' systolic pressure*
- assess the patient's conscious level using the Glasgow Coma Scale (GCS; *see* p. 351) *to identify an 'at risk' GCS score*
- assess the patient's hourly urine output if catheterized (*see* p. 91) or note the time and amount of urine passed by the patient *to identify an 'at risk' urinary output*
- assess the patient's body temperature (*see* p. 55) *to identify an 'at risk' temperature*
- if the patient's oxygen saturation is being monitored note the percentage (*see* p. 245) *to identify an 'at risk' saturation percentage*
- record the overall score and act immediately as directed by local policy. *Some hospitals may function with a medical emergency team, while other hospitals have a cardiac arrest team, which responds to peri-arrest situations. The higher the patient's score the more 'at risk' of cardiac arrest.* Identifying patients at risk is often viewed as the first act in the 'Chain of Survival', which highlights the actions linking a patient who has a cardiac arrest with survival (Resuscitation Council (UK) 2005).

2. USING THE ABCDE APPROACH

Indications for this nursing practice

A common method used to identify and treat problems is known as the ABCDE approach. This refers to Airway; Breathing; Circulation; Disability; Exposure.

The ABCDE approach is a systematic framework that allows the nurse to identify problems and to act on these without delay. The process is continuous and staff should reassess the casualty at each point where intervention takes place for signs of improvement or deterioration. Nurses should only work to their own level of clinical expertise and should be aware of their limitations. It is essential to call for help as soon as it is required and to acknowledge your limitations.

Airway

- the airway should be assessed to determine whether it is patent, partially obstructed or completely obstructed. *If a patient can give a verbal response, then it is likely that the airway is patent* (Garrioch 2000)
- if there is evidence of noise (e.g. stridor or wheeze) then the airway is partially obstructed. *Stridor often indicates an upper airway obstruction and wheeze usually indicates a lower obstruction*
- simple manoeuvres should be used to open the airway (Resuscitation Council (UK) 2006b). If the patient is conscious and assuming there is no neck injury, *the patient may attempt to optimise their own airway by sitting*

upright, if this is clearly not effective and the patient remains conscious, then lifting the chin forward may help. If the patient is unconscious the head-tilt-chin-lift manoeuvre can be used, or if neck injury is suspected, jaw thrust by experienced personnel

- if these manoeuvres are ineffective airway adjuncts may be considered (e.g. naso-pharyngeal airway in a conscious patient with a glossopharyngeal reflex or oro-pharyngeal airway in an unconscious casualty without glossopharyngeal reflex). Airway adjuncts should only be used by personnel experienced in their use (Resuscitation Council (UK) 2006b)
- if the airway is completely obstructed the patient may develop a 'see-saw' pattern of respiration, with a silent chest. See-saw respiratory pattern is confirmed by the abdomen moving in as the chest moves out and vice versa. ***This is an extreme clinical emergency and will require immediate, advanced airway management; an anaesthetist should be contacted immediately according to local protocol***.

Breathing

- when assessing breathing, the respiratory rate should be observed and particular attention should be paid to the effort of breathing displayed by the acute patient, tachypnoea and the use of accessory muscles of respiration should be noted and reported immediately. These are worrying signs
- other observations of breathing should include listening to the chest with a stethoscope and percussion of the chest by trained personnel. ***As a guide, it is suggested by early warning scoring systems that if the patient's respiratory rate is < 5 or > 36 help should be sought***
- any patient with an acute breathing problem should be administered high-flow oxygen initially (White 2000).

Circulation

- the nurse should observe the patient for signs of circulatory failure, an initial observation will determine if the patient is sweaty, clammy, pale, etc.
- the patient's pulse should be assessed and recorded noting the rate, regularity and volume ***to indicate cardiovascular function*** (*see* Practice 34)
- a blood pressure recording (*see* Practice 4) ***to determine the effectiveness of the cardiovascular system***
- changes in pulse and blood pressure should be reported to medical staff, according to local policy
- if the patient is clearly deteriorating and an adequately experienced clinician is available, the circulation should be accessed with intravenous cannulae ***to aid quick and easy administration of medications***
- if the equipment is available, the patient should be monitored with a cardiac monitor and pulse oximetry ***to provide objective physiological measurements***.

Disability

- disability relates to the neurological status of the patient
- ***a quick and easy way to determine how well the brain is being perfused is to assess the patient using the AVPU score***. This translates to the following (Resuscitation Council (UK) 2006a):
  — the patient is **A**lert

— the patient responds to **V**oice

— the patient responds to **P**ain

— the patient is **U**nresponsive

- if a patient's condition deteriorates from one level to a lower one this is indicative of a significant change in neurological status and should not be overlooked. An AVPU recording of 'P' or less indicates a Glasgow Coma Scale score of < 8 and means this patient's airway cannot be protected fully by the patient. *Expert help is required immediately*.

Exposure

- a top-to-toe examination of the patient *allows the nurse the opportunity to identify any obvious cause of condition change*. Problems identified should be dealt with immediately.

Table 8.2 provides a summary of the rapid assessment actions as described above. This assessment has to be swift and efficient to be effective. Problems *must* be dealt with as they arise. *Always* reassess after every action and if the patient's condition changes go back to ABCDE.

3. CONFIRMING CARDIAC ARREST

Cardiac arrest is the abrupt cessation of cardiac function and is the ultimate medical emergency. CPR is a dramatic, emergency exercise that aims to restore effective circulation and ventilation following cardiac arrest.

Causes of cardiac arrest include (Resuscitation Council 2006a):

- heart attack
- drowning
- choking
- bleeding
- drug overdose
- hypoxia.

Confirming cardiac arrest involves a sequence of steps, which can be remembered using the mnemonic 'Dr's ABC':

Danger – remove any obvious danger to the rescuer

Response – check the response of the patient by shaking them and asking, 'Are you alright?' (Fig. 8.1). If the casualty does not respond

Shout – and summon *help*

Airway – open the airway using the head-tilt-chin-lift manoeuvre (Fig. 8.2) if there is an obvious obstruction visible, remove this with suction or forceps. Dentures should remain in situ if they are well fitting as this creates a good seal during assisted ventilation

Breathing – While maintaining an open airway, position your ear over the mouth and nose and direct your eyes towards the chest to look for chest movement listen for breath sounds and feel for expired air (Fig. 8.3). Take no more than 10 seconds to do this. If the breathing is abnormal (occasional, noisy, laboured gasps) act as if it is absent. Agonal gasps will be evident in 40% of victims,

TABLE 8.2
Summary of rapid assessment of ABCDE

A	Check patency and maintain	• Position
		• Suction if required
		• Use adjuncts if required
		• If tolerates oral airway, may require intubation
B	Rate	• Give oxygen 15L via trauma mask
	Air entry	• REASSESS
	Effort of breathing	
	Colour	
	Percussion	
	Listen	
C	Rate	• Get access
	BP and pulse pressure	• Monitor
	Peripheral and central pulses:	• Support
	• Are the pulses present?	• Consider fluid challenge
	• Check amplitude skin perfusion:	
	• CRT (> 2 seconds)	
	• Temp	
	• Colour	
	• Mottling	
D	GCS: worrying if drops by 2 points or more	• Get **HELP**!!!
	• E = 4	• Airway may be at risk
	• V = 5	
	• M = 6	
	AVPU:	
	• Alert	
	• Responds to Voice	
	• Responds to Pain	
	• Unresponsive	
	If recorded as P or below GCS approximately 8 or less, therefore airway protection may be required	
E	Exposure:	• Examine patient
		• Top-to-toe assessment

do not confuse this with normal respiration (International Liaison Committee On Resuscitation 2005a)

Circulation – is checked by looking for obvious signs of life (movement, swallowing, etc.) if you are experienced in clinical assessment you may wish to combine the breathing check with a carotid pulse check. ***This combined assessment should take no longer than 10 seconds**.*

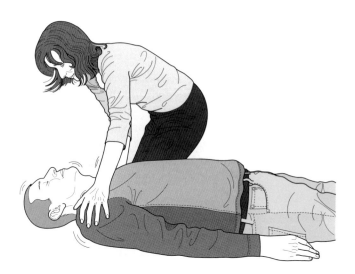

FIGURE 8.1
Shake and shout to check for response

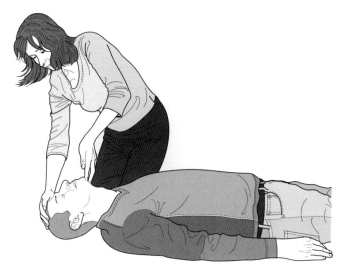

FIGURE 8.2
Open the airway

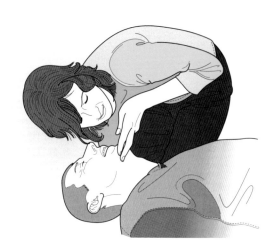

FIGURE 8.3
Look, listen and feel for signs of life

Clinical Nursing Practices

The diagnosis of cardiac arrest is confirmed by

- a sudden loss of consciousness
- evidence of abnormal breathing (e.g. slow, laboured, gasping, absence)
- the absence of signs of circulation.

As soon as the diagnosis is confirmed, ensure that appropriately experienced clinicians are alerted, and the emergency equipment is gathered. In hospital this will be the cardiac arrest team or equivalent. With as little delay as possible, commence chest compressions. This may involve sending a second person for help, to make best use of the elapsing time and gain support from skilled personnel.

4. INITIATING IN-HOSPITAL ADULT CARDIOPULMONARY RESUSCITATION

Equipment

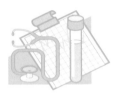

1. Suction equipment
2. Airway adjuncts such as an oropharyngeal (Guedel) airway, nasopharyngeal airway or laryngeal mask airway
3. Disposable face mask, e.g. Laderal pocket mask (for community use)
4. Ambu bag and face mask or similar equipment, with oxygen supply
5. Defibrillator or automated external defibrillator (AED)
6. Equipment for intubation (including endotracheal tubes, laryngoscope, bougie and connectors)
7. Emergency cardiac medications and equipment for intravenous access (*see* 'Intravenous therapy', p. 169)
8. Receptacle for soiled disposable items.

Guidelines for cardiopulmonary resuscitation (cpr)

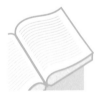

- once cardiac arrest has been confirmed, note the time. *A knowledge of the time elapsed is very important as the brain cells will begin to die from a lack of oxygen within 3 minutes*.

Chest compression

- place the patient in a supine position on a firm flat surface *to permit easy access to the patient's chest and airway*
- place one hand on top of the other, on the centre of the chest, at the lower half of the sternum (Fig. 8.4). The arms should be straight and the elbows locked, lean over the casualty with the shoulder positioned in line with the heel of the hand, keep the fingers off the ribs (Fig. 8.5). Press the chest by 4–5 cm aiming for a rate of 100 per minute. Give 30 compressions, followed by two ventilations (Resuscitation Council (UK) 2006a).

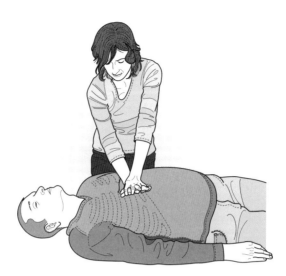

FIGURE 8.4
Place hands on centre of the chest, one on top of the other

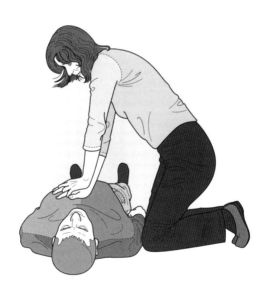

FIGURE 8.5
Arm position

Ventilation

- while maintaining an open airway, ventilate the patient, using an adjunct such as a pocket mask (Fig. 8.6) or bag–valve–mask device (Fig. 8.7) with supplementary oxygen (if available). Give two breaths, each inspiration should last for 1 second; *note the rising of the chest wall to confirm ventilation*. Each breath should create chest movement, similar to a normal breath
- the chest should fall fully prior to the second breath being delivered, *to avoid hyperventilation*
- the combination of compressions to ventilation should be a ratio of 30:2 (Fig. 8.8). If more than one healthcare provider is available, a two-person technique for ventilation and compressions should be used
- when the nurse tires during chest compressions, roles may be changed with minimal disruption to chest compressions (Resuscitation Council (UK) 2006a)

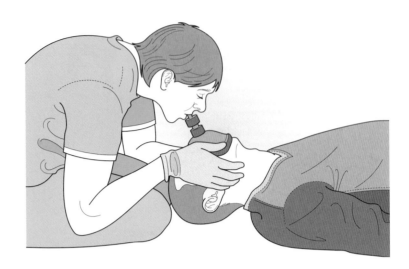

FIGURE 8.6
Pocket mask in use

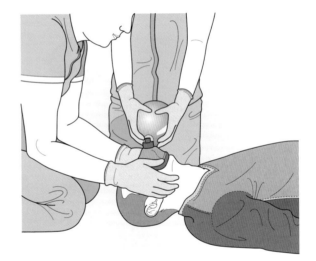

FIGURE 8.7
Bag–valve–mask (BVM)
technique

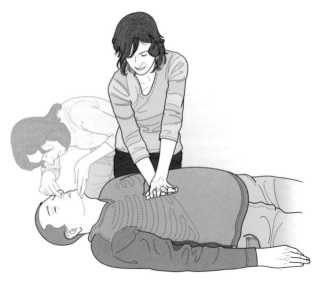

FIGURE 8.8
Combining mouth
to mouth with chest
compressions – single
rescuer

■ once an airway is secured, usually by an anaesthetist, with an endotracheal tube, chest compressions should continue uninterrupted at a rate of 100 per minute and the patient should be ventilated at a rate of 10 breaths per minute (Resuscitation Council (UK) 2006c).

Defibrillation

■ as soon as the defibrillator is available, it should be attached without delay and the patient should be monitored. The chest compressions should **not** be interrupted while attaching the defibrillator **to maintain tissue oxygenation**. When clinicians with defibrillation skills are available and if indicated the patient should be defibrillated immediately (International Liaison Committee On Resuscitation 2005b)

■ the use of automated external defibrillators (AED) is becoming more common in the healthcare environment. Once switched on the nurse should be guided by the voice prompt of the defibrillator and attach the monitoring pads to the bare chest. The staff should stand clear from the patient and bed while the defibrillator assesses the cardiac rhythm and remain clear while the shock is delivered **to prevent personnel acting as an 'earth' for the electric current. This would endanger the lives of those present and negate the AED effectiveness**. The nurse should only touch the patient when advised to by the AED.

An in-hospital resuscitation algorithm (Resuscitation Council (UK) 2006d) is shown in Figure 8.9.

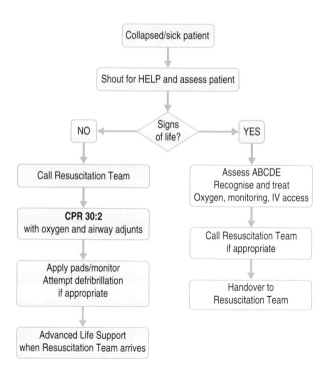

FIGURE 8.9
In-hospital resuscitation algorithm

Safety issues

- in an institutional setting, there may be difficulty accessing the patient due to equipment and furniture. If this is the case, the immediate area should be cleared as quickly as possible *to enhance access to the patient and promote staff and patient safety*
- if the patient is on the floor kneel by their side, if they are in bed alter the bed height to suit the rescuer or if the patient is on a chair, they should be lowered to the floor adhering to local moving and handling policy (*see* Practice 25) permitting patient access to allow CPR to be initiated.

Advanced life support

With the arrival of skilled personnel the resuscitation action may move into advanced life support. The Resuscitation Council UK (2006c) advanced algorithm is beyond the scope of this text, but is included for the reader's interest (Fig. 8.10).

Supplementary considerations

- consideration of the decision not to resuscitate a patient presents a difficult ethical problem for healthcare professionals. A transparent decision-making process using professional guidelines and involving all concerned should be implemented (Hatchett 2002). The process must be documented in the medical and nursing notes and, unless it is against the wishes of the patient, their family should be informed (Gibson 2004)
- if cardiac arrest cannot be reversed, consideration of potential organ transplantation should be discussed with the relatives. The personnel involved must have a knowledge of the various physiological, psychological, social, cultural, religious and spiritual issues surrounding organ donation and be a skilled communicator when raising this subject with distressed relatives (Lawton 2006).

FIGURE 8.10
Advanced life support algorithm
From Resuscitation Council (UK) 2006c, with permission

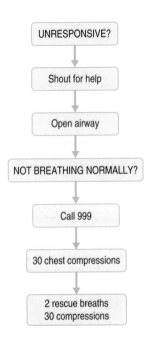

UNRESPONSIVE?

Shout for help

Open airway

NOT BREATHING NORMALLY?

Call 999

30 chest compressions

2 rescue breaths
30 compressions

5. INITIATING ADULT CARDIOPULMONARY RESUSCITATION IN A COMMUNITY CARE ENVIRONMENT

The guidelines described above for in-hospital CPR should be followed with some alterations (Fig. 8.11):

- contact the emergency medical services by telephoning for help *to seek skilled personnel assistance*
- it is advisable to carry an airway adjunct such as a pocket mask *to act as a barrier device*

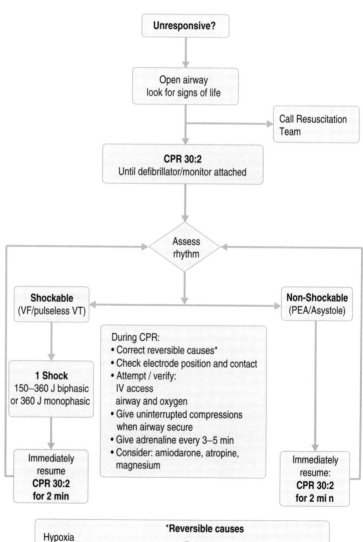

FIGURE 8.11
Adult basic life support algorithm
From Resuscitation Council (UK) 2006e, with permission

- there may be the exceptional occasion when airway adjuncts are not available, in these situations it will be necessary to consider giving mouth to mouth ventilation (see below)
- resuscitation should continue until expert help arrives, the casualty displays signs of life or the rescuer becomes exhausted (International Liaison Committee On Resuscitation 2005a).

Compression-only CPR

- if the nurse is unable or unwilling to do mouth to mouth ventilation, the patient should be given compression-only CPR. This involves following the steps for life support as described previously without stopping to ventilate. Compressions should be delivered continuously at a rate of 100 per minute (International Liaison Committee On Resuscitation 2005a).

Patient/carer education

Key points

As suggested by the Resuscitation Council (UK) (2005), the nurse has a role in encouraging and teaching the general population to develop skills in basic life support.

Following a successful resuscitation, the patient and relatives must be given information about the event and be permitted to discuss their feelings and anxieties about the emergency. Other patients within the clinical area will also require to be given an explanation of the events to assist in relieving some of their own anxieties.

Should the resuscitation be unsuccessful, the relatives must be informed of the outcome of CPR as soon as possible and be given all relevant information pertaining to the events that led up to the cardiac arrest and the measures implemented to treat their relative. Staff experienced in communicating 'bad' news to relatives must undertake the difficult task of informing the relatives of the death of their loved one. This should ensure the delivery of sensitive support and assistance to the relatives at this life-changing situation.

References

Garrioch M 2000 Airway management and ventilation. In: Royal College of Physicians and Surgeons of Glasgow (eds) Ill medical patients acute care and treatment course handbook. RCPSG, Glasgow, UK

Gibson T 2004 Cardiopulmonary resuscitation. In: Dougherty L, Lister S (eds) The Royal Marsden Hospital manual of clinical nursing procedures, 6th edn, Chapter 7. Blackwell Science, Oxford, UK

Hatchett R 2002 Caring for the patient with a cardiovascular disorder. In: Walsh M (ed) Watson's clinical nursing and related sciences, 6th edn. Baillière Tindall, Edinburgh

International Liaison Committee On Resuscitation (ILCOR) 2005a Part 2 Adult basic life support. Resuscitation 67(2–3): 187–201

International Liaison Committee On Resuscitation (ILCOR) 2005b Part 3 Defibrillation. Resuscitation 67(2–3): 203–211

Jevon P 2006 An overview of the new resuscitation guidelines. Nursing Times 102(3): 25–27

Lawton L 2006 The patient who experiences trauma. In: Alexander M, Fawcett J, Runciman P (eds) Nursing practice – hospital and home: the adult, 3rd edn. Churchill Livingstone, Edinburgh

Resuscitation Council (UK) 2005 Resuscitation guidelines 2005. Resuscitation Council UK, London

Resuscitation Council (UK) 2006a Recognition of the critically ill patient and prevention of cardiac arrest. In: Resuscitation Council (UK) (eds) Advanced life support course manual, 5th edn. Resuscitation Council (UK), London

Resuscitation Council (UK) 2006b Airway management and ventilation. In: Resuscitation Council (UK) (eds) Immediate life support course manual, 2nd edn. Resuscitation Council (UK), London

Resuscitation Council (UK) 2006c Advanced life support algorithm. In: Resuscitation Council (UK) (eds) Advanced life support course manual, 5th edn. Resuscitation Council (UK), London

Resuscitation Council (UK) 2006d In-hospital resuscitation. In: Resuscitation Council (UK) (eds) Advanced life support course manual, 5th edn. Resuscitation Council (UK), London

Resuscitation Council (UK) 2006e Lay rescuer basic life support. In: Resuscitation Council (UK) (eds) Immediate life support course manual, 2nd edn. Resuscitation Council (UK), London

White R 2000 Airway management and ventilation. In: Royal College of Physicians and Surgeons of Glasgow (eds) Ill medical patients acute care and treatment course handbook. RCPSG, Glasgow

Websites

Resuscitation Council UK: http://www.resus.org.uk

Royal College of Nursing: http://www.rcn.org.uk

Self assessment

1. Why would you use an EWSs?
2. How would you confirm a cardiac arrest?
3. What are your local processes for contacting the hospital resuscitation team when an emergency arises?
4. List three airway adjuncts that may be used during adult resuscitation.
5. What does an automated external defibrillator do?

Practice 9
Care of the Deceased Person

Learning outcomes	**By the end of this section, you should know how to:** ■ care for a deceased person.
Background knowledge required	Revision of local policy on the care of a deceased person Review of the religious and spiritual rites of care of a deceased person Revision of 'Personal Hygiene' (*see* p. 259) and 'Mouth Care' (*see* p. 205).
Indications and rationale for care of a deceased person	Before transfer to the mortuary or undertaker's premises, a deceased patient requires care that may be delivered by a professional carer, an undertaker or the appropriate person identified by the spiritual beliefs of the deceased. This care may also be referred to as the 'Last Offices'.

Equipment

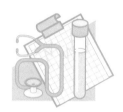

1. Disposable gloves
2. Equipment as for 'Personal Hygiene' (*see* p. 259)
3. Equipment as for 'Mouth Care' (*see* p. 205)
4. Incontinence pad or disposable napkin
5. Dressing pack
6. Waterproof dressing for open wounds if necessary
7. Hypoallergenic tape
8. Shroud
9. Two patient identification bands
10. Patient identification cards and/or notification of death cards appropriately completed with the patient's full name and other details as requested
11. Mortuary sheet or clean white sheet
12. Gauze bandage
13. Trolley for equipment
14. Receptacle for patient's clothing
15. Patient clothing list book
16. Patient valuables list book
17. Receptacle for patient's valuables
18. Receptacle for soiled linen
19. Receptacle for soiled disposable items.

Guidelines and rationale for this nursing practice 	Details of the practice can vary according to the patient's cultural background and religious practice, therefore awareness of specific requirements prior to, during or after death is essential (Roper et al 2000, McGhee 2002). A patient who dies suddenly and unexpectedly will require a post-mortem examination (Scottish Executive 2003).

Hand washing should take place before commencing and on completion of the practice.

- inform the medical practitioner when a patient is thought to have died **to confirm the diagnosis of death and comply with the legal requirements before the issue of a death certificate**. A senior nurse who is appropriately trained may also be permitted to verify the death of a patient or resident within the agreed local policy (Dimond 2004)
- ensure the patient's privacy and the privacy of the relatives **to prevent further distress to those persons present**
- ensure that the patient's relatives, if they are not present, are notified of the death. **This will allow the expressed wishes of the deceased to be implemented and funeral arrangements to be initiated**
- ensure relatives are adequately and kindly informed about immediate practicalities (Scottish Executive 2003, Department of Health 2005)
- assist and support bereaved relatives **as the professional carer is in a key position at this time** (Roper et al 2000)
- inform the charge nurse or deputy and portering staff or, in the patient's home, assist the carer to contact the undertaker **to make the initial arrangements for the transfer of the body to the mortuary or undertaker's premises**
- collect and prepare the equipment **to ensure all the equipment is available**
- wash the hands, apply an apron and gloves **to reduce the potential of cross infection** (Jeanes 2005)
- remove all the upper bed linen, leaving a sheet to cover the patient **to give easy access to the body**
- lay the patient flat, face up, with limbs in a natural position and arms by his or her side. **Rigor mortis occurs 2–4 hours following death; positioning the body after this time is difficult**
- remove any nursing or medical equipment **in order to reduce the 'clinical' appearance of the room**
- gently close the eyelids **to protect the tissues should the deceased or relatives give permission for corneal donation and also to improve the facial appearance** (Roper et al 2000)
- clean the patient's mouth and replace any dentures **to enhance the aesthetic appearance of the deceased and maintain hygiene**
- support the mandible in a closed position using a light pillow. An hour may elapse prior to the continuation of the practice, but this interval is not essential. **This will allow rigor mortis to develop prior to the completion of the practice**
- remove all tubes and drains, unless otherwise instructed, **to reduce the health hazard**
- re-dress all wounds with a waterproof dressing, **thereby reducing the potential problem of the leakage of body fluids**. Any drains or tubes left in position should also be covered with a padded waterproof dressing
- drains, tubes and dressings may be left in position during this practice if a patient dies unexpectedly, within 24 hours of surgery or receiving an anaesthetic, or within 24 hours if involvement in some from of trauma (Department of Health 2005)
- wash the patient as for 'Personal Hygiene' (*see* p. 259), **for general hygiene purposes**

- a male patient should be shaved *for aesthetic reasons*
- all jewellery, once removed, should be listed in the patient valuables book in the presence of two nurses, *to maintain the security of the deceased's belongings*. In the community, personal belongings should not be removed by the nurse unless a witness is present. Any action should be documented and signed
- apply identification bands and cards to the appropriate limbs and parts of the body as per local policy *to ensure continued identification of the deceased*
- apply an incontinence pad or disposable napkin, *which will reduce the health hazard from further body fluid leakage for staff who are in contact with the body*
- place the shroud or, at home, fresh bedclothes, in position *to enhance the appearance should relatives wish to view the deceased.*

Institution

- wrap the body in the sheet, ensuring complete coverage, and secure the sheet with adhesive tape or gauze bandage *to prevent exposure of the deceased during transfer to the mortuary*
- fix an identification card or notification of death card to the sheet using adhesive tape, *for ease of future identification*
- if there is a risk of infection, the body may be placed in a cadaver bag. The bag is labelled 'Danger of Infection' plus the name of the infection (Nicol et al 2004)
- list the patient's clothing, *thus creating a receipt for future use*
- place this clothing and the patient's valuables in a secure place *to ensure safe keeping until removal by the relatives*
- dispose of equipment safely *to reduce any health hazard*
- inform portering staff that the body is ready for collection, *this will permit the body to be cooled as soon as possible after death, thus slowing the decomposition process*
- on the arrival of portering staff with the mortuary trolley, ensure the privacy of the other patients *in an attempt to prevent further distress*
- other patients should be informed kindly and honestly that the patient has died and given support when needed (Lawton 2006)
- document the nursing practice appropriately *to provide a written record of the care given.*

Community

- cover the patient with a sheet *for aesthetic purposes*. Unless requested otherwise by the carer, leave the face uncovered
- remove any portable nursing material or equipment in order *to reduce the 'clinical' appearance of the room*
- following the removal of the body, arrange for the collection of any residual equipment, *thereby returning the home environment to 'normal'*
- document the nursing practice appropriately *to provide a written record of the care given.*

In undertaking this practice, nurses are accountable for their actions, the quality of care delivered and record-keeping according to the Code of Professional Conduct: Standards for Conduct, Performance and Ethics (Nursing and Midwifery Council 2004) and Guidelines for Records and Record Keeping (Nursing and Midwifery Council 2005).

Patient/carer education

Key points

It is important that families and carers are aware of what to do after a death and what support groups are available to them (Scottish Executive 2003). The bereaved relatives will require sensitive and compassionate care.

Any request to see the deceased should be arranged as soon as possible as this may assist the relatives during the grieving process; care should be taken to ensure that the patient looks as peaceful as possible, that the environment is cleared of equipment and that a chair is available.

Many nurses try not to show how much a patient's death has affected them, regarding their own distress as a sign of weakness (Smy 2004). The nurse may also need to assist and support his or her colleagues prior to, during and after the nursing practice.

References

Department of Health 2005 When a patient dies – advice on developing bereavement services in the NHS. Department of Health Publications, London

Dimond B 2004 The law and the certification, verification and registration of death. British Journal of Nursing 13(8): 480–481

Jeanes A 2005 Infection control. A practical guide to the use of hand decontaminants. Nursing Times 101(20): 46–48

Lawton L 2006 The patient who experiences trauma. In: Alexander M, Fawcett J, Runciman P (eds) Nursing practice – hospital and home: the adult, 3rd edn. Churchill Livingstone, Edinburgh

McGhee P 2002 Nursing with dignity. Nursing Times 98(9): 33–35

Nicol M, Bavin C, Bedford-Turner S et al 2004 Essential nursing skills. Mosby, London

Nursing and Midwifery Council 2004 Code of professional conduct: standards for conduct, performance and ethics. NMC, London

Nursing and Midwifery Council 2005 Guidelines for records and record keeping. NMC, London

Roper N, Logan W, Tierney A 2000 The Roper–Logan–Tierney model of nursing. Churchill Livingstone, Edinburgh

Scottish Executive 2003 What to do after a death in Scotland practical advice for times of bereavement, 7th edn. HMSO, Edinburgh

Smy J 2004 Supporting colleagues when patients die. Nursing Times 100(22): 70–71

Website

The Marie Curie website: http://www.mariecurie.org.uk/forhealthcareprofessionals/
This is a useful source for carers and healthcare professionals working in different care settings covering care pathways and spiritual needs.

Self assessment

1. What is 'Last Offices'?
2. What is essential to prevent cross-infection during this procedure?
3. How should the nurse deal with the deceased patient's personal belongings?

Practice 10
Catheterisation: Urinary

There are four parts to this section:

1 **Catheterisation**

2 **Catheter care**

3 **Bladder irrigation**

4 **Administration of catheter maintenance solutions**

The concluding subsection, 'Patient/carer education', and the 'Self-assessment questions' refer to the four practices collectively.

Learning outcomes

By the end of this section, you should know how to:
- prepare the patient for any of these four nursing practices
- collect and prepare the equipment
- carry out catheterisation, catheter care, bladder irrigation and administration of catheter maintenance solutions.

Background knowledge required

Revision of the anatomy and physiology of the urinary system and external genitalia
Revision of 'Wound Care' technique (*see* p. 381)
Revision of local policy regarding catheter selection, catheter bags and administration of catheter maintenance solutions.

1. CATHETERISATION

Indications and rationale for urethral catheterisation

An estimated 15–25% of patients admitted to hospital have a urinary catheter passed (Tenke et al 2004). Because of the invasive nature of this procedure, the National Institute for Clinical Excellence (NICE) states that you must be competent before undertaking this nursing practice (National Institute for Clinical Excellence 2003). This competency should minimise the risks to the patient of discomfort, pain and catheter-associated urinary track infection (CAUTI).

Urinary catheters can be inserted:
- *to re-establish a flow of urine in urinary retention*

- *to provide a channel for drainage when micturition is impaired*
- *to empty the bladder preoperatively*
- *to allow the monitoring of fluid balance in a seriously ill patient*
- *to facilitate bladder irrigation procedures*
- *to maintain a dry environment in urinary incontinence when all other forms of nursing intervention have failed*
- *for the administration of medication*
- *to promote comfort for terminally ill patients*.

Equipment

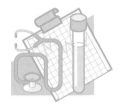

1. Trolley or adequate surface for equipment
2. Good light source, such as spotlight or torch
3. Sterile gloves
4. Clean apron
5. Sterile catheterisation or dressings pack
6. Mild soap and water and also sterile water-based solution for cleansing the genitalia
7. Sterile anaesthetic gel or water-soluble lubricant if anaesthetic gel is contraindicated
8. Sterile receiver
9. Sterile catheter of the type and size required
10. Appropriate equipment for catheter balloon inflation for non-pre-filled catheters only, e.g. syringe, needles and sterile water
11. Sterile closed drainage system if required, or catheter valve
12. Hypoallergenic tape
13. If requested, sterile specimen container appropriately labelled with a completed laboratory form and plastic specimen bag for transportation
14. Receptacle for soiled disposable items.

Catheters and catheter bags

Catheter type

The reason for urinary catheterisation can dictate the type and size of catheter (Fig. 10.1) to be used:

- a round-ended catheter can be used when a retained catheter is not required
- a Foley double-lumen, self-retaining catheter can be used when a short-term retained catheter is required
- a Foley triple-lumen, self-retaining catheter can be used when continuous bladder irrigation is required
- a Tiemann catheter can be used when the urethral canal is narrowed, for example when a male patient has an enlarged prostate gland; the shape of the catheter tip aids the passage of the catheter
- a whistle-tipped catheter can be used postoperatively to allow the passage of blood clots, particularly when bladder irrigation is not being utilised
- a silastic catheter can be used when a retained catheter is required for long-term use, as silastic is less irritant to the body tissue.

Sizes

The smallest Charrière size that will drain urine should be used (Tew et al 2005). A 10 ml balloon should be chosen unless under specialist advice (Stewart 2001). This

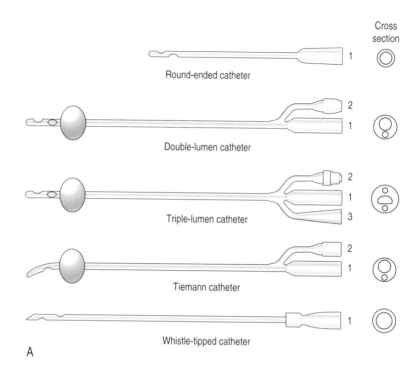

Cross section

Round-ended catheter   1

Double-lumen catheter   2 / 1

Triple-lumen catheter   2 / 1 / 3

Tiemann catheter   2 / 1

Whistle-tipped catheter   1

A

FIGURE 10.1
Catheterisation
A Examples of catheters (1 channel for urine flow; 2 channel for balloon inflation; 3 channel for irrigating fluid flow)
B Types of drainage bag
C Catheter valve

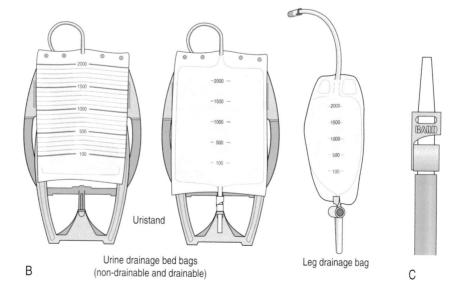

Uristand

Urine drainage bed bags
(non-drainable and drainable)

B

Leg drainage bag

C

is because the drainage eye of the catheter sits higher in the bladder with a 30 ml balloon, allowing residual urine to collect below the balloon, which in turn can lead to infection.

- 12–14 FG is a suitable size of catheter for female and male patients. Intermittent self-catheterisation catheters are usually 10–12 FG in size
- catheters are manufactured in female and male catheter lengths, male length catheters being approximately 42 cm long and female ones about 26 cm
- for routine use, select a catheter with a 10 ml balloon.

Materials

A variety of catheter materials is available, the choice being geared to the needs of the individual patient.

Short term (2–4 weeks):
- a latex catheter (these are rarely used)
- a PTFE-coated, latex Foley catheter.

Long term (up to 12 weeks):
- a silicone elastomer catheter – latex and silicone
- a hydrogel elastomer catheter – latex and hydrogel
- a polymer hydrogel catheter – latex and polymer hydrogel
- a 100% silicone catheter (latex free but there is a risk of diffusion of water from the balloon, therefore the water in the balloon must be checked regularly)
- a plastic nelaton catheter for intermittent self-catheterisation.

Only PVC and 100% silicone catheters contain no latex and must be used in patients with a latex allergy.

Catheter bags

There are three elements to be considered when choosing an appropriate catheter bag: the capacity, the length of the inlet tube and the type of outlet tap for emptying (Tenke et al 2004). The selection depends on the rationale for catheter use, patient preference and the patient's manual dexterity. The leg bag can be supported by leg straps or by a variety of garments such as net sleeves. A 'belly bag' can also be prescribed in place of a leg bag. Worn around the waist this product is manufactured for users who may, for example, have a bilateral amputation (National Health Service Quality Improvement Scotland 2004).

Guidelines and rationale for this nursing practice

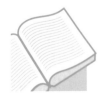

Female patient

- explain the nursing practice to the patient **to obtain consent and co-operation**
- collect and prepare the equipment **to ensure that all equipment is available and ready for use**
- ensure the patient's privacy **to reduce anxiety**
- observe the patient throughout this activity **to note any signs of distress**
- prepare and help the patient into a supine position with the knees bent, the hips flexed and the feet resting on the bed approximately 70 cm apart. **This position provides good access to and visualisation of the genitalia**

- place an incontinence pad or similar waterproof sheet under the patient's buttocks *to prevent any spillage of fluids onto the patient's bed linen*
- arrange the lighting *to assist with good visualisation of the genitalia*
- wash the hands and put on the gloves, *which will act as a barrier between the nurse's skin and the patient's tissues, thus reducing the incidence of contamination* (National Institute for Clinical Excellence 2003, National Health Service Quality Improvement Scotland 2004)
- open and arrange the equipment, maintaining sterility *to reduce contamination*
- cleanse the labia minora, swabbing from above downwards *to reduce the danger of cross-infection from the anal region*
- using the non-dominant hand, separate the labia minora to reveal the urethral meatus. Hold this position until catheter insertion has been completed in order *to prevent recontamination of the urethral meatus by the labia minora after cleansing*
- insert anaesthetic gel or water-soluble lubricant into the urethral meatus *to ease the passage of the catheter.* The use of an anaesthetic gel is indicated to reduce discomfort and damage to the urethra and to reduce the risk of infection (National Institute for Clinical Excellence 2003). Caution should be used if there is urethral bleeding as this may cause systemic absorption of the anaesthetic. The British National Formulary states that it should be used with caution in patients with cardiac conditions, liver problems and epilepsy (British Medical Association 2005). Allow the time specified by the manufacturer for the anaesthetic to work
- with the dominant hand, cleanse the urethral meatus *to prevent the introduction of micro-organisms into the urethra and/or bladder* and position the sterile receiver *to collect the urine from the catheter*
- insert the lubricated catheter into the urethra in an upward and backward direction, *which follows the anatomical route of the female urethra* (Fig. 10.2)
- avoid contamination of the surface of the catheter until a flow of urine has been established, *to prevent the introduction of micro-organisms*
- if it is not intended that the catheter should be left in situ, gently remove the catheter when the urine flow ceases
- if the catheter is to be retained, gently advance the catheter 4–5 cm and slowly inflate the balloon according to the manufacturer's directions. *The inflated balloon will maintain the catheter's position*
- a complaint of pain may suggest that the inflating balloon is still within the patient's urethra. Stop the inflation and withdraw the fluid inserted into the balloon. Advance the catheter another 4–5 cm and repeat the inflation process. *The length of a patient's urethra can vary so it is important to adjust practice to meet the individual patient's needs and prevent complications*
- attach a drainage system (Fig. 10.3) and properly manage all potential entry points of infection *to prevent the development of ascending infection* (Morrow 2006)
- anchor the catheter when appropriate by supporting the catheter and drainage tubing *to reduce trauma to the bladder neck and urethra, which could lead to pressure sore development.* Straps, e.g. G-straps are available to assist in this process

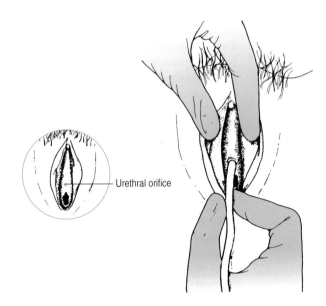

FIGURE 10.2
**Catheterisation:
inserting a catheter into
the female urethra**
From Roper et al 1985,
with permission

Urethral orifice

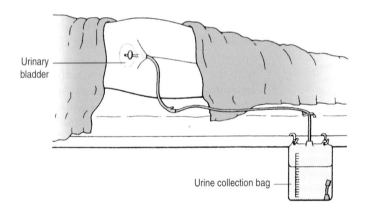

Urinary
bladder

Urine collection bag

FIGURE 10.3
**Closed bladder drainage
system showing the
drainage bag below the
level of the bladder**

- ensure that the patient is left feeling as comfortable as possible, thus
  maintaining the quality of this nursing practice
- dispose of the equipment safely *to reduce any health hazard*
- document the nursing practice appropriately, monitor the after-effects and
  report any abnormal findings immediately, *providing a written record and
  assisting in the implementation of any action should an abnormality
  or adverse reaction to the practice be noted.*

Male patient

This practice is usually carried out by a medical practitioner, a male nurse or a
female nurse who has achieved the required level of competence. A female nurse
may prefer to have a chaperone for this procedure.

- explain the nursing practice to the patient *to obtain consent and co-
  operation*

- collect and prepare the equipment *to ensure that all equipment is available and ready for use*
- ensure the patient's privacy *to reduce anxiety*
- observe the patient throughout this activity *to note any signs of distress*
- prepare and help the patient into a supine position. *This position provides good access to and visualisation of the genitalia*
- place an incontinence pad or similar waterproof sheet under the patient's buttocks *to prevent any spillage of fluids onto the patient's bed linen*
- arrange the lighting *to assist with good visualisation of the genitalia*
- wash the hands and put on gloves, *which will act as a barrier between the nurse's skin and the patient's tissues, thus reducing the incidence of contamination* (National Institute for Clinical Excellence 2003, National Health Service Quality Improvement Scotland 2004)
- open and arrange the equipment, maintaining sterility *to reduce contamination*
- withdraw the patient's foreskin with the non-dominant hand. Maintain this position until catheter insertion has been completed in order *to prevent recontamination of the urethral meatus by the foreskin after cleansing*
- with the dominant hand, cleanse the glans penis and urethral meatus *to prevent the introduction of micro-organisms into the urethra and/or bladder*
- insert the lidocaine gel and leave for the time specified by the manufacturer *to allow the local anaesthetic to act*
- position the sterile receiver and, with the non-dominant hand, gently grasp the shaft of the penis, raising it straight up *as this will aid the passage of the catheter along the length of the urethra*
- *as the male urethra is longer than the female*, insert the lubricated catheter into the urethral meatus for approximately 20–25 cm until a flow of urine is established (Fig. 10.4)

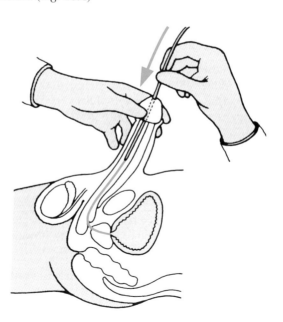

FIGURE 10.4
Catheterisation: inserting a catheter into the male urethra

- continue as for the female patient until the anchoring of the catheter
- replace the patient's foreskin over the glans penis or *a paraphimosis may develop*
- anchor the catheter, when appropriate, by supporting the catheter and drainage tubing *to reduce trauma to the bladder neck and urethra, which could lead to pressure sore development*. Straps, e.g. G-straps are available to assist in this process
- ensure that the patient is left feeling as comfortable as possible, *maintaining the quality of this nursing practice*
- dispose of the equipment safely *to reduce any health hazard*
- document the nursing practice appropriately, monitor the after-effects and report any abnormal findings immediately, *providing a written record and assisting in the implementation of any action should an abnormality or adverse reaction to the practice be noted*
- in undertaking this practice, nurses are accountable for their actions, the quality of care delivered and record-keeping according to the Code of Professional Conduct: Standards for Conduct, Performance and Ethics (Nursing and Midwifery Council 2004) and Guidelines for Records and Record Keeping (Nursing and Midwifery Council 2005).

Catheter-associated urinary track infection (CAUTI)

Catheterisation carries with it a significant risk of infection (Pratt et al 2001) and it is vital that informed consent is obtained prior to this procedure (Tew et al 2004). Guidelines exist to support you in the decision-making process to ensure appropriate reasons for catheterisation and to reduce infection risks (National Institute for Clinical Excellence 2003, Pellowe et al 2004).

Increased risk of CAUTIs:
- Prolonged catheterisation
- Female
- Diabetes
- Malnutrition
- Renal failure
- Older age.

Research into the prevention of CAUTIs continues to develop and the use of silver-alloy-coated catheters may be one option. It has been suggested that these catheters can reduce CAUTIs by up to 45% (Davenport & Keeley 2004, Department of Health 2004) by reducing bacterial adhesion onto the catheter. However, the Department of Health conclude that further research is required to audit the cost implications of the potential for reducing CAUTIs against the increased cost to supply the catheters. This discussion should lead to the development of local guidelines to ensure the appropriate use of these catheters.

Cranberry juice has also been advocated to prevent CAUTIs by reducing the alkalinity of the urine. There is, however, a lack of research to prove or disprove this theory (McMurdo et al 2005).

Appropriate management once the catheter is in situ will help to reduce the risk of infection, including:

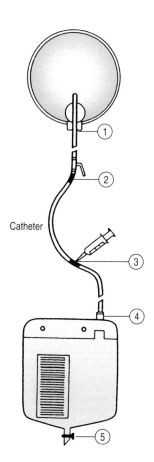

Catheter

Points at which pathogens can enter a closed urinary drainage system: 1 the urethral orifice; 2 the connection between the catheter and the drainage tube; 3 where the sample of urine is taken; 4 at the connection between the drainage tube and collecting bag; 5 at the drainage bag outlet
From Roper et al 1985, with permission

- Disturb closed drainage system only when indicated (Fig. 10.5)
- Cleanse meatus with mild soap and water daily
- Change leg/night bags when clinically appropriate or as per manufacturer's instructions
- Always follow infection-control guidelines (National Institute for Clinical Excellence 2003, Pellowe et al 2004).

2. CATHETER CARE

Indications and rationale for catheter care

Catheter care is the cleansing of the exposed part of a catheter; this may:

- ***help to reduce the risk of infection ascending via the catheter to other parts of the urinary system***
- ***remove any crusts or discharge from the catheter as these can harbour pathogenic micro-organisms***.

Equipment

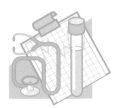

1. Gloves/apron
2. Disposable wipes
3. Mild soap and water
4. Flat surface for equipment
5. Receptacle for soiled disposable items.

Guidelines and rationale for this nursing practice

- explain the nursing practice to the patient **to obtain consent and co-operation**
- collect and prepare the equipment **to ensure that all equipment is available and ready for use**
- ensure the patient's privacy **to reduce anxiety**
- observe the patient throughout this activity **to note any signs of distress**
- help the patient into a suitable position **allowing the nurse easy, comfortable access to the patient**
- wash the hands and put on apron **to reduce cross-infection** (National Institute for Clinical Excellence 2003), apply gloves, and arrange the equipment, **allowing easy access during the practice**
- gently cleanse the external urethral meatus, using the swab only once and in only one direction, swabbing from above downwards in the female patient and away from the catheter–meatus junction **to reduce the risk of cross-infection**
- in a male patient, retract the foreskin before cleansing, **allowing clear access to the meatus**
- replace the foreskin following the completion of this nursing practice, **to prevent the development of a paraphimosis**
- gently swab the shaft of the catheter away from the catheter–meatus junction, **to remove any discharge away from the urethral orifice**
- ensure that the patient is left feeling as comfortable as possible, **maintaining the quality of this nursing practice**
- dispose of the equipment safely **to reduce any health hazard**
- document the nursing practice appropriately, monitor the after-effects and report any abnormal findings immediately, **providing a written record and assisting in the implementation of any action should an abnormality or adverse reaction to the practice be noted**
- in undertaking this practice, nurses are accountable for their actions, the quality of care delivered and record-keeping according to the Code of Professional Conduct: Standards for Conduct, Performance and Ethics (Nursing and Midwifery Council 2004) and Guidelines for Records and Record Keeping (Nursing and Midwifery Council 2005).

3.   BLADDER IRRIGATION

Indications and rationale for bladder irrigation

Bladder irrigation is the continuous washing out of the bladder using sterile fluid, usually only performed within a specialised clinical environment, e.g. urology. Continuous bladder irrigation can be carried out through a three-way urethral catheter or via a suprapubic and a urethral catheter:

- *to prevent the formation of blood clots after surgery to the urinary tract*
- *to aid the removal of blood clots and/or sediment in the bladder*
- *to clear an obstructed catheter*.

Equipment

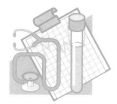

1. Sterile gloves/apron
2. Sterile dressings pack
3. Sterile normal saline
4. Sterile irrigating solution at 37.8°C, usually normal saline solution 0.9%
5. Sterile irrigation set
6. Sterile drainage bag with outlet tap
7. Trolley/adequate surface for equipment
8. Receptacle for soiled disposable items.

Guidelines and rationale for this nursing practice

- explain the nursing practice to the patient *to gain consent and co-operation*
- collect and prepare the equipment *to ensure that all equipment is available and ready for use*
- ensure the patient's privacy *to reduce anxiety*
- observe the patient throughout this activity *to note any signs of distress*
- help the patient into a comfortable position *allowing the nurse easy, comfortable access to the patient*
- wash the hands *to reduce cross-infection* (National Institute for Clinical Excellence 2003), apply gloves, and arrange the equipment, *allowing easy access during the practice*
- cleanse the irrigation inlet arm of the catheter with the antiseptic solution *to reduce cross-infection*
- insert the irrigation set connector into the cleansed inlet arm of the catheter *to permit the introduction of the irrigating fluid*
- attach the urine drainage bag if a drainage bag is not already in use. *This will act as a collection container for the returned irrigating fluid*
- empty the drainage bag *to allow accurate monitoring of the volume of returned irrigating fluid and urine output*
- open the valve of the irrigation set and regulate the flow to the prescribed rate, *complying with the medical practitioner's prescription*
- renew the irrigating fluid as stated on the patient's prescription and empty the drainage bag as required *to maintain the bladder irrigation*
- ensure that the patient is left feeling as comfortable as possible, *maintaining the quality of this nursing practice*
- dispose of the equipment safely *to reduce any health hazard*
- document the nursing practice, monitor the after-effects and report any abnormal findings immediately, *providing a written record and assisting in the implementation of any action should an abnormality or adverse reaction to the practice be noted*
- in undertaking this practice, nurses are accountable for their actions, the quality of care delivered and record-keeping according to the Code of Professional Conduct: Standards for Conduct, Performance and Ethics (Nursing and Midwifery Council 2004) and Guidelines for Records and Record Keeping (Nursing and Midwifery Council 2005).

4. ADMINISTRATION OF CATHETER MAINTENANCE SOLUTIONS

Indications and rationale for catheter maintenance solution

It is common for urinary catheters to block, usually because of a build up of mineral salts or encrustations from the urine on the catheter surface (Getliffe 2003). Careful assessment and proactive care is required to ensure appropriate management of this process as recurrent blocking will impact on both the quality of the patient's life and on professional time. It is important to note that catheters can also bypass because of bladder spasm, constipation and CAUTIs.

Bladder spasms occur when the bladder mucosa becomes clamped around the catheter, occluding the eyes of the catheter (Williams & Tonkin 2003). The urine cannot drain effectively and therefore follows the path of least resistance and leaks down the sides of the catheter causing the patient to experience an episode of incontinence. Usually urine can still be seen in the leg bag, and should return to normal flow once the spasm has worn off. A blockage will not resolve spontaneously without a catheter maintenance solution and on removal of the catheter deposits can usually be seen on it.

Proactive management of patients that experience frequent catheter blockages should help you to treat the cause of the blocking instead of undertaking crisis management when it does block (Williams & Tonkin 2003, National Health Service Quality Improvement Scotland 2004). By maintaining accurate documentation you will be able to assess the average duration that a catheter can remain in situ before it blocks. If a catheter blocks more frequently than every 2 weeks and the pH of the urine is found to be alkaline then the instillation of an acidic maintenance solution may help prevent further blockages (Getliffe 2003). Studies show that acidic catheter maintenance solutions (**not** saline and chlorhexidine) are effective in dissolving encrustations (Getliffe 2003) but care should be taken to ensure that the solution chosen has components aimed to reduce irritation to the bladder wall. There is a lack of evidence to direct you in the frequency for administering a catheter maintenance solution and it is therefore important that care is individualised for each patient.

Equipment

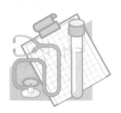

1. Sterile gloves/apron
2. Appropriate catheter maintenance solution
3. New leg bag/night bag to replace existing one
4. Alcohol-impregnated wipe
5. Sterile drape
6. Trolley/adequate surface for equipment
7. Receptacle for soiled disposable items.

Guidelines and rationale for this nursing practice

- explain the nursing practice to the patient *to gain consent and co-operation*
- collect and prepare the equipment required *to ensure that all equipment is available and ready for use*
- ensure the patient's privacy *to reduce any anxiety*
- observe the patient throughout this activity *to note any signs of distress*
- help the patient into a comfortable position *allowing the nurse easy, comfortable access to the patient*
- wash the hands *to reduce cross-infection* (National Institute for Clinical Excellence 2003) and arrange the equipment, *allowing easy access during the practice*
- place the sterile drape under the catheter *to prevent soiling the bed should any urine leak during this procedure*
- disconnect the drainage bag and discard *to prevent ascending infection should this bag be reconnected*
- cleanse the end of the catheter with the alcohol-impregnated wipe using a gloved hand. *This will reduce the number of micro-organisms present on the end of the catheter and lessen the risk of cross-infection*
- remove the protective cover from the catheter maintenance solution and administer as per the manufacturer's guidelines. *A sudden, fast introduction of the solution fluid may cause the patient extreme discomfort*
- monitor return from catheter maintenance solution, checking for cloudiness, evidence of blood or any other abnormalities. *Report any abnormalities to medical staff*
- ensure that the patient is left feeling as comfortable as possible, *maintaining the quality of this nursing practice*
- dispose of the equipment safely *to reduce any health hazard*
- document the nursing practice appropriately, monitor the after-effects and report any abnormal findings immediately, *providing a written record and assisting in the implementation of any action should an abnormality or adverse reaction to the practice be noted*
- in undertaking this practice, nurses are accountable for their actions, the quality of care delivered and record-keeping according to the Code of Professional Conduct: Standards for Conduct, Performance and Ethics (Nursing and Midwifery Council 2004) and Guidelines for Record and Record Keeping (Nursing and Midwifery Council 2005).

Additional information

The majority of patients who require urinary catheterisation will have their fluid intake and output recorded in a fluid balance chart. In addition to measuring the quantity of urine the nurse should note the colour. Pale pink or red through to brown is suggestive of blood in the urine (haematuria). Blood or sediment in the urine could indicate a malfunction of the renal or urinary system. It should be remembered that certain medicines or foods, such as beetroot, colour the urine.

**Patient/carer
education**

Key points

Patients and carers must be educated in the correct infection-control procedures to prevent CAUTIs.

The use of a urinary catheter is a deviation from the normal mechanism of micturition and can thus have an effect on the patient's self-esteem and body image. The nurse and carer must be sensitive to the needs of the patient and assist and support the patient during the period of adaptation to this change. Full sexual activity is not precluded by the presence of a catheter, and patients and their partners should be given leaflets and practical advice. Advice should also be given in relation to the practicalities of sleeping when wearing a leg and night bag.

As the patient moves during sleep, the catheter and/or tubing may become trapped, causing the patient to awaken from the discomfort caused by tension on the catheter. Night bags are made with a long length of tubing to allow the patient free movement and some manufacturers make night bags with 'extra long' tubing.

A patient at home will require information and education on when to renew both leg and night bags, how to receive supplies at home, and contact phone numbers so that they can access the appropriate healthcare professional if required.

References

British Medical Association 2005 British National Formulary 49. BMA, London

Davenport K, Keeley FX 2004 Evidence for the use of silver alloy coated urethral catheters. Journal of Hospital Infection 60(4): 298–303

Department of Health 2004 Bardex IC: silver alloy coated hydrogel catheters. Available at: http://www.hpa.org.uk/infections/topics az/rapid review/pdf/bardex2.pdf

Getliffe K 2003 Managing recurrent urinary catheter blockage: problems, promises and practicalities. Journal of Wound, Ostomy and Continence Nurses 30(3): 146–151

McMurdo MET, Bisset LY, Price RJG et al 2005 Does ingestion of cranberry juice reduce symptomatic UTIs in older people in hospital? A double blind, placebo controlled trial. Age and Aging 34(3): 256–261

Morrow 2006 Continence. In: Alexander M, Fawcett J, Runciman P (eds) Nursing practice – hospital and home: the adult, 3rd edn. Churchill Livingstone, Edinburgh

National Health Service Quality Improvement Scotland 2004 Healthcare associated infections in acute and community care. Scottish Executive, Edinburgh

National Institute for Clinical Excellence 2003 Infection control: prevention of healthcare associated infection in primary and community care. NICE, London

Nursing and Midwifery Council 2004 Code of professional conduct: standards for conduct, performance and ethics. NMC, London

Nursing and Midwifery Council 2005 Guidelines for records and record keeping. NMC, London

Pellowe CM, Pratt RJ, Loveday HP et al 2004 The epic project. Updating the evidence base for national evidence based guidelines for preventing healthcare associated infections in NHS hospitals in England: a report with recommendations. British Journal of Infection Control 5(6): 10–16

Pratt RJ, Pellowe C, Loveday HP 2001 The epic project: developing national evidence based guidelines for preventing health associated infection. Journal of Hospital Infection 47(Suppl) S3–S82

Roper N, Logan W, Tierney A 1985 The elements of nursing, 2nd edn. Churchill Livingstone, Edinburgh

Stewart E 2001 Urinary catheters: selection, maintenance and nursing care. In: Pope Cruickshank J, Woodward S (eds) Management of continence and urinary catheters. BJN Monograph. Quay Books, Salisbury, UK

Tenke X, Jackel M, Nagy E 2004 Prevention and treatment of catheter associated infections: myth or reality? EVA Update Series 2: 106–115

Tew L, Pomfret I, King D 2005 Infection risks associated with urinary catheterisation. Nursing Standard 20(7): 55–61

Williams C, Tonkin S 2003 Blocked urinary catheters: solutions are not the only solution. British Journal of Community Nursing 8(7): 321–324, 326

Websites

NHS Quality Improvement Scotland: http://www.nhshealthquality.org
Nursing and Midwifery Council: http://www.nmc.org
Multiple Sclerosis Resource Centre: http://www.msrc.co.uk
The Continence Foundation: http://www.continence-foundation.org.uk
Coloplast Ltd: http://www.coloplast.co.uk

Self assessment

1. List five reasons for an indwelling urinary catheter being inserted.
2. List four risk factors increasing the risk of CAUTIs in patients.
3. Describe the different types of catheters available.
4. What is the best size of catheter to use and why?
5. What are the indications for instilling a catheter maintenance solution?

Practice 11
Central Venous Pressure

There are two parts to this section:

1 Insertion of a central venous catheter

2 Measuring and recording central venous pressure

Learning outcomes	**By the end of this section, you should know how to:**
	▪ prepare and support the patient for this nursing practice
	▪ collect and prepare the equipment
	▪ assist the medical practitioner with safe insertion of the central venous catheter
	▪ monitor and record the central venous pressure (CVP)
	▪ care for the central venous catheter.

Background knowledge required	Revision of the anatomy and physiology of the cardiovascular system, especially the heart, main vessels and veins of the neck and upper thorax
	Revision of 'Intravenous therapy', especially part 4, the Hickman catheter (*see* p. 181)
	Revision of 'Aseptic technique' (*see* p. 386)
	Review of local policies and procedures in relation to CVP.

Indications and rationale for monitoring central venous pressure	A central venous line may be required for three main reasons:
	▪ ***to enable the rapid or high-volume fluid infusion of irritant substances*** (e.g. cytotoxic drugs or total parenteral nutrition)
	▪ ***to monitor the venous pressure***
	▪ ***to allow frequent venous blood monitoring***.

The CVP recording is the measurement of the pressure in the right atrium of the heart and is quantified in cmH_2O. Sixty per cent of the circulating blood volume is held within the venous system, the CVP being the product of blood volume and venous tone. The pressure recorded reflects the circulating fluid volume; ***this may need to be assessed in seriously ill patients in whom a close monitoring of fluid balance is needed***. It may be indicated:

▪ for the preoperative monitoring of patients who have suffered haemorrhage or trauma ***to monitor fluid balance closely***

▪ for postoperative monitoring following major surgery, especially when intravenous therapy or parenteral nutrition is being administered, ***to monitor fluid balance***

▪ for patients who have severe dehydration, for example after vomiting, diarrhoea or haemorrhage, ***to monitor fluid replacement therapy***

- for patients who have cardiogenic, bacteraemic or hypovolaemic shock, *as this will adversely affect the circulatory system as the cardiac output falls*
- for patients who have cardiac disease, *to monitor fluid overload*
- for patients who have renal disease, *to monitor fluid overload*
- for patients who have acute renal failure during haemodialysis or ultrafiltration procedures *to monitor fluid balance*.

1. INSERTION OF A CENTRAL VENOUS CATHETER

Outline of the procedure

This procedure is carried out by a medical practitioner using an aseptic technique. The procedure involves the passage of a catheter through the veins to the superior vena cava or the right atrium of the heart (Fig. 11.1). The catheter is then connected to the manometer and giving set, and an intravenous infusion is commenced (*see* 'Parenteral nutrition', p. 237).

The position of the patient

The position of the patient is important during this procedure and is dependent on the choice of the entry site for catheterisation. *Veins on the right side are usually selected because they provide easier access to the heart than do those on the left* (Royal College of Nursing 2003). There are three main entry sites (the first two being more frequently used; Royal College of Nursing 2003).

The subclavian vein

The patient lies supine with the arms by his or her side. The head of the bed is lowered by 10° *to lessen the danger of an embolus occurring*.

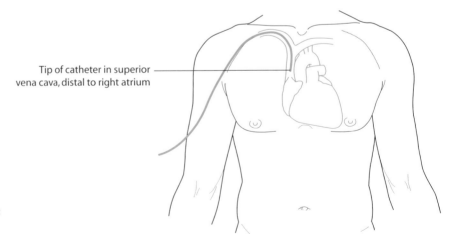

Tip of catheter in superior vena cava, distal to right atrium

FIGURE 11.1
Central venous pressure: position of the catheter in relation to the heart

The internal jugular vein

The patient lies supine, with no pillow, and with the neck extended. The head is rotated away from the site of entry and well supported in position. The head of the bed is lowered by 10°. ***This position is important to prevent an air embolus occurring***.

The median cephalic vein

The patient lies supine. The chosen arm is extended with the palm upwards and the elbow supported ***to ensure easy access to the entry site***.

Equipment

As for intravenous infusion (*see* p. 170).

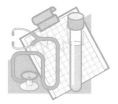

Additional equipment

1. Sterile gown
2. Sterile gloves
3. Minor operation sterile pack or sterile drape and towels
4. Waterproof protection for the bed
5. Alcohol-based antiseptic for cleansing the skin. Evidence suggests that alcohol-based chlorhexidine is more effective than iodine solution (Pellowe et al 2004)
6. Scissors or clippers to remove any body hair from the intended site of insertion (Royal College of Nursing 2003)
7. Venous pressure manometer set
8. Non-viscous sterile intravenous fluid, e.g. normal saline or dextrose 5% (which will be prescribed by the medical practitioner)
9. Appropriate sterile catheter depending on the site of entry used, e.g. a single-, double- or triple-lumen catheter (Fig. 11.2)
10. Sterile needles and black silk sutures
11. ECG monitoring equipment if required
12. Local anaesthetic and equipment necessary for its administration.

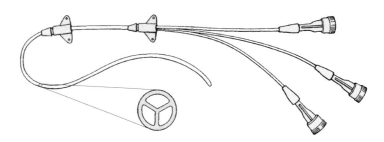

FIGURE 11.2
Triple-lumen catheter

Guidelines and rationale for this nursing practice

Refer to the section on 'Intravenous therapy' (*see* p. 169) for detailed guidelines.

- help to explain the procedure to the patient *to gain consent and co-operation, and to encourage participation in care*
- check whether the patient has an allergy to the skin-cleansing solution and choice of dressing *to avoid reactions*
- ensure the patient's privacy, *respecting his or her individuality*
- prepare the equipment and prime the administration set with the prescribed infusion fluid *in preparation for commencement of the infusion*
- help the patient into the correct position depending on the site of entry used *to ensure that access is safely achieved*
- observe the patient throughout this activity *to monitor any adverse effects*
- adjust the angle of the bed so that the patient's head is lowered if required *to increase venous engorgement and prevent an air embolus*
- protect the bed with waterproof material *as some fluid or blood may spill*
- assist the medical practitioner as required, *ensuring safe practice*
- remain with the patient *to help to maintain his or her position and reduce anxiety as far as possible*
- commence the infusion of the prescribed fluid once the catheter is in position and connected to the manometer and administration set. If a double- or triple-lumen catheter is used, the line designated for CVP recording is connected to the appropriate administration set and manometer, and labelled accordingly, *ensuring that all personnel have accurate information* (Nursing and Midwifery Council 2005)
- ensure that the patient is left feeling as comfortable as possible *so that he or she will tolerate the catheter in situ as long as necessary* (Royal College of Nursing 2003)
- dispose of the equipment safely *to prevent the transmission of infection*
- document the procedure appropriately, monitor the after-effects and report any abnormal findings immediately *to ensure safe practice and enable prompt appropriate medical and nursing care to be initiated as soon as possible*
- monitor and adjust the flow rate *to maintain the infusion at the rate prescribed* (*see* 'Intravenous therapy', p. 179).

A portable chest X-ray image is taken as soon as possible after catheter insertion *to check that the catheter is in the correct position*. Fluids will not be administered through the newly inserted central line until the correct position is verified. A temporary sterile dressing may be applied until this has been performed. The catheter is usually held in place with skin sutures *once it is judged to be correctly positioned*, and a sterile semipermeable, transparent and occlusive dressing is applied over the site *to maintain asepsis* (Royal College of Nursing 2003). The dressing should be changed ever 48 hours or if integrity is compromised (Royal College of Nursing 2003).

Arrhythmias occasionally occur *as a result of irritation of the heart by the passage of the catheter*, and observations may be supplemented by ECG monitoring. The rhythm usually returns to normal *once the catheter is in the correct position*.

2. MEASURING AND RECORDING CENTRAL VENOUS PRESSURE

The CVP is measured in cmH_2O, the range of normal being 3–10 cmH_2O. The CVP will be measured as advised by the medical practitioner.

Equipment

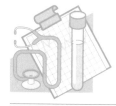

1. A central venous catheter, intravenous fluid and associated lines in situ (Fig. 11.3)
2. A venous pressure manometer (Fig. 11.3)
3. A spirit level.

Guidelines and rationale for this nursing practice

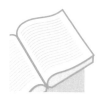

- explain the nursing practice to the patient **to gain consent and co-operation, and to encourage participation in care**
- ensure the patient's privacy **to respect individuality and maintain self-esteem**
- help the patient into the correct position (Fig. 11.3). It is preferable for the patient to lie flat **for absolute accuracy, as this position will stop any**

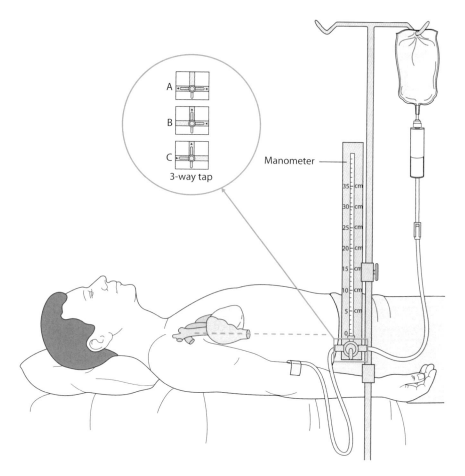

FIGURE 11.3
Measuring the central venous pressure
From Nicol et al 2003, with permission

upward pressure of the abdominal organs affecting the reading. If lying flat causes the patient any distress, an acceptable reading can, however, be obtained with the patient sitting comfortably at an angle of about 45°. His or her body should be straight, with the shoulders flat against the back of the bed; *the thorax must not be turned or twisted, or a false reading may result* (Woodrow 2002). The position chosen should be documented and used at each subsequent reading

- position the manometer. It should be supported on a pole *so that it is easily read*, while still allowing the patient freedom of movement in bed between readings. *To prevent disconnection*, there should be no strain on the lines or the catheter

- observe the patient throughout this activity *to monitor any adverse effects*

- assess the baseline. *The baseline is the pressure level above which the measurement of CVP is made*. This is level with the patient's right atrium, where the tip of the catheter is lying. The medical practitioner will note the level at an imaginary 90° angle between the sternal notch and the midline from the axilla. In some areas, it is the practice to use the sternal notch as a proxy for this point. With the patient's consent, this can be marked on his or her skin *to ensure consistency of baseline measurement*

- read the baseline. A spirit level is used to record the level on the manometer gauge that corresponds to the baseline level, which may be marked on the side of the patient's chest; *this ensures that measurement is as accurate as possible*

- turn off all other infusions. Ideally, only the CVP fluid should be infused through the CVP line, but other fluids are on occasion infused through the same line. *As the CVP is measured in centimetres of water, only fluids of similar specific gravity, for example normal saline, should be used*. The use of multiple-lumen lines overcomes this problem. The tap of the three-way stopcock should be at position A between recordings and before commencing the reading (*see* Fig. 11.3)

- flush the line *to ensure patency and to clear all other infusions* (Gabriel 2005)

- turn the tap on the three-way stopcock away from the patient and towards the infusion fluid, to position B (*see* Fig. 11.3); *this allows the manometer tube to refill with fluid*

- turn the tap towards the patient to position C (*see* Fig. 11.3); *this allows the establishment of a free flow of fluid between the manometer tube and the catheter*. The fluid in the manometer tube will fall to a level that *corresponds to the pressure in the right atrium or superior vena cava*. The fluid fluctuates *in relation to the patient's respiration* once it falls to the level for recording

- read the level of the lower fluctuation on the manometer gauge once the fluid in the tube is maintaining a steady level with a fluctuation of 0.2–1.0 cm. *This relates to the pressure in the right atrium*

- subtract the baseline reading from this figure, *the resultant figure being the measurement of CVP*

- if using an electronic monitor, ensure that it is zeroed according to the manufacturer's instructions, align the transducer with the right atrium and continue as before

- turn the tap on the stopcock back to position A (see Fig. 11.3) *to occlude the manometer and recommence the infusion fluid at the prescribed rate*

- ensure that the patient is left feeling as comfortable as possible *to help to reduce anxiety and promote the healing process*
- document the nursing practice appropriately, monitor the after-effects and report any abnormal findings immediately. *This ensures safe practice and enables prompt appropriate medical and nursing intervention to be initiated*. A single reading is not as valuable as monitoring a series of recordings. *These will show whether the CVP is rising, falling or remaining steady and give some indication of the patient's response to treatment*
- administration sets should be changed every 72 hours. However, should integrity be compromised then the set should be changed immediately (Royal College of Nursing 2003)
- in undertaking this practice, nurses are accountable for their actions, the quality of care delivered and record-keeping according to the Code of Professional Conduct: Standards for Conduct, Performance and Ethics (Nursing and Midwifery Council 2004) and Guidelines for Records and Record Keeping (Nursing and Midwifery Council 2005).

Pressure transducers

Pressure transducers are increasingly being used to monitor CVP. The principles of the practice, the care of the patient and the care of the lines are exactly the same. The pressure transducer, continuous flush device and administration set are substituted for the manometer set. The monitoring set is connected to either 0.9% normal saline or fluids with the same specific gravity. The addition of heparin to the fluid has been shown to maintain patency and reduce bacterial colonisation (Department of Health 2001). The set is connected to a bedside monitor screen and the CVP measurement is displayed. When a reading is taken, the height of the transducer, which may be supported on a pole, or fastened to the patient's arm, is adjusted to be level with the assessed baseline, as previously described. The monitor may be programmed to assess the reading in mmHg. The normal recording parameters may have to be adjusted (see the manufacturer's instructions). The pressure transducer and monitoring set should be changed every 96 hours (National Institute for Clinical Excellence 2003).

Additional information

Because of increased pulmonary pressure the CVP value is raised in patients who have respiratory disease and is significantly raised in patients with bronchospasm. It also increases in patients with congestive cardiac failure because of the increase in circulatory fluid volume.

Patient/carer education

Key points

In partnership with the patient and/or carer, ensure that they are competent to carry out any practices required. Information should be given on an appropriate point of contact for any concerns that may arise.

The reason for CVP monitoring and its importance for treatment and care should be explained to the patient. This practice will normally only take place in an institutional setting.

The importance of maintaining the catheter in situ should be emphasised, and the dangers of disconnection explained, so that the patient does not pull the lines or dislodge the dressing.

All patients should understand the importance of reporting to the nursing staff any redness, swelling or pain at the infusion site, even after the line has been removed, as this may indicate a developing infection.

References

Department of Health 2001 Guidelines for preventing infection associated with the insertion and maintenance of central venous catheters. Journal of Hospital Infection 47(Suppl): S47–S67

Gabriel J 2005 Vascular access: indications and implications for patient care. Nursing Standard 19(26): 45–52

National Institute for Clinical Excellence 2003 Infection control: prevention of healthcare-associated infection in primary and community care (clinical guidelines 2). NICE, London

Nicol M, Bavin C, Bedford-Turner S et al 2003 Essential nursing skills, 2nd edn. Mosby, London

Nursing and Midwifery Council 2004 Code of professional conduct: standards for conduct, performance and ethics. NMC, London

Nursing and Midwifery Council 2005 Guidelines for records and record keeping. NMC, London

Pellowe CM, Pratt RJ, Loveday HP et al 2004 The epic project. Updating the evidence base for national evidence based guidelines for preventing healthcare associated infections in NHS hospitals in England. Journal of Hospital Infection 5(6): 10–16

Royal College of Nursing 2003 Standards for infusion therapy. RCN, London

Woodrow P 2002 Central venous catheters and central venous pressure. Nursing Standard 16(26): 45–52, 54

Self assessment

1. What are the main indications for measuring central venous pressure?
2. Consider the processes required to measure and record central venous pressure.
3. List the main entry sites that are used for the insertion of an intravenous catheter.

Practice 12

Chest Drainage: Underwater Seal or Chest Drainage System

There are three parts to this section:

1　Insertion of an underwater seal chest drain

2　Changing a chest drainage bottle

3　Removal of an underwater seal chest drain

Learning outcomes

By the end of this section, you should know how to:
- support and prepare the patient for these three nursing practices
- collect and prepare the equipment necessary to insert a chest drain and connect it to underwater seal drainage, change a chest drainage bottle and assist with removal of an underwater seal chest drain
- assist the medical practitioner in parts 1 and 3
- care for the patient who has a chest drain connected to underwater seal drainage.

Background knowledge required

Revision of the anatomy, physiology and pathology of the respiratory system, including the structures of the chest wall
Revision of 'Aseptic technique' (*see* p. 386).
Revision of local policy on chest drainage.

1.　INSERTION OF AN UNDERWATER SEAL CHEST DRAIN

Indications and rationale for insertion of an underwater seal chest drain

Chest drainage refers to a closed system of drainage that allows air or fluid to pass in one direction only, from the pleural space to either a collecting bottle or flutter valve system. It may be required in a variety of situations when ventilation is impaired, such as traumatic injuries, malignancy, post-thoracic surgery or following spontaneous collapse of the lung (pneumothorax). Chest drainage may therefore be used to remove air, blood, fluid or pus from the pleural space to improve ventilation capacity.

Chest drains may also be inserted to allow drug administration to occur, for example in lung cancer.

The choice of drainage system will depend upon the clinical status and underlying condition of the patient, the nature of the expected drainage and whether the drain is being inserted perioperatively or in a ward or outpatient unit. Underwater seal drainage bottles are at risk of being knocked over, inhibit patient mobilisation and need to be monitored on an inpatient basis. Flutter valve systems are useful for draining air though they cannot be used for draining fluid. The flutter valve system has the advantage of allowing mobilisation.

The drain insertion site will also vary according to the clinical status of the patient. Confirmation of the insertion site should be made following clinical examination and chest X-ray in all cases, apart from tension pneumothorax when it would be a priority to insert the drain quickly. Sometimes the drain is inserted with the aid of imaging such as ultrasound (Laws et al 2003). For many of the indications for chest drain insertion, the site will be the third, fourth or fifth intercostal space in the mid axillary line.

Position of the patient

During insertion, the patient's clinical status will determine the optimum position to be adopted. It is often sitting upright and the patient may use a table with a pillow to rest on.

Outline of the procedure

Using an aseptic technique, the medical practitioner cleanses the patient's skin with iodine or an alcohol-based antiseptic (as per local skin preparation policy), over the selected site of entry for the drain, injects a local anaesthetic and waits for it to take effect. The method of drain insertion will vary depending on the size of drain required. The aim is to avoid excessive force that may cause damage to intrathoracic structures. Sometimes an introducer is used, or blunt dissection of the subcutaneous tissue using forceps may be used for larger sizes of drainage tube. Once the tube is in place, the medical practitioner connects the drain to the equipment already prepared by the nurse. A suture is inserted round the entry site of the drain to seal the site off when the drain is eventually removed. A purse-string suture should not be used (Laws et al 2003). A sterile transparent dressing is placed over the site to help to prevent infection of the small wound (Fig. 12.1).

Equipment

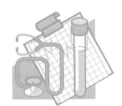

1. Trolley
2. Sterile dressings pack
3. Sterile gloves
4. Iodine preparation or alcohol-based antiseptic (as per local policy on skin cleansing)
5. Local anaesthetic and equipment for its administration
6. Sterile scalpel and blade and/or Spencer Wells forceps
7. Sterile black silk suture
8. Sterile chest drain and introducer
9. Sterile drainage equipment, e.g. Pleurovac or Argyle double-seal system
10. Two pairs of tubing clamps
11. Receptacle for soiled disposable items
12. Sharps box.

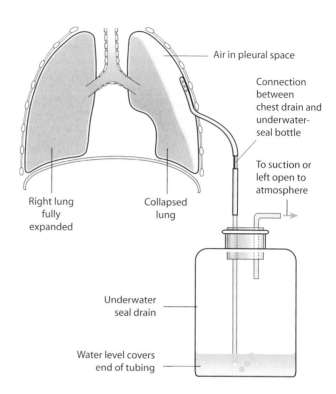

Air in pleural space

Connection between chest drain and underwater-seal bottle

To suction or left open to atmosphere

Right lung fully expanded

Collapsed lung

Underwater seal drain

Water level covers end of tubing

FIGURE 12.1
Underwater seal chest drainage system
From Brooker & Nicol 2003, with permission

Guidelines and rationale for this nursing practice

- help to explain the procedure to the patient *to gain informed consent and co-operation. Patients should be encouraged to be active partners in care*
- ensure the patient's privacy *to help maintain dignity*
- administer a pre-medication if prescribed by the medical staff *to help to reduce the patient's anxiety*
- administer analgesia as prescribed *to minimize pain during and after the procedure*
- collect the equipment, *for efficiency of practice*
- help the patient into the position suggested by the medical staff *to allow best access to the site for insertion of the drain*
- observe the patient throughout this activity *to detect signs of discomfort, distress or adverse effects*
- ensure that the drainage equipment is assembled correctly and ready for connection to the drain when required, *for efficient practice*
- open the sterile equipment and help the medical practitioner as requested
- seal all connections *to ensure that they are airtight, as this is necessary for maximum functioning of the drain*
- ensure that the collection equipment is always below the level of the patient's chest *so that there is no reflux into the pleural space* (Fig. 12.2)

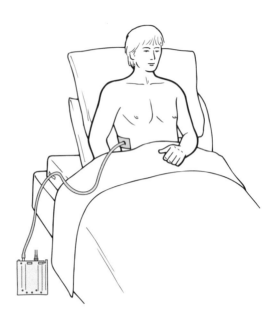

FIGURE 12.2
Patient with underwater seal chest drainage

- ***to allow the apparatus to start functioning***, release the clamps when the drain is connected and when you are satisfied that there are no air leaks at the connections
- check that the apparatus is functioning; the fluid should be oscillating in the long underwater tube in time with the patient's respiration indicating patency of the tube. If positive suction is required, connect the short rod of the drainage bottle to the long rod of a second drainage bottle using tubing. The short rod of this second drainage bottle is then connected by tubing to a suction machine, the pressure of which has been decided by the medical practitioner
- apply a sterile transparent dressing to the wound site ***to help to prevent infection and to facilitate observation of the site***
- ensure that the patient is left feeling as comfortable as possible, ***to maintain the quality of this practice***
- dispose of the equipment safely ***to comply with health and safety and infection-control requirements***
- document the procedure appropriately, monitor the after-effects and report any abnormal findings immediately ***to ensure safe practice and enable prompt, appropriate medical and nursing intervention to be initiated***
- monitor vital signs ***to assess response to intervention***
- observe and record amount, type and consistency of drainage ***to monitor patient's progress and maintain fluid balance***
- in undertaking this practice, nurses are accountable for their actions, the quality of care delivered and record-keeping according to the Code of Professional Conduct: Standards for Conduct, Performance and Ethics (Nursing and Midwifery Council 2004) and Guidelines for Records and Record Keeping (Nursing and Midwifery Council 2005).

2. CHANGING A CHEST DRAINAGE BOTTLE

Indications and rationale for changing a drainage bottle

As drainage from the pleural space accumulates and approaches the three-quarters-full level, the drainage bottle has to be changed:

- **to enable the equipment to continue functioning efficiently** as increased volume in the bottle may cause resistance to drainage (Allibone 2003).

Equipment

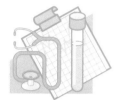

1. Sterile drainage bottle, cap, glass or plastic rods and tubing or a disposable set
2. 500 ml of sterile water or normal saline
3. Receptacle for soiled disposable items.

Guidelines and rationale for this nursing practice

- collect and prepare the equipment **for efficiency of practice**
- explain this practice to the patient **to encourage active participation in care**
- observe the patient throughout this activity **to detect signs of discomfort, distress or adverse effects**
- clamp off the chest drain, one close to the chest wall and one below the connection to the drainage tubing to **prevent any backflow of air or fluid** (Parkin 2002)
- disconnect the tubing
- connect the fresh tubing and apparatus
- ensure that all the connections are airtight and that the drainage bottle is below chest level **so that it will function correctly**
- release the clamps and check the oscillation of the fluid in the underwater tube **to confirm that the apparatus is functioning correctly**
- ensure that the patient is left feeling as comfortable as possible **to maintain the quality of this practice**
- dispose of the equipment safely **for the protection of others**
- document this nursing practice and report abnormal findings immediately **so that action can be taken to relieve any problems**
- observations and recording of vital signs should be performed following the procedure **to monitor the patient's progress**
- observation and monitoring of drainage should continue **to monitor patient's progress and maintain fluid balance**
- in undertaking this practice, nurses are accountable for their actions, the quality of care delivered and record-keeping according to the Code of Professional Conduct: Standards for Conduct, Performance and Ethics (Nursing and Midwifery Council 2004) and Guidelines for Records and Record Keeping (Nursing and Midwifery Council 2005).

Clinical Nursing Practices

3. REMOVAL OF AN UNDERWATER SEAL CHEST DRAIN

Indications and rationale for removal of an underwater seal chest drain

Underwater seal drainage is a temporary measure and is removed:
- when radiological examination demonstrates that the patient's lung has fully reinflated
- when air or fluid no longer drains and when breath sounds have improved.

Equipment

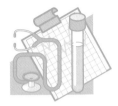

1. Trolley
2. Sterile dressings pack
3. Sterile stitch-cutter
4. Sterile artery forceps
5. Receptacle for soiled disposable items.

Guidelines and rationale for this nursing practice

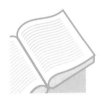

Two nurses, one of whom must be qualified, or the nurse and a medical practitioner are required to carry out this practice.
- explain the nursing practice to the patient *to gain consent and co-operation. Patients should be encouraged to be active partners in their care*
- ensure the patient's privacy *to maintain dignity and a sense of self*
- administer analgesia if it is prescribed by the medical practitioner *to manage pain*
- collect the equipment *for efficiency of practice*
- prepare and assist the patient into a suitable position that is as comfortable as possible *to allow clear access to the drain site*
- observe the patient throughout this activity *to detect any signs of discomfort and distress*
- remove the dressing from the drain site
- tell the patient to take 3 deep breaths and then hold their breath while the drain is removed *to equalize intrapulmonary pressure*
- when the drain has been removed, smoothly and firmly, the assistant will quickly tie the previously placed suture *to close the wound and form an airtight seal around the wound*
- tell the patient to breath normally
- order a chest X-ray *to ensure that the lung is functioning normally*
- ensure that the patient is left feeling as comfortable as possible, *to maintain the quality of this practice*
- dispose of the equipment safely *for the protection of others*
- document the nursing practice, monitor the after-effects and report any abnormal findings immediately *to provide a written record and assist in the implementation of any action should an abnormality or adverse reaction to the practice be noted*
- in undertaking this practice, nurses are accountable for their actions, the quality of care delivered and record-keeping according to the Code of Professional Conduct: Standards for Conduct, Performance and Ethics (Nursing and Midwifery Council 2004) and Guidelines for Records and Record Keeping (Nursing and Midwifery Council 2005).

Additional information

Ensure that the tubing is not being compressed or kinked by the patient lying on it, as this will cause the equipment to function inefficiently. It is imperative that the drainage bottle is kept below the level of the patient's chest, unless double-clamped, or there may be a backflow of fluid into the pleural cavity.

When the drain is being removed, care must be taken to prevent a pneumothorax (i.e. the entry of air into the pleural space).

Because of breathlessness, the patient may have difficulty in talking. A pencil and paper may help communication with staff and visitors, and the nurse call system should always be to hand to summon assistance if necessary.

Analgesics may be prescribed to help relieve any pain or discomfort.

If the equipment is functioning correctly, the patient's respiratory rate should gradually return to the normal range after the drain has been inserted.

The patient's respiration should be closely monitored after the removal of the drain so that the potential complication of pneumothorax can be quickly detected.

Some assistance with washing and dressing may have to be given to those who are attached to underwater seal drainage equipment as their mobility is reduced. Light, loose clothing should be worn so that breathing is not unduly impaired.

Movement will be restricted by the equipment, but the patient should be encouraged to be as independent as possible.

The patient's normal sleeping pattern may be altered because of difficulty with breathing and because of the presence of the equipment, so the nurse should take measures that help to induce sleep.

Patient/carer education

Key points

The patient should be given clear information about the procedure to ensure they are able to give informed consent and to encourage their participation in care. The patient and carers should be informed of the need to keep the drainage system below the level of the chest. Specific information about mobilising safely should also be given. Written educational leaflets should also be available. The patient should be encouraged to report any problems such as pulling of the tube or increased dyspnoea. Adequate pain relief should be available to the patient. Patients should be informed of the nursing observations that will be made when the chest drain is in place to alleviate anxiety.

References

Allibone L 2003 Nursing management of chest drains. Nursing Standard 17(22): 45–56

Brooker C, Nicol M 2003 Nursing adults: the practice of caring. Mosby, Edinburgh

Laws D, Neville E, Duffy J 2003 BTS guidelines for the insertion of a chest drain. Thorax 58: 53–59

Nursing and Midwifery Council 2004 Code of professional conduct: standards for conduct, performance and ethics. NMC, London

Nursing and Midwifery Council 2005 Guidelines for records and record keeping. NMC, London

Parkin C 2002 A retrospective audit of chest drain practice in a specialist cardiothoracic centre and concurrent review of chest drain literature. Nursing in Critical Care 7(1): 30–36

Websites

British Thoracic Society: http://www.brit-thoracic.org.uk

Thorax Online: http://www.thorax.bmjjournals.com

Self assessment

1. Describe the indications for chest drain insertion.
2. Consider what you would say to a patient to prepare them for chest drain insertion.
3. What aspects of the procedure might pose an infection control risk?
4. What observations would you make on the patient who has a chest drain in place?
5. How would you know if the chest drainage system could be removed?

Practice 13
Eardrops: Instillation of

Learning outcomes	**By the end of this section, you should know how to:**
	▪ prepare the patient for this nursing practice
	▪ collect and prepare the equipment
	▪ instil drops safely and effectively into the patient's ear.

Background knowledge required	Revision of the anatomy of the ear
	Revision of 'Administration of medicines', especially checking the medication against the prescription (*see* p. 13).

Indications and rationale for instilling eardrops	The instillation of eardrops involves dropping a prescribed solution into the external auditory canal from a dropper. This may be required:
	▪ **to soften wax before syringing**. If the wax has become impacted, syringing the external canal with solution will be ineffective unless the wax has first been softened (Aung & Mulley 2002)
	▪ **to reduce inflammation and relieve discomfort**
	▪ **to combat infection**.

Equipment 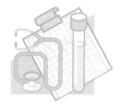	1. Prescribed eardrops
	2. Cotton wool balls
	3. Receptacle for soiled disposable items.

Guidelines and rationale for this nursing practice	▪ explain the practice to the patient **to ensure understanding and gain consent and co-operation**
	▪ wash hands **to reduce the potential of cross infection** (Jeanes 2005)
	▪ collect and prepare the equipment **for efficiency of practice**
	▪ ensure the patient's privacy **to preserve dignity and a sense of self**
	▪ assist the patient to sit in an upright position with the head tilted slightly away from the affected ear **so that the drops inserted will run the length of the canal**
	▪ observe the patient throughout this activity **to detect any signs of discomfort**
	▪ check the drug prescription with the label on the eardrops **to ensure that the correct drops are administered**
	▪ check the expiry date on the bottle of eardrops **as expired medication may be ineffective**
	▪ verify which ear should receive the drops, **to avoid errors**

- pull the pinna of the ear gently in an upward and backward direction in adults, and a downward and backward direction in children, *to straighten the external canal*
- insert the prescribed number of eardrops into the canal
- release the pinna
- position a piece of cotton wool at the entrance to the canal if this is local policy
- dispose of the equipment safely *for the protection of others*
- document this nursing practice appropriately, monitor the after-effects and report any abnormal findings immediately *to provide a written record and assist in the implementation of any action should an abnormality or adverse reaction to the practice be noted*
- in undertaking this practice, nurses are accountable for their actions, the quality of care delivered and record-keeping according to the Code of Professional Conduct: Standards for Conduct, Performance and Ethics (Nursing and Midwifery Council 2004), Guidelines for Records and Record Keeping (Nursing and Midwifery Council 2005).

Patient/carer education
Key points

In partnership with the patient and/or carer, ensure that they are competent to carry out any practices required. Information should be given on an appropriate point of contact for any concerns that may arise.

If the patient is expected to self-administer the drops, it will be necessary to teach this technique and ensure proficiency.

References

Aung T, Mulley GP 2002 Removal of ear wax. British Medical Journal 325(7354): 27
Jeanes A 2005 Infection control. A practical guide to the use of hand decontaminants. Nursing Times 101(20): 46–48
Nursing and Midwifery Council 2004 Code of professional conduct: standards for conduct, performance and ethics. NMC, London
Nursing and Midwifery Council 2005 Guidelines for records and record keeping. NMC, London

Website
Nursing and Midwifery Council: http://www.nmc-uk.org

Self assessment

1. List the three main reasons for administering ear drops.
2. What equipment is required when administering ear drops?
3. Why is the patient required to sit in an upright position during administration of ear drops?
4. Why is it necessary to check the expiry date on the bottle of ear drops prior to administration?
5. In what direction should the ear be gently pulled in an adult prior to administering ear drops?

Practice 14
Ear Syringing

Learning outcomes	**By the end of this section, you should know how to:**
	▪ prepare the patient for this procedure
	▪ collect and prepare the equipment
	▪ syringe a patient's ear.

Background knowledge required	Revision of the anatomy and physiology of the external and middle ear
	Review of local policy for this procedure.

Indications and rationale for syringing an ear	Impacted cerumen (ear wax) can cause hearing loss, social withdrawal and perforated ear drums (Guest et al 2004). Ear syringing is the removal of this cerumen from the external auditory canal with water or a prescribed solution using specialized equipment. Because of the complications and contraindications related to this procedure it should only be performed by an appropriately trained professional (Harkin 2000).

This may be required:
- *to clear the external canal of an obstruction that may be blocking it*
- *to wash out softened wax that may be impeding the transmission of sound waves to the tympanic membrane.*

Outline of the procedure	Using an auriscope, the external canal and ear drum are examined. If the tympanic membrane is intact and no other abnormalities are detected, the practice of syringing the ear can be carried out. It is sometimes not possible to visualise the tympanic membrane at this stage because of the impacted wax and in this case the patient should be prescribed an appropriate softener, to be instilled as prescribed, to allow the cerumen to be irrigated effectively. Despite the range of softeners, it should be noted that there is a lack of research to support the rationale of choice behind each available make (Guest et al 2004, Hand & Harvey 2004). Under these circumstances, cost and patient compliance must be considered by the prescriber during their assessment.

For some patients the used of a softener for four days may be all that is required for effective removal of the impacted cerumen (Hand & Harvey 2004). However, if cerumen persists following this treatment and if there is no history of a ruptured ear drum, the ear can then be syringed. Although this practice is still called 'ear syringing', in practice the use of a metal syringe to irrigate cerumen has been condemned due to the number of cases of damage caused to ear drums, e.g. perforation of the tympanic membrane (Coopey 2001). Over a five-year period in the 1990s, 19% of cases settled by the Medical Defence Union were caused by incorrect ear syringing.

A machine called a Propulse II (Fig. 14.1) is now routinely used for this procedure. This is an electronically operated apparatus with a control dial to ensure a safe and constant delivery of warm water at the optimum pressure for ear irrigation. The use of 'individual use' jet tips ensures adherence to infection-control guidelines and the machine is cleansed on a daily basis following the manufacturer's guidelines. Ears should not be syringed in the following cases:

- evidence of a purulent or bloodstained discharge indicating a perforated ear drum
- evidence of otitis media in the last six weeks
- patients with a cleft palate (due to increased risk of infection due to poor development of the facial bones)
- previous ear surgery, unless patients have been discharged from ENT for more than 18 months (Harkin 2000).

Equipment

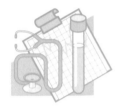

1. Propulse II machine
2. One-use Jet Tips
3. Auriscope with disposable earpieces
4. Waterproof protection for the patient
5. Water (at body temperature)
6. Thermometer
7. Receiver for return flow.

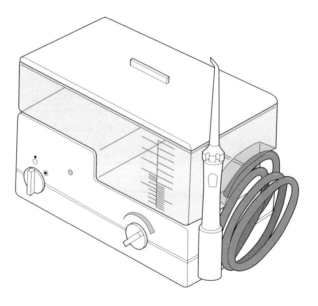

Propulse II electronic ear irrigator

Guidelines and rationale for this nursing practice

- help to explain the procedure to the patient *to ensure that the practice is understood and to gain consent and co-operation*
- assemble and prepare the equipment *to increase the efficiency of the practice*
- ensure the patient's privacy *to help to maintain dignity and a sense of self*
- assist the patient to sit in an upright position with the head tilted slightly to the affected side *to aid the return flow of the solution*
- observe the patient throughout this activity *to detect any signs of discomfort or distress*. Any reports of severe dizziness or pain and the procedure should be stopped immediately, and medical assistance requested if symptoms do not resolve
- arrange the waterproof protection around the patient's neck and shoulders *to prevent the patient's clothes becoming damp or damaged*
- place the receiver for the return flow under the patient's ear and ask for the patient's assistance in holding it in place
- after examining the external canal, insert the jet tip and direct the flow of water at a direction of 'one o'clock' for the left ear and 'eleven o'clock' for the right ear
- continue until the return flow is clear of debris. A maximum of two reservoirs of water should be used per ear.
- dry the patient's ear
- ensure that the patient is left feeling as comfortable as possible and check for improved hearing
- dispose of the equipment safely *for the protection of others*
- document the procedure appropriately, monitor the after-effects and report any abnormal findings immediately *to provide a written record and assist in the implementation of any action should an abnormality or adverse reaction to the practice be noted*
- in undertaking this practice, nurses are accountable for their actions, the quality of care delivered and record-keeping according to the Code of Professional Conduct: Standards for Conduct, Performance and Ethics (Nursing and Midwifery Council 2004) and Guidelines for Records and Record Keeping (Nursing and Midwifery Council 2005).

Additional information

The patient may experience feelings of slight dizziness when this practice is being carried out. This should settle fairly quickly if they rest for a while after the procedure.

There should be an immediate improvement in the patient's hearing. If a hearing aid is used ensure it is working satisfactorily before the patient leaves.

Patient/carer education
Key points

Information should be given on an appropriate point of contact for any concerns that may arise following this procedure.

It should be explained to the patient that tinnitus (noises in the ear) or dizziness may be experienced for a short time after the procedure (Harkin 2000). If the patient wears a hearing aid this should be placed back in the patient's ear and tested for effectiveness.

If the syringing was carried out to relieve impacted wax and improve hearing, the possibility of the condition recurring must be explained.

A maintenance dose of one drop of olive oil per week into each ear may slow the reoccurrence of impacted cerumen. Remind the patient/carer against the habit of using a cotton bud to clean the ear.

References

Coopey S 2001 Ear syringing: a case for clinical governance. Journal of Community Nursing 15(1): 20–22

Guest JF, Greener MJ, Robinson AC et al 2004 Impacted cerumen: composition, production, epidemiology and management. Quarterly Journal of Medicine 97(8): 477–488

Hand C, Harvey I 2004 The effectiveness of topical preparations for the treatment of earwax: a systematic review. British Journal of General Practice 54: 862–867

Harkin H 2000 Evidence based ear care. Primary Health Care 10(8): 25–29

Nursing and Midwifery Council 2004 Code of professional conduct: standards for conduct, performance and ethics. NMC, London

Nursing and Midwifery Council 2005 Guidelines for records and record keeping. NMC, London

Websites
ENT Nursing: http://www.entnursing.com/
The Primary Ear Care Centre: http://www.earcarecentre.com
Royal National Institute for Deaf: http://www.rnid.org.uk

Self assessment

1. Describe three potential complications for the patient with impacted cerumen.
2. At what angle should the jet tip be inserted into each ear for maximum irrigation?
3. Why was the use of a metal syringe for ear irrigation condemned?
4. What is the maximum volume of warm water to be irrigated into each ear during one session?
5. What sensations may the patient experience after this procedure?

Practice 15
Enema

Learning outcomes	**By the end of this section, you should know how to:**

- prepare the patient for this nursing practice
- have an understanding of criteria used to diagnose constipation
- collect and prepare the equipment
- administer an enema
- describe the various enema preparations and their modes of action.

Background knowledge required

Revision of the anatomy and physiology of the colon, rectum and anus

Revision of 'Administration of medicines', particularly checking the medicine against the prescription (*see* p. 13)

Understand common causes of constipation and know appropriate health education advice for the prevention of constipation.

Indications and rationale for administering an enema

An enema is the introduction of liquid into the rectum by means of a tube. It is used:

- **to relieve severe constipation**. Potential complications of unresolved constipation include abdominal pain and distension; confusion; nausea and vomiting; overflow diarrhoea; abdominal obstruction or perforation
- **to evacuate the bowel prior to surgery or investigation**
- **to administer medication**.

An appropriately trained nurse prescriber has the ability to assess, diagnose and prescribe an appropriate enema to rectify severe constipation. This is a specialised extended role, recognised by a registerable qualification with the Nursing and Midwifery Council. An awareness of the Rome II criteria for constipation (see Table 15.1) offers guidance to the practitioner when diagnosing constipation, as will a digital rectal examination (see Practice 35).

Equipment

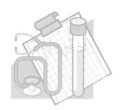

1. Flat surface/tray/trolley
2. Prescribed enema (warmed to body temperature)
3. Protective covering for the bed
4. Water-soluble lubricant
5. Disposable gloves
6. Apron
7. Medical wipes/tissues
8. Commode/bedpan/access to toilet facilities
9. Receptacle for soiled disposable items.

TABLE 15.1

Rome II criteria for constipation (adults)

A diagnosis of constipation requires two or more of the following symptoms to be present for at least three months (not necessarily consecutive) in the preceding twelve months:

1. Straining at defecation for at least a quarter of bowel movements

2. Lumpy and/or hard stools for at least a quarter of bowel movements

3. A sensation of incomplete evacuation for at least a quarter of bowel movements

4. Less than three bowel movements a week

5. Manual manoeuvres to facilitate a quarter of bowel movements (e.g. digital evacuation or support of the pelvic floor)

6. Loose stools not present and insufficient criteria met for irritable bowel syndrome

From Drossman 2000, with permission of the Rome Foundation.

Types of enema

There are three main kinds of enema (Fig. 15.1):

1. Medication

Enemas containing medication that should be retained as long as possible and should be inserted very slowly over half an hour.

2. Evacuant

Stimulant enemas that are usually returned, with faecal matter and flatus, within a few minutes; solutions containing phosphates or sodium citrate are commonly used.

3. Retention

Enemas that soften and lubricate the faeces and should be retained for a specified time; they usually contain arachis or olive oil. They may be inserted, for example, at bedtime to be retained overnight for maximum efficiency of action. The speed of introduction of the fluid will have an impact on peristalsis: the faster the introduction, the greater the effect, and therefore they should be administered slowly.

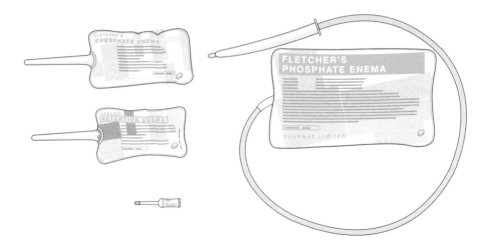

FIGURE 15.1
Examples of disposable enemas

Microenemas

These are also available as they cause less discomfort to patients when administered. The other enemas can be obtained with long delivery tubes to facilitate self-insertion by patients. Prior to the administration of any enema the nurse should check that the patient is not allergic to latex, phosphate or peanuts (arachis oil enemas contains peanut oil).

Guidelines and rationale for this nursing practice

- explain the nursing practice to the patient *to gain consent and co-operation and to check for any previous rectal problems*
- assemble and prepare the equipment *for efficiency of practice*
- warm the enema by immersing it in a jug of water. Mallett & Dougherty (2000) advocate a temperature of 40.5–43.5°C thereby reducing the risk of bowel spasm and shock (Addison 2000)
- if necessary, allow the patient to empty the bladder first *to reduce discomfort during the procedure* (Mallett & Dougherty 2000)
- ensure the patient's privacy and help the patient into the left lateral position *to allow ease of access to the anal sphincter*
- place the protective covering under the patient's buttocks *to contain any soiling or leakage*
- put on disposable gloves and apron
- the foot of the bed may be elevated to an angle of 45° when a retention enema has been administered, *in order to facilitate retention* (Mallett & Dougherty 2000)
- lubricate the end of the enema tube *to ease entry into the rectum*, and ask the patient to take deep breaths *to encourage relaxation and reduce discomfort on the insertion of the enema*. If any persistent resistance is felt or the patient experiences pain, discontinue procedure immediately and seek assistance. Care should be taken when there are haemorrhoids or fissures present at the anus and to avoid damaging the rectal mucosa when inserting the tube of the enema into the rectum
- squeeze a small amount of fluid down the tube to expel the air, *as air in the rectum will cause discomfort*
- insert the tube into the rectum in an upward and slightly backward direction for about 7.5 cm, *following the natural line of the rectum*
- administer the solution gently and slowly *to minimise any discomfort*, squeezing the bag and rolling it up so that all the contents are administered (Nicol et al 2000)
- observe the patient throughout this activity *to detect any signs of discomfort or distress*
- remove the tube when the prescribed amount has been administered
- dry the anal area *to prevent any irritation*
- the protective covering may be left in place *to help prevent soiling of bed linen by leaking faecal matter*
- provide toileting facilities when required. Access to a toilet is preferable *as it reduces the patient's embarrassment*
- ensure that the patient is left feeling as comfortable as possible, *maintaining the quality of this nursing practice*
- dispose of the equipment safely *for the protection of others*

- document this nursing practice appropriately, monitor the after-effects and report any abnormal findings immediately ***to provide a written record and assist in the implementation of any action should an abnormality or adverse reaction to the practice be noted***
- in undertaking this practice, nurses are accountable for their actions, the quality of care delivered and record-keeping according to the Code of Professional Conduct: Standards for Conduct, Performance and Ethics (Nursing and Midwifery Council 2004) and Guidelines for Records and Record Keeping (Nursing and Midwifery Council 2005).

Patient/carer education

Key points

If the enema is being administered to relieve constipation, advice should be given on how to prevent reoccurrence. The long-term use of laxatives, opiates, anticholinergics, iron, antidepressants and anti-Parkinsonian medicines have been implicated in increased risk of constipation The nutritional status of the patient, e.g. their diet, who provides their meals, and oral hygiene should be included in a full assessment. It may be appropriate to offer dietary information leaflets to patients and carers to assist them in maintaining both a high-fibre diet and an adequate fluid intake. Patients who have limited mobility have a greater tendency to experience constipation.

If this procedure is performed within a patient's home it may be appropriate for the nurse to leave prior to an effective result from the enema. Under these circumstances the nurse should tell the patient how long the enema requires to be retained for maximum effectiveness, and should ensure that further contact is made with the patient to ensure a satisfactory result was achieved. It may be appropriate to teach the patient or carer how to self-administer an enema if this process is likely to reoccur. Information should be given on an appropriate point of contact for any concerns that may arise.

References

Addison R 2000 How to administer enema and suppositories. Nursing Times 96(6 Suppl): 3–4

Drossman DA 2000 Rome II: the functional gastrointestinal disorders. Degnon Associates: McLean, VA

Mallett J, Dougherty L (eds) 2000 Royal Marsden manual of clinical nursing procedures, 5th edn. Blackwell Science, London

Nicol M, Bavin C, Bedford-Turner S et al 2000 Essential nursing skills. Mosby, London

Nursing and Midwifery Council 2004 Code of professional conduct: standards for conduct, performance and ethics. NMC, London

Nursing and Midwifery Council 2005 Guidelines for records and record keeping. NMC, London

Website

Rome Criteria – The Functional Gastrointestinal Disorders: http://www.romecriteria.org

Self assessment

1. Discuss the Rome II criteria for constipation.
2. Describe three types of enema.
3. Describe the optimum length of time each type of enema should remain in situ prior to evacuation.
4. List the equipment required for the administration of an enema.

Practice 16
Exercises: Active and Passive

Learning outcomes	**By the end of this section, you should know how to:** ■ prepare the patient for this nursing practice ■ carry out active and passive exercises.
Background knowledge required	Revision of the anatomy and physiology of the musculoskeletal system.
Indications and rationale for active and passive exercises	Active and passive exercises (Fig. 16.1) are muscle and joint movements carried out ***to assist circulation, maintain muscle tone and prevent the development of joint contracture***. These exercises can be performed by the patient (active) or by the nurse or carer helping the patient (passive), and are indicated: ■ following an anaesthetic or surgery ■ during a period of reduced mobility such as bed-rest ■ during prolonged inactivity resulting from the effects of disease or trauma.
Equipment 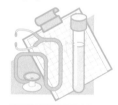	It may be necessary to include safety equipment, for example bed sides, to prevent a bed-fast patient falling out of bed during passive exercises.
Guidelines and rationale for this nursing practice	These guidelines could be used by the nurse to teach a patient's carer(s) to become involved in this practice. ■ explain the nursing practice to the patient ***to gain consent and co-operation*** ■ ensure the patient's privacy ***to reduce anxiety and/or embarrassment*** ■ observe the patient throughout this activity ***to note any signs of distress or discomfort*** ■ wash the hands ***to reduce the risk of cross-infection*** ■ help the patient into a comfortable position. The patient's position may need to be altered during the nursing practice ***to permit easy, comfortable access to each limb during the exercise programme*** ■ assist the patient to move the cervical spine and trunk through their normal range of movement, ***preventing damage and strain to any joint or muscle*** ■ taking each limb separately, assist the patient to move all the joints of the limb through their normal range of movement, ***allowing the patient and nurse***

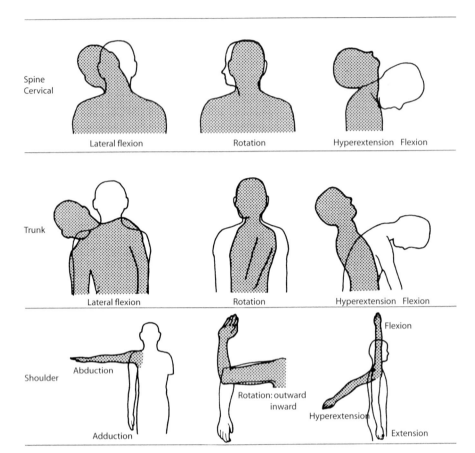

FIGURE 16.1
**Passive (assisted)
exercises for the bed-
fast patient: spine,
cervical; trunk; shoulder;
hips; arm and hand;
knee; wrist; ankle;
fingers; toes**
From Roper et al 1985,
with permission

*to concentrate fully on the limb's movement and thus preventing
damage to any tissue*
- maintain open communication with the patient and/or carer during this
  practice *to enable an identification of progress in joint movement*
- ensure that the patient is left feeling as comfortable as possible, *to ensure
  quality of patient care*
- document the nursing practice appropriately, monitor the after-effects and
  report any abnormal findings immediately, *providing a written record and
  assisting in the implementation of any action should an abnormality
  or adverse reaction to the practice be noted*
- in undertaking this practice, nurses are accountable for their actions, the
  quality of care delivered and record-keeping according to the Code of
  Professional Conduct: Standards for Conduct, Performance and Ethics (Nursing
  and Midwifery Council 2004) and Guidelines for Records and Record Keeping
  (Nursing and Midwifery Council 2005).

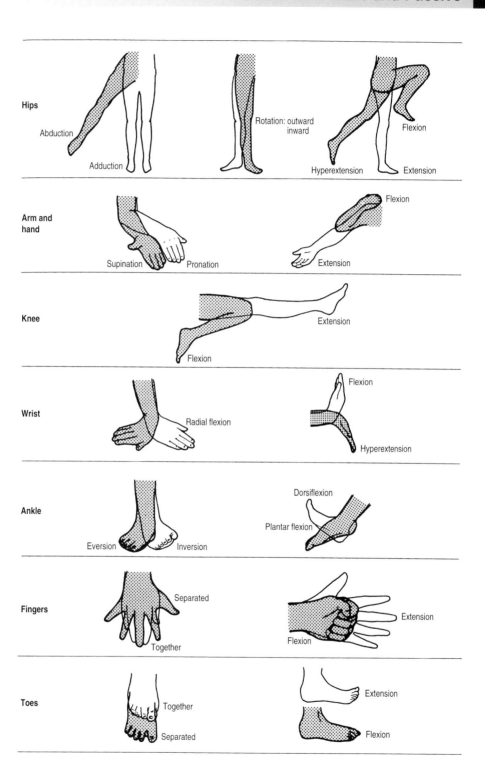

FIGURE 16.1   CONT'D

Patient/carer education

Key points

In partnership with the patient and/or carer, ensure that they are competent to carry out any practices required. Information should be given on an appropriate point of contact for any concerns that may arise.

Discuss with the patient and relatives the necessity and benefit of implementing this practice on a regular basis. A plan should be jointly agreed by the patient, carer and nurse for the most appropriate time for these exercises to be carried out. This plan may continue after the patient's discharge from hospital. Responsibility for this practice can help to empower patients in their own care.

Should an abnormality or adverse reaction be noted, inform the patient of the action taken and any subsequent treatment.

References

Nursing and Midwifery Council 2004 Code of professional conduct: standards for conduct, performance and ethics. NMC, London

Nursing and Midwifery Council 2005 Guidelines for records and record keeping. NMC, London

Roper N, Logan W, Tierney A 1985 The elements of nursing, 2nd edn. Churchill Livingstone, Edinburgh

Website

Nursing and Midwifery Council: http://www.nmc-uk.org

Self assessment

1. In what circumstances are active and passive exercises carried out?
2. Why is it necessary for the nurse to observe the patient throughout this procedure?
3. Why is it important to communicate with the patient during this procedure?
4. When should you document and report any abnormal findings found during the procedure?
5. Why is it important to include the patient in assessment of planning of this procedure?

Practice 17
Eye Care

There are four parts to this section:

1 **Eye swabbing**

2 **Eye irrigation**

3 **Instillation of eyedrops**

4 **Instillation of eye ointment**

Learning outcomes	**By the end of this section, you should know how to:**
	▪ prepare the patient for these four nursing practices
	▪ collect and prepare the equipment
	▪ carry out eye swabbing, eye irrigation, the instillation of eyedrops and the instillation of eye ointment.

Background knowledge required	Revision of the anatomy and physiology of the eye.
	Revision of 'Administration of medicines' (*see* p. 13) and 'Aseptic technique' (*see* p. 381).

1. EYE SWABBING

Indications and rationale for eye swabbing	▪ *to soothe the eye when a patient is suffering from an insensitive or diseased eye*
	▪ *to precede the instillation of an eyedrop or the application of an eye ointment*
	▪ *to remove eye discharge and/or crusts*.

Equipment	1. Sterile eye dressings pack containing a gallipot, small and other gauze swabs, or gauze swabs and a disposable towel
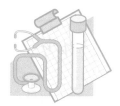	2. Sterile swabbing solution, usually normal saline solution, to soften any crusted discharge
	3. Good light source
	4. Trolley or tray for equipment
	5. Receptacle for soiled disposable items.

Guidelines and rationale for this nursing practice

- explain the practice to the patient **to gain consent and co-operation**
- wash the hands **to reduce cross-infection** (Jeanes 2005)
- collect and prepare the equipment **to ensure that all the equipment is available and ready for use**
- ensure the patient's privacy **to reduce anxiety**
- prepare the patient by helping him/her into a comfortable position, either lying down or seated with his/her head inclined backwards, **to allow the patient to maintain the position during the practice and permit easy access to the patient's eyes**
- observe the patient throughout this activity **to note any signs of distress**
- position the light source **to allow maximum observation of the patient's eyes without the beam shining directly into them**
- open and arrange the equipment **in preparation for the practice**
- wash and dry the hands **to reduce the risk of cross-infection** (Jeanes 2005)
- place the disposable towel around the patient's neck **to catch any spillages and protect the patient's clothing**
- lightly moisten a cotton wool or gauze swab in the prescribed solution. **Excess moisture will cause the patient's face to be soaked with the cleansing solution**
- ask the patient to close his or her eyes in order **to reduce the risk of corneal damage** (Watts 1998)
- gently swab from the inner canthus to the outer canthus of the eye, using each swab only once. **This decreases the risk of cross-infection from one eye to the other or infection of the lacrimal punctum. (If both eyes are being swabbed, the healthy eye should be treated first as this again reduces the risk of cross-infection)**
- gently dry the patient's eyelids **to remove excess moisture**
- ensure that the patient is left feeling as comfortable as possible, **maintaining the quality of this nursing practice**
- dispose of the equipment safely **to reduce any health hazard**
- document the nursing practice appropriately, monitor the after-effects and report any abnormal findings immediately, **providing a written record and assisting in the implementation of any action should an abnormality or adverse reaction to the practice be noted**
- in undertaking this practice, nurses are accountable for their actions, the quality of care delivered and record-keeping according to the Code of Professional Conduct: Standards for Conduct, Performance and Ethics (Nursing and Midwifery Council 2004) and Guidelines for Records and Record Keeping (Nursing and Midwifery Council 2005).

2. EYE IRRIGATION

Indications and rationale for eye irrigation

Irrigation involves the continuous washing of the eye surface with fluid:
- **to aid the removal of a corrosive substance from the eye.**

Equipment

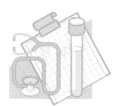

1. Waterproof sheet
2. Cotton towel
3. Sterile eye dressings pack containing a gallipot, small and other gauze swabs and a disposable towel
4. Irrigation fluid, e.g. sterile water or sterile normal saline
5. Lotion thermometer
6. Irrigating utensil, e.g. undine or intravenous giving set
7. Receiver for the irrigating fluid
8. Trolley or adequate surface for equipment
9. Receptacle for soiled disposable items.

Guidelines and rationale for this nursing practice

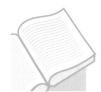

- explain the nursing practice to the patient *to gain consent and co-operation*
- wash the hands *to reduce cross-infection* (Jeanes 2005)
- collect and prepare the equipment *to ensure that all the equipment is available and ready for use*
- ensure the patient's privacy *to reduce anxiety*
- observe the patient throughout this activity *to note any signs of distress*
- warm the irrigating fluid to 37.8°C, *ensuring the comfort of the patient when the irrigating fluid is applied*
- help the patient into a suitable position, either sitting or lying with the head and neck well supported, *to allow the patient to maintain the position throughout the practice and permit easy access to the eyes*
- apply the waterproof sheet and towel around the patient's neck *to absorb any spillage*
- help the patient to turn his or her head to the side of the affected eye *to prevent any (or further) damage to the other eye by the corrosive substance when irrigation is commenced*
- wash and dry the hands *to reduce cross-infection* (Jeanes 2005)
- position the receiver below the affected eye against the patient's cheek *to collect the used irrigating fluid*
- remove any discharge from the eye with a gauze swab *to prevent contamination of the eye when the irrigation commences*
- explain to the patient that the flow of fluid is about to begin, *allowing the patient to prepare for the introduction of the fluid*
- hold the eyelids apart with the first and second fingers *as the natural defence mechanism of closing the eyes when an object approaches closely will interfere with the practice*
- direct the flow from the irrigator onto the patient's cheek *to check that the temperature is comfortable for the patient*
- hold the irrigator 2.5 cm above the eye *to allow the easy direction of the flow of fluid over the eye and prevent further damage to the eye*
- direct a steady flow of irrigating fluid from the inner canthus to the outer canthus of the eye, *allowing the fluid to cover the whole of the eye surface*
- ask the patient to move the eye up, down and all around *to ensure that the whole eye is irrigated*
- remove the equipment from the patient and ensure that the patient is left feeling as comfortable as possible, *maintaining the quality of this practice*
- dispose of the equipment safely *to reduce any health hazard*

- document the nursing practice appropriately, monitor the after-effects and report any abnormal findings immediately, *providing a written record and assisting in the implementation of any action should an abnormality or adverse reaction to the practice be noted*
- in undertaking this practice, nurses are accountable for their actions, the quality of care delivered and record-keeping according to the Code of Professional Conduct: Standards for Conduct, Performance and Ethics (Nursing and Midwifery Council 2004) and Guidelines for Records and Record Keeping (Nursing and Midwifery Council 2005).

3. INSTILLATION OF EYEDROPS

Indications and rationale for the instillation of eyedrops

Instillation involves the introduction of a liquid into a cavity drop by drop. In certain disease conditions and following injury, eyedrops are prescribed:

- *to apply a local anaesthetic topically prior to diagnostic investigations, e.g. tonometry, the removal of a foreign body or minor surgery*
- *to apply topically an antibiotic or anti-inflammatory medicine*
- *to apply topically a muscle constrictor or dilator to the eye*
- *to apply topically an artificial lubricant for the eye*.

Equipment

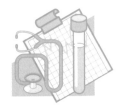

1. Sterile eye dressings pack containing a gallipot, small gauze swab and other gauze swabs and a disposable towel
2. Sterile solution, usually normal saline, for swabbing settings
3. Eyedrops to be administered
4. Automatic dropper for self-administration
5. Light source
6. Trolley or tray for equipment
7. Receptacle for soiled disposable items.

Guidelines and rationale for this nursing practice

- explain the nursing practice to the patient *to gain consent and co-operation*
- wash the hands *to reduce cross-infection* (Jeanes 2005)
- collect and prepare the equipment *to ensure that all the equipment is available and ready for use*
- ensure the patient's privacy *to reduce anxiety*
- observe the patient throughout this activity *to note any signs of distress*
- help the patient into a comfortable position *to allow easy access to the patient's eye and permit the patient to maintain the position throughout the practice*
- position the light source *to provide good visualisation of the eye*
- check the medicine prescription against the label on the eyedrops *to ensure that the correct medication will be administered*
- check the expiry date on the bottle of eyedrops, *ensuring the administration of stable medication*
- verify which eye should receive the drops *to ensure that the correct eye receives the medication*

- wash and dry the hands **to reduce cross-infection** (Jeanes 2005)
- swab the eye clean if a discharge is present in order **to remove contaminated debris**
- hold a swab in the non-dominant hand under the lower lid margin **to remove excess moisture after instillation of the drops**
- ask the patient to look up and evert the lower lid, **preventing the patient being aware of the approaching dropper**
- hold the dropper in the dominant hand **to provide controlled application**, about 2 cm above the eye, and allow one drop to fall into the lower conjunctival sac (Fig. 17.1)
- ask the patient to close the eye **to remove excess moisture**
- ensure that the patient is left feeling as comfortable as possible, **maintaining the quality of this practice**
- dispose of the equipment safely **to reduce any health hazard**
- document the nursing practice appropriately, monitor the after-effects and report any abnormal findings immediately, **providing a written record and assisting in the implementation of any action should an abnormality or adverse reaction to the practice be noted**
- in undertaking this practice, nurses are accountable for their actions, the quality of care delivered and record-keeping according to the Code of Professional Conduct: Standards for Conduct, Performance and Ethics (Nursing and Midwifery Council 2004) and Guidelines for Records and Record Keeping (Nursing and Midwifery Council 2005).

4. INSTILLATION OF EYE OINTMENT

Indications and rationale for the instillation of eye ointment

In certain disease conditions, and following injury, eye ointment is prescribed:
- **to instil a medicine topically in place of eyedrops when a prolonged action of the medicine is required**
- **to form a protective film over the corneal surface of the eye**
- **to act as a soothing agent for the patient suffering from an inflamed eye or lid margin**.

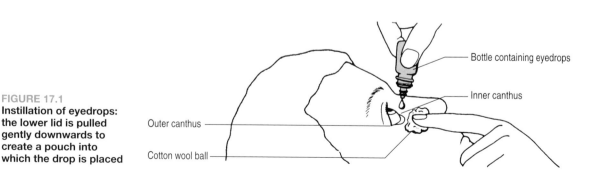

FIGURE 17.1
Instillation of eyedrops: the lower lid is pulled gently downwards to create a pouch into which the drop is placed

Bottle containing eyedrops

Inner canthus

Outer canthus

Cotton wool ball

Clinical Nursing Practices

Equipment

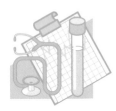

1. Sterile eye dressings pack containing a gallipot, small and other gauze swabs and a disposable towel
2. Sterile solution, usually normal saline, for swabbing settings
3. Eye ointment to be administered
4. Trolley or tray for equipment
5. Light source
6. Receptacle for soiled disposable items.

Guidelines and rationale for this nursing practice

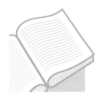

- explain the nursing practice to the patient *to gain consent and co-operation*
- wash the hands *to reduce cross-infection* (Jeanes 2005)
- collect and prepare the equipment *to ensure that all the equipment is available and ready for use*
- ensure the patient's privacy *to reduce anxiety*
- observe the patient throughout this activity *to note any signs of distress*
- help the patient into a comfortable position *to allow easy access to the patient's eye and permit the patient to maintain the position throughout the practice*
- position the light source *to provide good visualisation of the eye*
- check the medicine prescription against the label on the tube of eye ointment *to ensure that the correct medication will be administered*
- check the expiry date on the tube of ointment *to ensure the administration of stable medication*
- verify which eye should receive the ointment, *ensuring that the ointment is inserted into the correct eye*
- wash and dry the hands *to reduce cross-infection* (Jeanes 2005)
- swab the eye clean *to remove all traces of the previously instilled ointment and/or discharge*
- hold a swab in the non-dominant hand under the lower lid margin *to remove excess ointment after instillation*
- ask the patient to look up and evert the lower lid *to prevent the patient seeing the approaching nozzle, which may cause the eyelid to close*
- hold the tube of ointment in the dominant hand *to permit good control of the insertion of the ointment*
- with the nozzle of the tube 2.5 cm above the lower lid, squeeze the tube *to allow a ribbon of ointment to run into the lower conjunctival sac from the inner to the outer canthus* (Fig. 17.2)
- ask the patient to close the eye *to remove excess ointment*
- inform the patient that he or she may experience blurred vision for a few minutes following the instillation of the ointment *until the oily/greasy base disperses over the eye*
- ensure that the patient is left feeling as comfortable as possible, *maintaining the quality of this practice*
- dispose of the equipment safely *to reduce any health hazard*
- document the nursing practice appropriately, monitor the after-effects and report any abnormal findings immediately, *providing a written record and assisting in the implementation of any action should an abnormality or adverse reaction to the practice be noted*

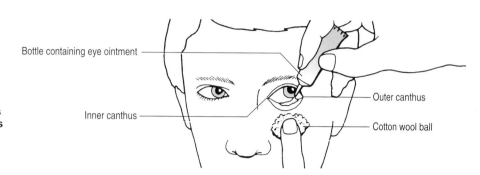

FIGURE 17.2
Instillation of eye ointment: the lower lid is pulled gently downwards to create a pouch into which the ointment is placed

Bottle containing eye ointment

Inner canthus

Outer canthus

Cotton wool ball

- in undertaking this practice, nurses are accountable for their actions, the quality of care delivered and record-keeping according to the Code of Professional Conduct: Standards for Conduct, Performance and Ethics (Nursing and Midwifery Council 2004) and Guidelines for Records and Record Keeping (Nursing and Midwifery Council 2005).

Patient/carer education
Key points

In partnership with the patient and/or carer, ensure that they are competent to carry out any practices required. Information should be given on an appropriate point of contact for any concerns that may arise.

The patient/carer may need to be taught one or all parts of this nursing practice. A patient who requires to use the automatic dropper will need adequate information and practice to ensure the skilled use of the equipment.

The nurse should ensure that the patient at home stores the medication safely and correctly.

The nurse has a responsibility to provide and encourage the education of the general population in the first-aid measures needed following contamination of the eye by a corrosive substance.

References

Jeanes A 2005 Infection control. A practical guide to the use of hand decontaminants. Nursing Times 101(20): 46–48
Nursing and Midwifery Council 2004 Code of professional conduct: standards for conduct, performance and ethics. NMC, London
Nursing and Midwifery Council 2005 Guidelines for records and record keeping. NMC, London
Watts A 1998 Cleaning the eyelids. Nursing Times 94(38 Suppl): 1–2

Website
Nursing and Midwifery Council: http://www.nmc-uk.org

Self assessment

1. In what circumstances should eyes be swabbed?
2. What equipment is required for eye swabbing?
3. Why is eye irrigation carried out?
4. In what direction should fluid flow during eye irrigation?
5. Why is it necessary to observe the patient during any of the procedures described in this section?

Practice 18
Gastric Aspiration

Learning outcomes	**By the end of this section, you should know how to:** ■ prepare and support the patient for this nursing practice ■ collect and prepare the equipment ■ pass a nasogastric tube ■ aspirate the stomach contents.
Background knowledge required	Revision of the anatomy and physiology of the nose, pharynx, oesophagus and stomach.
Indications and rationale for gastric aspiration	Gastric aspiration is used ***to keep the stomach empty of contents*** by passing a tube into it and applying some form of suction. It is usually performed in the following circumstances: ■ obstruction of the bowel ■ paralytic ileus ■ preoperatively for gastric or some abdominal surgery, e.g. perforated gastric ulcer or oesophageal and gastric varices ■ postoperatively, e.g. partial gastrectomy or cholecystectomy.

Equipment

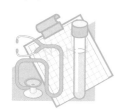

1. Trolley
2. Disposable gloves
3. Protective covering for the patient
4. Denture dish
5. Equipment for cleaning nostrils, if required
6. Nasogastric tube
7. Lubricant, e.g. iced water or water-soluble jelly
8. Water to sip
9. Catheter-tipped syringe
10. Litmus paper
11. pH indicator strips or paper
12. Receiver for aspirated fluid
13. Receptacle for soiled disposable items
14. Hypoallergenic tape
15. Stethoscope
16. Suction pump
17. Drainage bag or spigot
18. Fluid balance chart.

The size of tube selected depends on the size and age of the patient, the most commonly used sizes for the average adult are 14 and 16 FG.

Clinical Nursing Practices

Guidelines and rationale for this nursing practice

- collect and prepare the equipment and ensure it is in good working order **to promote safety and efficiency of practice**
- wash your hands **to promote infection control** (Jeanes 2005)
- explain the nursing practice to the patient and ensure that they understand **to gain consent and co-operation. Patients should be encouraged to be active partners in their care**
- **explain to the patient that there is a slight risk of a nose bleed during the procedure** (Rushing 2005)
- ensure the patient's privacy **to maintain dignity and a sense of self**
- help the patient into as comfortable and relaxed a position as possible, sitting upright and leaning forwards either in bed or on a chair **for ease of insertion of the tube**
- observe the patient throughout this activity **to detect any signs of discomfort or distress**
- measure the approximate distance from the patient's nose to his or her stomach and mark it on the nasogastric tube **so that you will have an indication of when the tube is in the region of the stomach**
- put on gloves
- remove the patient's dentures, if present, and place them in a labelled container
- ask the patient to blow the nose and sniff each nostril in turn, or clean the nostrils if necessary **to facilitate the passage of the tube**
- ascertain whether the patient has any nasal defect, tenderness or history of nasal surgery and change to the other nostril if the first nostril appears to be blocked. **Do not use great force as this may damage the nasal mucosa**
- lubricate the tube
- ask the patient to relax as much as possible while the tube is being passed. **This eases the passing of the tube**
- insert the tube and slide it gently but firmly inwards and backwards along the floor of the nose to the nasopharynx
- encourage the patient to swallow and breathe through his or her mouth when the tube reaches the pharynx, keeping the chin down and the head forward in order to assist the passage of the tube. **This is to try to overcome the gag reflex, which is present in the pharynx. Swallowing helps the tube to pass down by peristalsis**
- if the tube is sticking rotate slowly and advance towards the ear, do not force, or pull back gently and begin again. Ask the patient to open their mouth **to ensure the tube is not coiling at the back of the throat**
- if the patient starts to cough or there is a change in their respiratory status or they become cyanosed remove tube **as this suggests that the tube has entered the respiratory passages**
- when the tube has reached the measured distance, confirm, by testing (see below), that it is in the stomach
- secure the tube to the nose with tape when there is confirmation that it is in the stomach
- aspirate the stomach contents. Either continuous or intermittent aspiration will be ordered by the medical practitioner
- ensure that the patient is left feeling as comfortable as possible, **to maintain the quality of this practice**
- dispose of the equipment safely **for the protection of others**

- document this nursing practice appropriately, monitor the after-effects and report any abnormal findings immediately **to provide a written record and assist in the implementation of any action should an abnormality or adverse reaction to the procedure be noted**
- in undertaking this practice, nurses are accountable for their actions, the quality of care delivered and record-keeping according to the Code of Professional Conduct: Standards for Conduct, Performance and Ethics (Nursing and Midwifery Council 2004) and Guidelines for Records and Record Keeping (Nursing and Midwifery Council 2005).

Additional information

The recommended test to confirm the presence of the tube in the stomach is the aspiration of some of the stomach contents using a catheter-tipped syringe and their testing for acidity with litmus paper, pH indictor strips or paper with a range of 0–6 with half-point graduation (National Patient Safety Agency 2005). If the aspirate is from the stomach, the acidity will turn blue litmus paper pink. Use the indicator chart supplied with the pH strip to match the colour change to the strip, **to identify the pH of the stomach contents and correct placement of the tube**. pH indicator strips or paper must be kept clean and dry and stored in a sealed container **to ensure their reliability**. If it is not possible to aspirate sufficient stomach content for testing, a chest X-ray will be required to confirm the position of the tube.

Continuous aspiration can be carried out by some form of pump, the recommended suction pressure being 20–25 mmHg. A lower pressure is ineffective and a greater pressure can damage the lining of the stomach. Sometimes, usually postoperatively, a drainage bag and tubing may be attached to the end of the nasogastric tube. If the drainage bag is placed lower than the patient's stomach, the stomach contents will siphon into the bag.

Intermittent aspiration can be performed by pump or catheter-tipped syringe. Between aspirations, a clean spigot should be inserted in the end of the tube.

The presence of the tube may predispose to dry mucous membranes in the nose and mouth, so frequent oral and nasal hygiene will be necessary.

Patient/carer education

Key points

In partnership with the patient and/or carer, ensure that they are competent to carry out any practices required. Information should be given on an appropriate point of contact for any concerns that may arise.

Explaining why the tube is needed will help the patient to cope with the discomfort it causes.

The importance of not interfering with the tube should be explained to the patient, but if pain or extreme discomfort is experienced, he or she should tell someone. Monitoring of the position of the tube should be routinely carried out to ensure it has not moved out of the stomach. It should also be explained that, because the patient is unable to eat or drink, he or she may experience a dry mouth but that staff will help by giving mouthwashes, ice to suck, etc.

References

Jeanes A 2005 Infection control. A practical guide to the use of hand decontaminants. Nursing Times 101(20): 46–48

National Patient Safety Agency 2005 Patient and carer briefing: Checking the position of nasogastric feeding tubes. NPSA, London (Available from http://www.npsa.nhs.uk)

Nursing and Midwifery Council 2004 Code of professional conduct: standards for conduct, performance and ethics. NMC, London

Nursing and Midwifery Council 2005 Guidelines for records and record keeping. NMC, London

Rushing J 2005 Inserting a nasogastric tube. Nursing 35(5): 90–92

Website

National Patient Safety Agency: http://www.npsa.nhs.uk

Self assessment

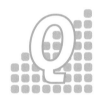

1. What are the indications for nasogastric tube insertion?
2. What would you do if the nasogastric tube stuck on insertion?
3. What are the recommended tests for checking the position of nasogastric tubes?
4. What are the complications of nasogastric tube insertion?

Practice 19
Infection Prevention and Control: Principles of

Prevention and control of infection is essential to protect patients and healthcare staff in any care setting – hospital, community or the patient's own home. Prevalence studies in the UK indicate that about 9% of hospital patients acquire an infection during their stay resulting in considerable personal and institutional cost (Walker 2002).

The principles of prevention of infection and control of spread of communicable disease looks at proactive measures that should be practised every day in every setting and consists of three sections:

1 **Safe practices**

2 **Safe environment**

3 **Procedures for coping with the unexpected**

Learning outcomes	**By the end of this chapter you should be able to:** ▪ apply standard infection control precautions to any care setting ▪ demonstrate to patients, relatives/carers and colleagues the different methods of hand hygiene ▪ be able to explain in simple terms the differences between cleaning, decontamination and sterilisation ▪ report an incident or accident that might result in an infection, e.g. sharps injury.
Background knowledge required	Revision of Standard Infection Control Precautions (*see* 'Isolation', p. 187). Review local policy regarding the management of outbreak of infection. Review local policy regarding the reporting of an incident and/or accident. Access and complete your local hand hygiene training. Review local policies regarding disinfection and sterilisation.
Indications and rationale for infection prevention and control processes	Many patients will have a pre-existing infection when they present to the healthcare worker in the clinic, at the ward or in an emergency situation. Some infected persons will not be aware of their status, e.g. those with undiagnosed blood-borne virus infection; and others may fear the stigma of their condition, e.g. patients with pulmonary tuberculosis. However, patients will not always appear 'sick' and in the early stages of incubation the symptoms of infection may appear vague, misleading or be absent. ***Healthcare workers should not make assumptions about infection risks and must consistently use standard infection control precautions***. Infection Prevention and Control policies are often closely linked to Risk Management policies and Occupational Health policies, such as:

- standard infection control precautions
- outbreak of infection management policy
- reporting incidents and accidents.

1. SAFE PRACTICES

Principles for these practices

Personal health and hygiene

- *healthcare workers have legal responsibilities to their clients under the Health & Safety at Work Act (1974), and if handling food or drink they have a 'duty of care' under the General Food Hygiene Regulations* (Department of Health 1995). They must not knowingly spread biological hazards that include gastrointestinal and skin infections. Staff illness must be reported to the local Occupational Health Service, if available, and medical advice sought if gastrointestinal symptoms ('enteric illness') do not resolve or diminish after 48 hours
- certain communicable infections, e.g. salmonella, must be notified under Public Health Legislation and Food Hygiene Regulations and the individual may be required to submit formal 'clearance' specimens prior to resuming duties (Department of Health and Social Security 1984, 1985) *to ensure appropriate public health measures can be implemented on a reactive and proactive basis*
- the nurse must maintain high standards of personal hygiene through daily bathing or showering and keeping hair clean and restrained while at work in clinical settings or food-service environments *to ensure they are not the direct or indirect source of cross-infection*.

Uniform issues

- workplace clothing is provided in most clinical settings and *acts as a form of corporate identification as well as ensuring staff have items suitable for undertaking diverse duties, e.g. Accident & Emergency Nurse Practitioners usually wear long sleeved water repellent tops and 'pyjama type' bottoms*
- clean uniforms should be available daily and extra stock kept to utilise *if the nurse becomes soiled during the course of the shift*. The fabrics of the clothing should be chosen for durability and temperature resilience
- items should be laundered on as hot a wash as the materials will tolerate. Some faecal organisms will survive low-temperature washing and so thermal disinfection by ironing is recommended following washing and drying (Patel et al 2006).

Personal protective clothing

- items that are provided to protect the nurse undertaking specialised clinical procedures are deemed by the Health and Safety Executive to be 'personal protective equipment' (PPE)
- formal risk assessment and monitoring must be undertaken to ensure compliance and suitability, e.g. disposable aprons, masks, face visors, gowns and hats used for isolation care, theatre lists and decontamination purposes

■ nurses must ensure that they are aware of the local policies for PPE and any special requirements such as testing respirator masks used when caring for patients with possible SARS or multiple resistant TB (Gamage 2005).

Hand hygiene

Hands carry infection from person to person, place to place and family to family. Researchers consistently find that nurses fail to wash their hands when working in clinical settings that they deem to be 'low risk' and need frequent reminders to improve practice. The World Health Organization programme (2005) 'Clean hospitals, clean healthcare' emphasises the key role of this often undervalued activity. The USA Centers for Disease Control (Centers for Disease Control 2002) guidelines, the NHS Education Scotland guidelines (NHS Education Scotland 2005) and the Department of Health/NPSA guidance in the 'Wash your hands' campaign (Department of Health 2005) all stress the value of hand hygiene. The forms of hand hygiene (Fig. 19.1) are:

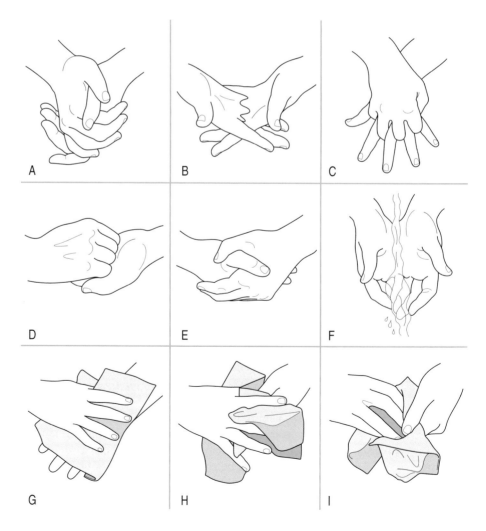

FIGURE 19.1
Handwashing technique

Social handwashing

- ensure that hand jewellery is minimised to only a plain wedding ring, remove your wristwatch and roll up sleeves *to ensure the whole hand is washed*
- wet the hands and using liquid soap and warm running water, or a bowl of freshly run water, wash hands thoroughly and check that all surfaces are washed especially the outer aspect of the thumb and smallest finger *to ensure all skin surfaces have been washed*
- dry well using a disposable paper towel.

Aseptic handwashing

- using an antimicrobial preparation for aseptic handwashing *will remove 'transient' or temporary micro-organisms acquired from the environment and contact with other persons from the surface of the nurse's skin*. Some aseptic preparations, e.g. chlorhexidine gluconate, also have a residual effect reducing the 'resident' or deep-seated skin flora, which continues for some hours after application and repeated use increases the effects
- in order to prevent antimicrobial resistance aseptic handwashing should be reserved for high-risk situations, e.g. where there are outbreaks of infection
- aseptic handwashing should be performed at a clinical washhand basin where elbow- or wrist-operated taps can be turned off without touching the tap surfaces.

Surgical scrubbing

- the correct technique for washing the hands and forearms (to the elbow) with the approved antimicrobial preparation should be taught to new staff who should then practice under supervision until deemed competent
- single use or sterile nailbrushes may be used to clean gently under the nails but care must be taken not to damage the nailbed that could lead to infection of the damaged surface
- special deep sinks with elbow- or foot-operated mixer taps are usually used for 'scrubbing' to minimise splash contamination of the uniform or environment and prevent recontamination of clean skin.

Alcohol hand rub

- alcohol handgel/rub may be used for rapid decontamination of visibly clean skin, after coming out of an isolation area where hands are washed before leaving the room or following social handwashing (Scottish Executive Health Department 2005)
- the gel or alcohol rub should be rubbed in until all surfaces are dry using the same hand washing technique as that used for plain soap.

Skin care

- nurses must report any possible allergic reactions to soap or gloves to their Occupational Health Service *to ensure an accurate health record of the employee*
- if special products are prescribed to an individual with a known skin condition, e.g. psoriasis or eczema, the product should be labelled for that nurse only and kept in a convenient area in the workplace
- advice should be given by the manager of the workplace about any special precautions or exclusions from duties, e.g. if the individual has an acute infected skin condition they may not be able to work with patients with MRSA

or to handle foods directly (Health and Safety at Work Act 1974, Health Services Advisory Committee 1999)

- all staff must cover cuts, wounds and septic lesions whilst at work **to prevent cross-infection**. Waterproof, impermeable dressings or gloves may be worn if appropriate (*see* 'Isolation nursing' p. 187).

Safe equipment

- all equipment purchased and used for healthcare must be 'fit for purpose'. At the most basic level this means that simple reusable items such as commodes should be designed to be cleaned and disinfected between uses
- technical items must be supplied with manufacturer's guidance and marked clearly to indicate if the equipment is for single use, single-patient use or multiple use and can be reprocessed
- single-patient use indicates that an item can be reused by one patient only, e.g. a nebuliser which can be washed in fresh warm water and detergent solution between uses and air-dried (Medical Devices Agency 2000)
- single-use items should always display the symbol (Fig. 19.2) indicating no second use or reprocessing (even for the same patient) on the external packaging
- medical devices are specialised items of equipment such as catheter bags. These products are regulated by legislation and monitored by national and international agencies such as the Medical Healthcare Regulation Agency (MHRA) in the United Kingdom.

2. SAFE ENVIRONMENT

Principles for these practices

Patient placement

- this is one of the key practices relating to prevention and control of infection. In modern hospitals elective high-risk surgery patients are usually segregated from persons with known infections (*see* 'Isolation nursing' p. 187)

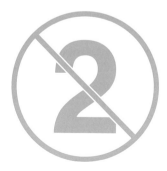

FIGURE 19.2
Universal symbol for single use

- in deciding where a patient with a known or suspected infection should be nursed it is important to consider the transmission route of the pathogen. A person with a wound that is not weeping and covered with an occlusive dressing may not present a major risk to the hospital ward, but a patient with a productive cough and untreated pulmonary tuberculosis could infect susceptible patients and staff
- enteric illness may quickly spread in a large open ward where commodes are used behind curtains and a single room with en suite toilet and handwashing facilities are recommended (NHS Estates 2002, Scottish Executive Health Department 2002, Department of Health 2003).

'Isolation' facilities

- single rooms or special wards used for persons with known or suspected infection or those who have compromised immunity and need protection from other patients
- 'cohort' nursing may be requested in a ward where a cluster or group of patients are all diagnosed with similar symptoms arising from suspected or confirmed infections. The patients will be placed in a geographical area with a designated team of staff to care only for them in order to minimise the potential for cross-infection to unaffected individuals. Precautions used will depend on the presenting symptoms, suspected organism and the patient (Healthcare Infection Control Practices Advisory Committee 2004).

Cleaning

- the first and most essential step in maintaining a safe environment for patient care is to remove organic matter that has adhered to or settled on surfaces (NHS Scotland National Healthcare Associated Infection Task Force 2004)
- a fresh solution of warm water and detergent and clean cloth, mop or cleaning brush is required. If the water is too hot it will lead to some fluids and protein-containing matter binding to the surface and make cleaning difficult. If the solution becomes cold it will not remove some sticky particles
- detergent is a chemical solution with surfactant properties designed to loosen grease into the surrounding water and make cleaning more effective. The product will also affect unprotected skin by removing natural oils and leaving the skin dry
- nurses and healthcare workers must remember always to wear gloves to protect their skin from the adverse effects of detergents and other chemicals and cleaning materials. The type of gloves depends on the environment, the type of chemical, any allergies the individual may have and local policy guidelines.

Decontamination

- this term describes the methods used to render safe equipment and environments that may have been soiled by infective matter
- the first step is to pre-clean the item or area to remove organic matter, followed by the application of an approved disinfectant solution to reduce the microbial load, and sterilisation (if appropriate for the item or area)
- disinfectants all have unwanted side effects. Some solutions such as glutaraldehyde have toxic respiratory and skin side effects and must be used with great care within specially ventilated contained areas. Some older

iodine- and chlorine-based disinfectants have acidic formulations and can cause skin damage, discolouration of fabric surfaces and corrosion of metallic surfaces
- when using a disinfectant check:
  — the chemical manufacturer's dilution recommendations
  — the expiry date
  — any special precautions, e.g. wear eye-protection and heavy-duty gloves
  — the item or area to be disinfected, can this product be used on this equipment?
  — how long the product should remain on the surface being decontaminated prior to rinsing it off and drying the area thoroughly.

Sterilisation

- if an item of medical equipment, e.g. a sterile urinary catheter is to be placed within a sterile body cavity it is important not only to remove organic matter but also spores that can survive disinfection
- sterilisation methods include wet steam under pressure in an autoclave (porous loads), e.g. theatre instrument trays packed for planned operations; dry heat and ionising radiation, e.g. packs of sterile needles and syringes
- some specialist units may alternatively use ethylene oxide gas or hydrogen peroxide plasma (cannot process long tubular devices)
- all sterile items should be carefully wrapped and labelled with the date, method and site where processed and expiry date
- items must be stored in a clean, dry area in cupboards or special containers to prevent dust accumulating on the outer wrappers
- benchtop steam sterilisers have traditionally been used in community settings to process small instruments used for podiatry, family planning clinics and dental instruments
- maintenance of benchtop sterilisers must be rigorous to ensure that the machine is working correctly and the patient is not exposed to infection. Daily, weekly and monthly tests must be performed and results recorded in addition to the engineering checks. The healthcare worker processing the items has legal liability for any mistakes or inadequate sterilisation (NHS Scotland National Healthcare Associated Infection Task Force 2004)
- following several highly publicised cases of inadequate sterilisation leading to infection, many practices and clinics now use items that are single use or reprocessed in area decontamination units with more sophisticated machinery.

In the United Kingdom sterilisation processes and equipment were extensively reviewed following the identification of vCJD linked to BSE. The reports of the working groups in Scotland (Health Department Letter 2001a, 2001b) highlighted the need to categorise procedures into 3 types to reduce the risk of CJD:
  — **high**-risk procedures, which are linked to neurological operations where the dura, trigeminal and dorsal root ganglia are pierced or the pineal and pituitary glands, optic nerve or retina
  — **medium**-risk procedures, where contact is made with the eye, lymphatic systems, tonsils or olfactory epithelium
  — **low**-risk procedures, were deemed to be invasive and included contact with cerebral fluid.

Note: This classification was particular only for CJD and not other healthcare associated infections (HAIs).

Spaulding devised an HAI risk-assessment system based on classification of the type of procedure, the infection status of the previous patient and the immune status of the present patient:

- — *critical* activities are those where devices enter a body cavity or tissue that is normally sterile, e.g. needles penetrating the blood supply
- — *semi-critical* procedures are those where an instrument has contact with intact mucous membrane but not sterile areas, e.g. vaginal speculae
- — *non-critical* devices only have contact with intact skin, e.g. stethoscopes.

Waste segregation

- ▪ it is important for all nurses and healthcare workers to be aware of the legislation that relates to waste arising from the clinical care given to patients in any setting
- ▪ there are international classifications agreed by the United Nations and the World Health Organization and implemented by member nations through national legislation
- ▪ the classification of waste is based upon the risk of the materials being infectious and the infectivity of suspected or known pathogens (Advisory Committee on Dangerous Pathogens 2003)
- ▪ within healthcare settings waste-disposal bags are usually colour coded to indicate the waste type, the infection risk and disposal stream:
  - — *yellow* bags for high-risk infectious material arising from an infectious disease unit. This waste would usually be incinerated
  - — *orange* bags for clinical waste such as used swabs and soiled dressings that can be disinfected by microwave and steam processing
  - — *black* bags for 'domestic or general' rubbish generated in hospitals and clinics that goes to landfill sites for burial
  - — *recycling containers* for paper, clean empty glass containers and metal cans
  - — *sharps boxes* for used needles and syringes (may be orange or yellow depending on waste disposal used)
  - — *special waste* containers for various items, e.g. pharmaceutical waste, which is incinerated and hazardous waste including mercury, radioactive waste and items that are toxic or corrosive and which require highly specialised disposal.
- ▪ sharps containers (Fig. 19.3) are provided in many shapes, sizes and designs and they should be 'fit for purpose' and large enough to ensure that items can be fully enclosed but small enough to require regular changing and not to be left for months half used. Boxes should be taken to the patient-treatment area when sharps are to be used, e.g. on the medication trolley or carried on a 'near patient tray' to the bedside. Having the disposal box available encourages staff to dispose of used needles and syringes immediately and reduces the risk of needlestick injury. Surveys of injuries have found that accidents commonly arise from incorrect disposal, e.g. during a cardiac arrest or when the used needles and syringes are mixed with other waste and placed in a plastic bag (Infection Control Nurses Association 2003)
- ▪ community waste generated in a client's own home must be carefully risk assessed by the care team and a discrete but clear record, e.g. using a 'biohazard' sticker, kept noting any known infection, any special precautions required

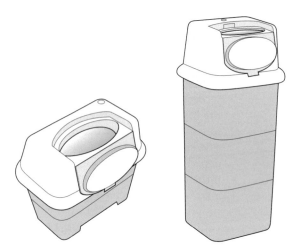

FIGURE 19.3
Sample of sharps containers

and the disposal method recommended. In rural areas there are particular challenges in transporting 'high-risk' items such as used sharps (needles, lancets, blades, etc.). Some health authorities permit very small quantities of waste to be transported in a special container in the healthcare worker's car, e.g. a small sharps box. Alternatively the nurse or case manager may need to arrange a secure storage place and regular uplift of full containers

▪ it is extremely important that all healthcare workers are taught the correct assembly, partial closure and full closure of their locally supplied sharps container(s) to ensure patient safety. The container must be dated when first used and when closed to ensure that there is a 'cradle to grave' audit trail in the event of an incident. Compliance with national legislation, e.g. the Environmental Protection Act 1990, and subsequent regulations is essential (Health and Safety Executive 1990, 1991, 1996, Health Services Advisory Committee 1999).

3.   PROCEDURES FOR COPING WITH THE UNEXPECTED

Principles for these practices

Blood and body fluid spills

▪ the nurse or careworker must be familiar with the local policy for cleaning and disinfection (*see* Cleaning and Decontamination above)

▪ Standard Infection Control Precautions (*see* 'Isolation nursing' p. 187) require that healthcare wastes are consistently treated with care because the infectivity of the fluids is often not known

▪ spills should be contained, cleaned and, if visible blood is present and the surface is suitable, the area disinfected with a chlorine-releasing agent, rinsed and dried. If possible, patients and the public should be kept away from the soiled area while it is being cleaned to protect them from exposure to possible infection and slip hazards.

'Needlestick' injuries

- staff working in a team setting should be immediately assisted to leave the patient and perform their own first aid:
  - — the wound should be washed as soon as possible with soap or antiseptic solution in warm running water and encouraged to bleed
  - — the area should then be dried and a clean dressing applied as per routine occupational injury policy
- the injured staff member should then report the injury immediately to their line manager and the occupational health service to enable an enhanced risk assessment to be taken and immediate referral to an accident and emergency department if deemed necessary
- if the needlestick injury has been sustained whilst caring for a patient with a known or suspected blood-borne virus infection the local post-exposure prophylaxis policy (PEP) will be implemented. The staff member will be offered confidential counselling and a blood sample checked for immunity to hepatitis B (HBV) infection. Baseline blood samples may also be requested from the patient in order to quantify the risk of HBV and HIV but the patient is entitled to refuse consent for tests. Local guidelines should be followed and appropriate documentation completed, e.g. Incident Form.

Floods

- floods are usually major spills or widespread soiling with dirty water and excrement due to blockage of sewers caused either by blockages in the local sanitation systems, e.g. bedpan macerators blocked by items that will not flush away; or 'back-pressure' in the extended system due to a rise in the water table
- patients need to be protected from potentially contaminated water and swift action is needed to move them away from the immediate danger area and contain the site to ensure that other staff are aware of the risk
- implement the local alert call and ensure that the emergency services are given the correct location of the problem
- evacuation of the patients should be undertaken with care and the nurse should ensure that any soiled clothing or footwear, patient or staff, is changed as soon as feasible. Neither food nor drinks should be touched by persons with soiled hands as this will help to prevent accidental ingestion of water-borne or faecal infections
- any contaminated skin should be cleansed and dried carefully with clean water and soap
- initially bottled water may be required for drinking and cleansing wipes for skincare.

Fire

- the consequences of a fire in healthcare premises are usually similar to flooding with the potential of water saturation, mould and algae growing in damp carpets and/or plaster and patients having to be moved in haste to temporary accommodation
- prevention of infection may be very difficult in non-clinical settings such as halls or hotels used as temporary accommodation centres. Attention to personal and environmental hygiene can be critical to preventing infections developing in vulnerable frail patients.

Outbreaks of infection

- an 'outbreak' is declared when the number of cases of a particular infection increases outside normal parameters. For some highly dangerous communicable diseases this may only mean one or two cases, e.g. viral haemorrhagic illnesses such as Ebola fever from Africa. In other circumstances wards and infection-control teams may have a baseline infection rate established using statistical process methodology and an outbreak is defined as the exceeding of the upper limit

- most hospitals, wards and departments have 'Outbreak of Infection Plans', which detail the actions that must be taken and the responsibilities of the key personnel and are based on government advisory documents such as the Scottish Infection Control Manual (Scottish Office 1998). It is the professional responsibility of the nurse to familiarise themselves with the local policy and location of any special equipment such as disposable gowns and masks

- an Outbreak Control Team (OCT) is usually required to co-ordinate the actions of all staff in the affected area and ensure that they have sufficient resources to undertake the care of affected patients. Documentation of discussions, advice taken and relevant clinical care planned and given is essential: these records may later be presented at a formal investigation or court of law if any patient dies during the outbreak (Department of Health 2000)

- in a community setting, e.g. an older persons' care home, the Public Health Medical Officer with responsibility for communicable disease control will lead the OCT investigating the outbreak with the assistance of the Community Infection Control Nurse and Environmental Health Officer from the local council. Staff working in care homes must also ensure that they follow their local outbreak plan and any special guidance from the Public Health Department. Documentation is equally vital, not only to demonstrate 'due diligence' in care of patients for any future legal case but also to facilitate accurate communication during shift changes and possible staff shortages due to illness

- outbreaks in non-healthcare premises are also investigated under the co-ordination of the Public Health Department, using a standardised risk-management approach (Scottish Executive Health Department 2003). There are also specific policies for investigating outbreaks related to ships docking in ports, aeroplanes bringing in flights with passengers who have become ill on the flight, and leisure industry incidents such as hotel functions (Scottish Executive Health Department 1999, Health Protection Scotland 2005).

References

Advisory Committee on Dangerous Pathogens 2003 Infection at work: controlling the risks. A guide for employers and the self-employed on identifying, assessing and controlling the risks of employment in the workplace. Health and Safety Executive, London

Centers for Disease Control 2002 Guidelines for hand hygiene in healthcare settings. Centers for Disease Control, Atlanta, GA, USA

Department of Health 1995 General food hygiene regulations. HMSO, London

Department of Health 2000 An organisation with a memory: report of an expert group on learning from adverse events in the NHS. HMSO, London

Department of Health 2003 Winning ways: working together to reduce healthcare associated infection in England. Department of Health, London

Department of Health 2005 Wash your hands. Department of Health, London

Department of Health and Social Security 1984 Public Health (Control of Disease) Act. HMSO, London

Department of Health and Social Security 1985 Public Health (Infectious Diseases) Regulations. HMSO, London

Gamage B 2005 Protecting healthcare workers from SARS and other respiratory pathogens: a review of the infection control literature. American Journal of Infection Control 33(2): 114–121

Health Department Letter 2001a The 'old' working group report. SEHD, Edinburgh

Health Department Letter 2001b The 'Glennie' working group report. SEHD, Edinburgh

Health Protection Scotland 2005 The identification and management of outbreaks of Norovirus infection in tourist and leisure industry settings: guide for NHS boards and local authorities. Joint Working Group Report. HMSO, Edinburgh

Health and Safety Executive 1996 The Special Waste Regulations. HSE, Sudbury, UK

Health and Safety at Work Act 1974. HMSO, London

Health and Safety Executive 1990 Environmental Protection Act. HSE, Sudbury, UK

Health and Safety Executive 1991 The Controlled Waste (Registration of Carriers & Seizure of Vehicles) Regulations. HSE, Sudbury, UK

Healthcare Infection Control Practices Advisory Committee (HICPAC) 2004 Draft guideline for isolation precautions: preventing transmission of infectious agents in healthcare settings. Centers for Disease Control, Atlanta, GA, USA

Health Services Advisory Committee 1999 Safe disposal of clinical waste. HMSO, London

Infection Control Nurses Association 2003 Reducing sharps injury: prevention and risk management. ICNA, London

Medical Devices Agency 2000 Single use medical devices: implications and consequences of reuse. MDA, London

NHS Education Scotland 2005 Promoting hand hygiene in healthcare: a short self-directed web-based learning package for healthcare workers. NHS Education Scotland, Edinburgh (Available online: http:nes-hai.info/)

NHS Estates 2002 Infection control in the built environment. HMSO, London

NHS Scotland National Healthcare Associated Infection Task Force 2004 Cleaning services specification. SEHD, Edinburgh

Patel SN, Murray-Leonard J, Wilson APR 2006 Laundering of hospital staff uniforms at home. Journal of Hospital Infection 62(1): 89–93

Scottish Executive Health Department 1999 The investigation and control of outbreaks of foodborne disease in Scotland. HMSO, Edinburgh

Scottish Executive Health Department 2002 Watt Group report: a review of the outbreak of salmonella at the Victoria Infirmary, Glasgow between December 2001 and January 2002 and the lessons that may be learned by both the Victoria Infirmary and the wider NHS family in Scotland. SEHD, Edinburgh

Scottish Executive Health Department 2003 Managing incidents presenting actual of potential risks to the public health. Guidance on the roles and responsibilities of incident control teams. HMSO, Edinburgh

Scottish Executive Health Department 2005 Alcohol based hand rubs and infection control. SEHD, Edinburgh.

Scottish Executive Health Department and NHS Scotland 2001 Working group report. Managing the risk of healthcare associated infection in NHS Scotland. HMSO, Edinburgh

Scottish Office 1998 Infection control manual. HMSO, Edinburgh

Walker A 2002 Hospital acquired infection and bed use in NHS Scotland. Robertson Centre for Biostatistics, University of Glasgow, Glasgow

World Health Organization 2005 Global patient safety challenge. WHO, Geneva

Websites

Health Protection Scotland: http://www.show.scot.nhs.uk/hps

Infection Control Nurses Association: http://www.icna.co.uk

Nursing and Midwifery Council – Professional Body: http://www.nmc-uk.org
Royal College of Nursing publications: http://www.rcn.org.uk

Self assessment

1. Hand hygiene: review your local training programme and practice the correct technique with a colleague to observe.
2. An audit of sharps boxes in your department highlights concerns about 'overfilling' and the potential for needlestick injury. Describe three actions that you might take.
3. Find local guidance relating to outbreaks of Norovirus and see if there is an audit tool that could be used in your workplace?

Practice 20
Intrapleural Aspiration

Learning outcomes

By the end of this section, you should know how to:
- prepare the patient for this nursing practice
- collect and prepare the equipment
- assist the medical practitioner during chest aspiration.

Background knowledge required

Revision of the anatomy and physiology of the respiratory system
Revision of 'Aseptic technique' (*see* p. 381).

Indications and rationale for this nursing practice

The lungs are covered by the visceral pleura, the inner chest wall being lined by the parietal pleura. Between these pleura lies a thin layer of serous fluid the surface tension of which holds the two pleural linings together. As a result, the lung follows the movement of the chest wall, the lung volume being determined by the size of the thorax.

An increase in the amount of fluid in the space upsets this mechanism. Chest aspiration involves the introduction of a needle into the pleural cavity between the visceral and parietal pleura. It may be performed for the following reasons:
- ***to examine a specimen of the pleural fluid as an aid to the diagnosis of disease, e.g. tuberculosis or carcinoma***
- ***to relieve dyspnoea, by removing excess pleural fluid***
- ***to introduce medication, e.g. antibiotics, into the pleural cavity.***

Outline of the procedure

Using an aseptic technique, the medical practitioner washes and dries his or her hands, cleanses the patient's skin over the selected site of entry of the aspiration needle, injects a local anaesthetic and waits for it to take effect. The aspiration needle is then inserted into the cavity between the visceral and parietal layers of the pleura. After withdrawing the stilette from the needle, specimens of fluid can be obtained from the cavity for laboratory investigation, and the remaining fluid can be allowed to drain out. Should there be a large amount of fluid to be aspirated, it may be necessary to interrupt the drainage process for 2–3 hours before recommencing. If the fluid is purulent, it may have to be aspirated by attaching a large syringe to the needle. A patient with a large pleural effusion may require the insertion of an indwelling catheter to facilitate ongoing drainage (Grodzin & Baik 1997).

At the end of the procedure, the aspirating needle is withdrawn, a sterile plastic spray is applied to the wound puncture, and an adhesive dressing is placed over it.

Equipment

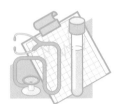

1. Trolley
2. Sterile dressings pack
3. Sterile gloves
4. Alcohol-based antiseptic for skin cleansing
5. Local anaesthetic and equipment for its administration
6. 50 ml sterile syringe
7. Sterile aspiration needles
8. Sterile two-way tap with a length of sterile tubing
9. Sterile bowl for collecting fluid
10. Sterile specimen bottles and an appropriately labelled laboratory form
11. Plastic specimen bag for transportation
12. Sterile plastic spray and adhesive dressing
13. Receptacle for soiled disposable items.

Guidelines and rationale for this nursing practice

- help to explain the procedure to the patient, *ensuring that he or she has some understanding of the procedure, and obtain consent and co-operation*
- ensure the patient's privacy *to help maintain dignity and a sense of self*
- wash hands *to prevent cross-infection* (Jeanes 2005)
- collect the equipment *for efficiency of practice*
- administer a sedative, if prescribed by the medical staff, *to help to relieve stress and anxiety in the patient*
- help the patient into a back-fastening gown *so that there is ease of access to the site for aspiration*
- assist the patient to sit up with arms extended over a bed table on which a pillow has been placed for the head to rest on. If this is not comfortable for the patient, lying in bed on the unaffected side should still allow good access to the needle site. *The medical practitioner requires unobstructed access to the site of needle insertion*
- observe the patient throughout this activity *to detect any signs of discomfort or distress*
- wash the hands and apply an apron *to reduce cross-infection* (Jeanes 2005)
- open the sterile equipment as it is required by medical staff
- remain with the patient and help to maintain the chosen position as required. *Continuing explanation and support will help the patient through this procedure*
- observe the patient's respirations and attend to any complaints of pain during the procedure. *This may indicate that the needle has penetrated through the pleura and into the lung*
- ensure that the patient is left feeling as comfortable as possible, *to maintain the quality of this practice*
- dispose of equipment safely *for the protection of others*
- immediately despatch the labelled specimen container, in a plastic specimen bag, to the laboratory, along with the completed laboratory form. *Immediate despatch ensures that the specimen arrives in optimal condition for any tests required*
- document this nursing practice appropriately, monitor the after-effects and report any abnormal findings immediately *so that measures to overcome these can be instigated as soon as possible*

- in undertaking this practice, nurses are accountable for their actions, the quality of care delivered and record-keeping according to the Code of Professional Conduct: Standards for Conduct, Performance and Ethics (Nursing and Midwifery Council 2004) and Guidelines for Records and Record Keeping (Nursing and Midwifery Council 2005).

Patient/carer education
Key points

In partnership with the patient and/or carer, ensure that they are competent to carry out any practices required. Information should be given on an appropriate point of contact for any concerns that may arise.

A detailed explanation and step-by-step guidance through the procedure should help the patient to maintain co-operation.

If medication has been instilled into the cavity, the patient should be helped to turn into different positions over the next couple of hours to facilitate its dispersal.

References

Grodzin C, Baik R 1997 Indwelling small pleural catheter needle thoracentesis in the management of large pleural effusions. Chest 111(4): 981–988

Jeanes A 2005 Infection control. A practical guide to the use of hand decontaminants. Nursing Times 101(20): 46–48

Nursing and Midwifery Council 2004 Code of professional conduct: standards for conduct, performance and ethics. NMC, London

Nursing and Midwifery Council 2005 Guidelines for records and record keeping. NMC, London

Self assessment

1. Why may a patient present with a pleural effusion?
2. Identify three potential complications during or after an intrapleural aspiration.
3. How would you assist the patient to reduce the anxiety created by the practice?

Practice 21
Intravenous Therapy

There are four parts to this section:

1 Commencing an intravenous infusion

2 Priming the equipment for intravenous infusion

3 Maintaining the infusion for a period of time

4 Care of a Hickman catheter for long-term intravenous therapy

Learning outcomes	**By the end of this section, you should know how to:** ■ prepare and support the patient for these nursing practices, both at home and in an institutional setting ■ collect and prepare the equipment ■ assist the medical practitioner with the safe insertion of an intravenous cannula or catheter ■ maintain an intravenous infusion as prescribed.
Background knowledge required	Revision of the anatomy and physiology of the cardiovascular system, with special reference to the circulation of the blood, and body fluids Revision of 'Aseptic technique' (*see* p. 386) Review of local policy in relation to intravenous therapy in both community and institutional care.
Indications and rationale for intravenous infusion	An intravenous infusion is the introduction of prescribed sterile fluid into the blood circulation; it may be indicated for the following reasons: ■ *to maintain a normal fluid, nutrient and electrolyte balance when the patient is unable to maintain adequate intake by mouth and nasogastric feeding is inappropriate*, e.g.: — a patient during the preoperative and postoperative periods — a patient who has had surgery involving the alimentary system — a patient who has malabsorption problems ■ *to replace severe fluid loss in emergency situations*, e.g.: — a patient who has severe haemorrhage and haemorrhagic shock — a patient who has severe burns or scalds — a patient dehydrated by vomiting or diarrhoea usually associated with enteric infection ■ to administer medication when other routes are not appropriate or when there is a need for a rapid-onset action or accurate titration of the dose, e.g.: — analgesic medication for effective pain relief — chemotherapy for the treatment of patients with malignancy.

1. COMMENCING AN INTRAVENOUS INFUSION

Outline of the procedure

Intravenous therapy is prescribed by the medical practitioner and initiated by a doctor or a nurse who has undertaken specialist training and is deemed competent to carry out this procedure. The non-specialist nurse may be required to help with the procedure, to maintain the infusion safely for a period of time and to undertake removal of the cannula.

Using an aseptic technique, the competent practitioner chooses a suitable vein site for access, body hair should be clipped as necessary and the site cleansed with antiseptic lotion such as a chlorhexidine and alcohol-based solution, which is allowed to dry fully before the skin is punctured (Pellowe et al 2004). Shaving body hair is no longer recommended as it has been suggested that it can increase bacterial colonisation of the skin (Royal College of Nursing 2003). A topical preparation of local anaesthetic, i.e. Emla cream, can be applied to the skin surface approximately 2 hours prior to the procedure, or Ametop, which can be applied 10 minutes before the procedure (Scales 2005).

A sterile cannula is inserted into the vein so that the prescribed infusion fluid can enter the patient's blood circulation. The infusion fluid flows into the cannula through an administration set that will have been primed ready for use. The cannula is secured in position and covered by a sterile dressing. The flow of infusion fluid is maintained, and the containers of fluid replaced as prescribed, until the intravenous infusion is discontinued (Royal College of Nursing 2003).

Short-term intravenous therapy

Sites chosen for intravenous cannulation

The metacarpal veins and the dorsal venous arch at the back of the hand or the superficial veins of the wrist or lower arm such as the cephalic or basilica veins (Scales 2005) are chosen for short-term infusions expected to last for a few hours or days. Cannulation increases the risk of venous thrombosis in the veins used for access; if this occurs in the smaller branches of the peripheral veins following an infusion, it is still possible to use the larger branches of the same vein at a later date if required. The veins of the lower limbs are rarely used because of the increased risk of thrombosis as a result of a slower venous flow. The non-dominant limb should be used if possible to minimise the patient's discomfort and promote independence.

Long-term intravenous therapy

For long-term intravenous infusions lasting for several days or weeks, a long catheter is inserted into the subclavian or internal jugular vein so that the tip of the catheter lies in the superior vena cava (*see* 'Care of a Hickman catheter', p. 181 and 'Central venous pressure', p. 107).

Equipment

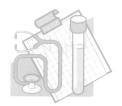

1. Trolley or tray
2. Sterile dressings pack, if required
3. Sterile cannula sizes 18–22 gauge depending on fluids to be infused
4. An antiseptic solution such as chlorhexidine in alcohol for cleansing the skin (as per local policy)
5. Non-sterile gloves/apron
6. Sterile administration set
7. Prescribed sterile infusion fluid
8. Sterile semipermeable cannula dressing
9. Infusion stand
10. Tourniquet
11. Hypoallergenic tape
12. Receptacle for soiled disposable items.

Additional equipment if required

Scissors for clipping any body hair
Local anaesthetic and equipment for its administration
Air inlet for glass containers
Holder for glass containers (bottle holder)
Continuous infusion pump and appropriate cassette (*see* Fig. 21.3, p. 174)
Syringe driver and appropriate-sized syringe.

Infusion fluids

The most commonly prescribed fluids are:
normal saline (sodium chloride 0.9%)
dextrose 5% in water
Ringer's lactate/Hartmann's solution
plasma or plasma expanders, e.g. Haemaccel or Gelofusine
blood (*see* 'Blood transfusion', p. 47)
parenteral nutrients (*see* 'Parenteral nutrition', p. 240).

Most prescribed fluids are commercially prepared in sterile containers, being labelled 'FOR INTRAVENOUS INFUSION'. They may also be prepared by the hospital pharmacy. The containers used for these preparations are frequently soft plastic bags protected by an outer covering (see the manufacturer's instructions), although glass bottles or semi-rigid plastic containers (Polyfusors) are still used for some preparations.

Cannulae

Various cannulae (Fig. 21.1) are available and are prepared commercially in sterile packs. Size 18–14 gauge can be used for the administration of fluids very quickly such as in a resuscitation event. However, smaller gauge cannulae are preferred, as they cause less damage to the inner vessel wall. A gauge 22 would be sufficient size to deliver maintenance therapy as it can deliver up to 42 ml min^{-1} or 2.5 L h^{-1}, (Scales 2005). Those chosen by the competent practitioner have an inner needle surrounded by a plastic cannula. The needle is withdrawn once the vein has been punctured, allowing blood to flow back. Once the cannula is safely in situ, the infusion fluid is connected and the cannula secured in position. Some cannula packs include an accompanying syringe, e.g. Medicut. Small winged needles

Clinical Nursing Practices

FIGURE 21.1
Intravenous infusion:
cannulae in common use
A Cannula used when
intravenous drugs are to
be administered with the
infusion or post-infusion
B Cannula used
preoperatively for short-
term infusion

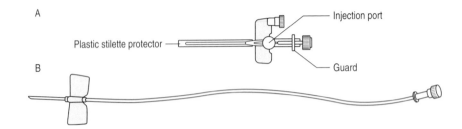

are used for access to scalp veins in babies and young children, and for elderly patients who have fragile veins.

Administration sets

Administration sets are commercially prepared in sterile packs. The set contains specialised sterile tubing with, at one end, a rigid trocar protected by a sterile sheath. At the other end is a similarly protected Luer connector nozzle. Towards the trocar end, the tubing widens into a drip chamber. An adjustable roller clamp surrounds the tubing below the drip chamber, which allows the flow of fluid to be regulated at the prescribed flow rate. Blood administration sets include a filter and should be changed at the end of transfusion or at 24 hours (Royal College of Nursing 2003). Simple administration sets are available without a filter, for the infusion of crystalloid fluids (Fig. 21.2). These should be changed every 72 hours (Royal College of Nursing 2003).

Specialised
administration sets
(burette sets)

A specialised administration set is used for infusions when a volumetric infusion pump is not available and a more accurate control of flow rate is needed. The burette can also be used to mix and administer drug infusions, which should be infused over short periods of time. They are also particularly important in reducing the risk of fluid overload when infusions are prescribed for babies or young children. The burette set has a calibrated drip chamber with one roller clamp above and one roller clamp below. The drip chamber is filled with the amount of fluid prescribed in millilitres per hour, and this amount of fluid is infused during 1 hour. The flow rate will depend on the drop factor and the amount prescribed (see the manufacturer's instructions). For the infusion to continue, the drip chamber has to be refilled as prescribed each time it has emptied.

Volumetric infusion
pumps

Some volumetric infusion pumps are used with specific sterile cassettes (e.g. Accuset) as well as a normal administration set so that an accurate flow of fluid can be maintained during the infusion. When primed and connected, these can be set to infuse fluid within a range of 1–999 ml h^{-1}. Other volumetric infusion sets simply use a specifically adapted administration set. The infusion is controlled by a column of electronically controlled rollers that adjust the flow rate as required, constantly monitoring the rate, total volume infused and infusion pressure. This equipment must be mechanically serviced as per the manufacturer's guidelines and local policy.

Syringe pumps

Syringe pumps are used to deliver drug infusions over a prescribed period of time. Patient controlled analgesia (PCA) is delivered via a syringe pump (Fig. 21.3).

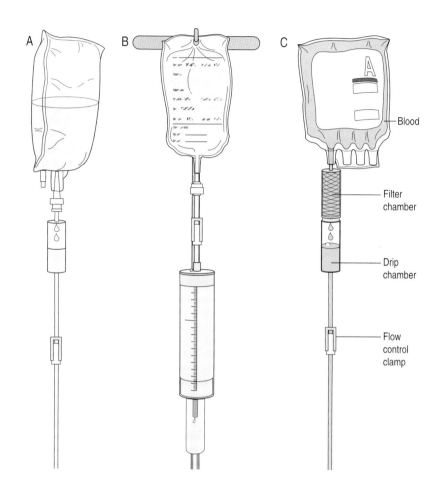

A   B   C

Blood

Filter
chamber

Drip
chamber

Flow
control
clamp

FIGURE 21.2
**A Standard
administration set
B Blood administration
set
C Burette**
From Nicol et al 2003, with
permission

**Guidelines and
rationale for this
nursing practice**

- help to explain the nursing practice to the patient *to gain consent and co-
  operation and encourage participation in care*
- ensure the patient's privacy, *respecting his or her individuality*
- help to collect and prepare the equipment. Wash hands using appropriate
  procedure (Jeanes 2005) and wear non-sterile gloves *to prevent
  contamination with body fluids* (Royal College of Nursing 2003)
- check the prescribed infusion fluid with a registered nurse or medical
  practitioner. *This is a legal requirement and part of professional
  practice*
- prime the administration set with the infusion fluid, maintaining asepsis, *so
  that it is ready once the cannula is in position*
- place the infusion fluid on the stand beside the patient, check that it is running
  freely and that all air has been expelled from the system. *This prevents any
  danger of air embolus*. If not connected immediately, the end should be
  protected by replacing the sterile cap *to prevent contamination*
- help the patient into as comfortable a position as possible *so that he or she
  will tolerate the intravenous therapy without distress*

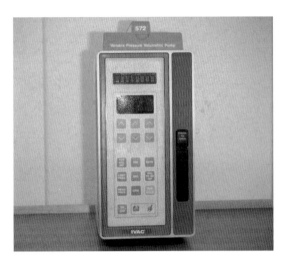

FIGURE 21.3
Infusion pump

- observe the patient throughout this activity *to monitor any adverse effects as well as any improvement in condition*
- expose and support the area for cannulation *to facilitate access*
- help to prepare the sterile equipment as required, *to maintain a safe environment*
- apply pressure around the limb above the cannulation site as directed using a tourniquet. *This will retain more blood in the veins and facilitate cannulation*
- release the pressure as directed once the venous cannula is correctly positioned and the infusion lines are connected, *to commence the flow of fluid to the veins*
- regulate the flow rate as prescribed *to maintain the prescribed fluid intake*
- help the competent practitioner to secure the dressing and tubing *to maintain asepsis and prevent disconnection of the tubing and cannula* (Fig. 21.4)
- apply a splint to the limb *if the site of the infusion requires the limb to be immobilised*. This is not routine practice
- ensure that the patient is left feeling as comfortable as possible *so that he or she will continue to tolerate the intravenous therapy. Comfort helps to reduce stress levels and promotes healing*
- dispose of equipment safely *to prevent the transmission of infection*
- document this nursing practice appropriately, monitor the after-effects and report any abnormal findings immediately, *ensuring safe practice and enabling prompt, appropriate medical and nursing intervention to be initiated as soon as possible*
- maintain the infusion at the prescribed flow rate *for continuation of the treatment*. To reduce the risk of infection, administration sets should be

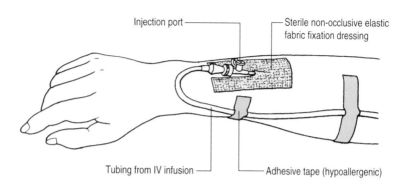

Injection port — Sterile non-occlusive elastic fabric fixation dressing

Tubing from IV infusion — Adhesive tape (hypoallergenic)

FIGURE 21.4
Anchoring the tubing with adhesive tape

changed as per local policy and immediately following the infusion of blood products (Royal College of Nursing 2003). On-going care involves regular monitoring of the site to identify localised infection, infiltration of fluid into the surrounding tissue or the development of thrombophlebitis. Royal College of Nursing (2003) and Scales (2005) advocate the formal monitoring of cannulation sites daily using a graded 5-point assessment tool (Fig. 21.5)

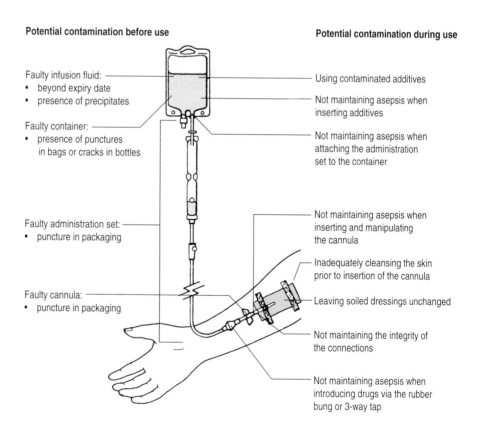

Potential contamination before use

Faulty infusion fluid:
• beyond expiry date
• presence of precipitates

Faulty container:
• presence of punctures in bags or cracks in bottles

Faulty administration set:
• puncture in packaging

Faulty cannula:
• puncture in packaging

Potential contamination during use

Using contaminated additives

Not maintaining asepsis when inserting additives

Not maintaining asepsis when attaching the administration set to the container

Not maintaining asepsis when inserting and manipulating the cannula

Inadequately cleansing the skin prior to insertion of the cannula

Leaving soiled dressings unchanged

Not maintaining the integrity of the connections

Not maintaining asepsis when introducing drugs via the rubber bung or 3-way tap

FIGURE 21.5
Potential routes for contamination associated with intravenous infusion

- all the equipment connections should be inspected for disconnections, flaws or leakage **to prevent contamination or an air embolus**. The tubing should be inspected to check there are no air bubbles
- fluid balance charts should be accurately maintained **to enable assessment of the patient's state of hydration**
- in undertaking this practice, nurses are accountable for their actions, the quality of care delivered and record-keeping according to the Code of Professional Conduct: Standards for Conduct, Performance and Ethics (Nursing and Midwifery Council 2004) and Guidelines for Records and Record Keeping (Nursing and Midwifery Council 2005).

2. PRIMING THE EQUIPMENT FOR INTRAVENOUS INFUSION

This is the preparation of the prescribed infusion fluid by running it through the administration set. Asepsis should be maintained during this part of the practice **to prevent any internal or exposed areas being contaminated**.

Equipment

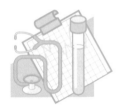

1. Prescribed intravenous infusion fluid
2. Sterile administration set
3. Sterile gallipot
4. Receptacle for soiled disposable items
5. Infusion stand
6. Chlorhexidine and alcohol-based antiseptic solution and swabs
7. Sterile air inlet
8. Bottle holder for use with glass container
9. Trolley or tray.

Guidelines and rationale for this nursing practice

- check the infusion fluid, which is prescribed by the medical practitioner. Each container of fluid is checked by two people, one of whom must be a registered nurse or a medical practitioner (*see* 'Administration of medicines', p. 14), **for safe practice**
- check the following details against the patient's own documentation and the label on the infusion fluid **to make sure that the correct prescribed infusion is given**:
  — the patient's name and unit number
  — the date of the prescription
  — the type of infusion prescribed
  — the amount of infusion prescribed
  — the container labelled 'FOR INTRAVENOUS INFUSION'
  — the expiry date of the infusion fluid
  — the time prescribed for commencement of the infusion
  — the time to be taken for completion of the infusion
  — the signature of the medical practitioner
- check the fluid for cloudiness, sediment or discoloration. The container should be checked for flaws, leaks or evidence of contamination. Any suspect fluid or

containers must be discarded immediately according to healthcare provider's policy **to prevent any introduction of infection or contamination and to maintain a safe environment**

- include the serial number of the fluid as well as the signature of the nurse or medical practitioner checking the infusion prescription in the documentation. **If the patient suffers any adverse effects, the particular infusion can then be identified**

- establish the identity of the patient by appropriate means, e.g. identification bracelet, thus **maintaining safe practice.**

When using a soft plastic container (bag)

- perform the appropriate handwashing technique and wear non-sterile gloves **to prevent infection** (Jeanes 2005)
- remove the outer plastic covering of the container **in preparation for use**
- remove the sheath covering the entry channel without contaminating the inside, thus **maintaining asepsis**
- remove the administration set from its package **in preparation for use**
- close the flow control clamp **to prevent any uncontrolled flow of fluid**
- remove the protective sheath from the trocar of the administration set, maintaining asepsis **in preparation for insertion**
- insert the trocar firmly through the seal of the container's entry channel **so that fluid flows into the first part of the administration set** (Fig. 21.6)
- invert the container and hang it on the infusion pole **so that gravity will aid the flow**
- gently squeeze the chamber of the administration set **to allow it partly to fill**
- temporarily remove the protective sheath covering the Luer connector at the end of the administration set and hold it over a sterile container (e.g. gallipot) **to prevent any contamination**
- slowly release the flow-control clamp **to allow the fluid to fill the rest of the tubing**
- eliminate any air bubbles from the fluid in the tubing by running some fluid into a sterile container if necessary, **to prevent any danger of air embolus**
- close the flow control clamp **to stop the flow of fluid**

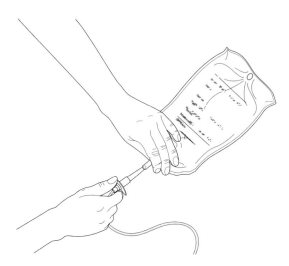

FIGURE 21.6
Inserting the spike of the administration set into the new infusion bag
From Nicol et al 2003, with permission

- replace the protective cover on the Luer connector nozzle *to prevent any infection*
- place the free end of the tubing in the notch provided on the flow-control clamp *to keep the Luer connector nozzle protected from contamination*
- place the primed equipment on the infusion stand beside the patient's bed *ready for connection to the intravenous cannula*.

The equipment should only be primed immediately prior to the infusion *to minimise the risk of infection. If contamination occurs or the container is punctured while priming the equipment, the infusion and the administration set are discarded and the procedure recommenced*.

When using a glass container (bottle)

- maintain an aseptic technique as before
- remove the seal from the top of the checked infusion fluid bottle *to expose the rubber bung*
- clean the rubber bung with chlorhexidine in alcohol-based solution and allow it to dry completely, *to prevent the transmission of infection*
- prepare the administration set as before
- push the trocar firmly through the rubber bung *to access the fluid*
- remove the sterile air inlet from its outer package and remove the protective sheath from the needle
- insert the needle of the air inlet through the rubber bung *to equalise the pressure in the bottle and thus facilitate the flow of fluid*
- hang the inverted bottle on the infusion stand, using a bottle holder if required, and, if necessary, support the end of the air inlet above the level of the fluid in the bottle *to allow the fluid to flow freely*
- proceed to prime the equipment as before.

When using a semi-rigid plastic container (Polyfusor)

- maintain an aseptic technique as before
- remove the outer package of the checked infusion fluid
- snap off the end of the entry channel *to maintain asepsis*
- prepare the administration set as before
- insert the trocar into the entry channel and twist it for a firm fit *to gain access*
- invert the container and hang it on the infusion stand *so gravity will aid the flow*
- proceed to prime the equipment as before (no air inlet being required for this container).

3. MAINTAINING THE INFUSION FOR A PERIOD OF TIME

The number of drops per minute required for each particular infusion has to be accurately calculated *in order to maintain the flow of infusion at the prescribed rate*. Volumetric pumps are now used routinely.

Guidelines and rationale for this nursing practice

Calculating the flow rate of infusion fluids

All administration sets include details of the number of drops delivered per millilitre for that particular set, this being known as the drop factor. Some sets include within the pack a scale of drops per minute for a given time. Using this information, an accurate assessment of the flow rate needed can be calculated (Fig. 21.7).

Formula used for calculation

$$\frac{\text{Total volume of infusion fluid} \times \text{Drop factor (}\textit{see}\text{ administration set)}}{\text{Total time of infusion in minutes}}$$

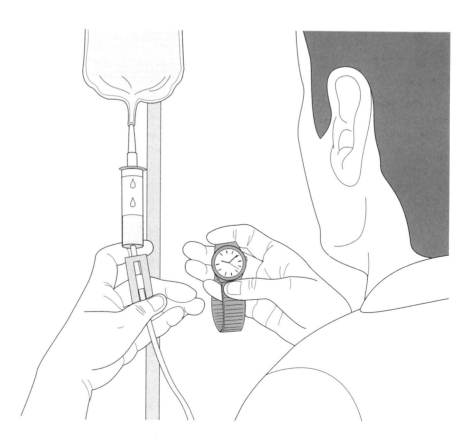

FIGURE 21.7
Setting the flow rate
From Nicol et al 2003, with permission

Example

Total volume of fluid = 500 ml

Time for completion = 4 hours, i.e. 240 minutes (4 × 60)

Drop factor = 15

$$\frac{500 \times 15}{240}$$

= 31.25 = 30 drops (approximately)

Thus the number of drops required to maintain the infusion at the required rate is 30 per minute when the drop factor is 15 drops ml^{-1}.

The position of the cannula in the vein and the movement of the patient's limbs may have an effect on the flow rate. *It is therefore important to assess visually the rate of fall of fluid in the infusion container as well as to regulate the number of drops required per minute*. For example, when the time for completion is 4 hours, one quarter of the fluid should have been infused after 1 hour and half the fluid after 2 hours.

Changing the infusion container

Within 24 hours, the empty container can be replaced with a full container of prescribed infusion fluid without changing the administration set depending on the duration of infusion. The containers should be exchanged before the level of fluid drops below the point of the trocar in the neck of the container. Preparation for changing a container should begin while a small amount of fluid remains in the infusion container; *this prevents the formation of air bubbles in the system and the danger of air embolus*.

Guidelines and rationale for this nursing practice

- explain the nursing practice to the patient *to gain consent and co-operation*
- perform handwashing *and maintain asepsis during this practice as before*
- check the prescribed infusion fluid
- prepare the new container of infusion fluid as for priming the equipment
- temporarily turn off the infusion by closing the roller clamp
- remove the trocar of the administration set from the empty container and insert it into the new infusion fluid, maintaining asepsis. A new air inlet should be used when changing glass bottles *to reduce the risk of infection*
- recommence the infusion as soon as possible at the prescribed flow rate
- maintain observations as before
- dispose of the used container safely *to prevent the transmission of infection*
- document the nursing practice appropriately, monitor the after-effects and report any abnormal findings immediately *to ensure safe practice and enable prompt appropriate medical and nursing intervention to be initiated as soon as possible*
- in undertaking this practice, nurses are accountable for their actions, the quality of care delivered and record-keeping according to the Code of Professional Conduct: Standards for Conduct, Performance and Ethics (Nursing and Midwifery Council 2004) and Guidelines for Records and Record Keeping (Nursing and Midwifery Council 2005).

Removal of the intravenous cannula

This is performed using an aseptic technique when intravenous infusion is discontinued or when a new site for access is needed to continue an infusion. Cannula should be removed between 72–96 hours following insertion, depending on usage.

- explain the procedure to the patient **to obtain consent and co-operation**
- ensure the patient's privacy, **respecting his or her individuality**
- close the flow clamp **to discontinue infusion of the fluid**
- prepare a trolley and sterile dressings as required **to maintain a safe environment**
- apply non-sterile gloves **to protect against blood-borne infection**
- expose the site of insertion of the cannula, **maintaining asepsis**
- hold a sterile swab lightly over the entry site using the non-dominant hand and slowly withdraw the cannula with the dominant hand, applying pressure once it has been removed **to reduce any bleeding**
- retain pressure on the puncture site as required **until the bleeding stops, maintaining asepsis**
- cover the site with a small sterile dressing, e.g. Airstrip, **to prevent infection**
- dispose of equipment safely **to prevent the transmission of infection**
- resume the observation of the site as appropriate **to monitor the healing process**
- document the nursing practice appropriately, monitor the after-effects and report any abnormal findings immediately, **ensuring safe practice**
- in undertaking this practice, nurses are accountable for their actions, the quality of care delivered and record-keeping according to the Code of Professional Conduct: Standards for Conduct, Performance and Ethics (Nursing and Midwifery Council 2004) and Guidelines for Records and Record Keeping (Nursing and Midwifery Council 2005).

The tip of the cannula is occasionally sent to the laboratory for microbiological investigation. If this is ordered, the tip must be cut off with sterile scissors, put into an appropriately labelled sterile specimen container, maintaining asepsis, and sent to the appropriate laboratory with the completed laboratory form (*see* 'Specimen collection', p. 303).

4. CARE OF A HICKMAN CATHETER FOR LONG-TERM INTRAVENOUS THERAPY

General indications and rationale for use of a Hickman catheter

These are as for Central Venous Pressure (*see* p. 107).

Specific indications and rationale for use of a Hickman catheter

The use of a Hickman catheter may be chosen by the medical practitioner for continuous or intermittent intravenous therapy for a period of months or even for as long as 3 years (Fig. 21.8).

The patient may be at home or in an institutional setting (Simcock 2001). This method is chosen because the radio-opaque silastic catheter, which is usually

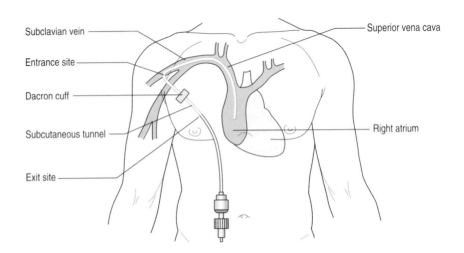

FIGURE 21.8
Hickman catheter in situ

'tunnelled', can safely remain in situ for a long period if efficient care of the catheter is maintained. Patient education should help patients to become independent in their own care so that they can be discharged home with a long-term catheter in place, under the supervision of the community team (Simcock 2001).

A Hickman catheter may be required for:

- the administration of medicines, for example chemotherapy to give repeated doses of cytotoxic medication for the treatment of malignant disease such as leukaemia, over a period of weeks. Cytotoxic medication can cause damage to the peripheral vessels, but *central venous access allows the irritant medication to be diluted rapidly in the circulating fluid of the large veins and transported safely round the body*
- long-term parenteral nutrition (*see* 'Parenteral nutrition', p. 237). Nutrients in the parenteral feeding regime may also irritate the lining of the peripheral blood vessels; *access via a central line prevents irritation as the nutrients are infused directly into the central veins*
- taking blood samples over a period of time *to monitor the progress of treatment*, for example in children or adults with malignant disease *to prevent repeated venepuncture*
- poor peripheral venous access due to intravenous drug abuse.

Skin-tunnelled catheters

A Hickman catheter will remain in situ for a period of time. The distal end of the catheter is usually tunnelled subcutaneously so that the entry site to the vein is separated from the skin exit site, thus reducing the risk of infection entering the circulation from the catheter insertion site. This is particularly important for patients receiving chemotherapy as both the disease and the treatment may cause immunosuppression, further reducing resistance to infection (Royal College of Nursing 2003).

A Hickman catheter has a Dacron cuff at the distal end, around which fibrous tissue will form, anchoring the catheter in position and ensuring safer long-term use.

| Outline of the procedure | *See* 'Insertion of a central venous catheter' (p. 108) and 'Parenteral nutrition' (p. 237). |

Equipment

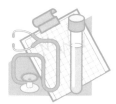

Equipment for insertion of a Hickman catheter

This is as for 'Intravenous therapy' (p. 170) and 'Insertion of a central venous catheter' (p. 108). This procedure is usually performed in theatre.

In addition:
1. Hickman catheter – a flexible, radio-opaque, silicone tube, approximately 90 cm long, incorporating a Dacron cuff at the distal end
2. Injectable cap with a Luer lock for access to the line.

Equipment for care outside the hospital setting

1. Equipment for dressing the entry site if required (semipermeable occlusive transparent polyurethane dressing; Royal College of Nursing 2003).
2. Instruction sheet or booklet to reinforce the patient education commenced prior to transfer
3. Suitable container for storing equipment
4. Spare Luer lock caps. Most Hickman catheters have two ports, blood line and drug line (see the manufacturer's instructions)
5. Sterile 5 ml syringe
6. Sterile 19 G needle for drawing up the heparin
7. Prepared heparinised saline (local policy may vary)
8. Chlorhexidine in alcohol antiseptic solution and swabs
9. Approved container for the disposal of sharps.

All the above should be available in the patient's home and continuously replaced as required for as long as the treatment continues. It is helpful if all the equipment is stored in a suitable container and used only for the care of the catheter so that a safe environment can be obtained.

Guidelines and rationale for this nursing practice

These guidelines are applicable to the nurse and also to the patient or carer as the patient develops confidence in his or her own care.
- help to explain the procedure to the patient **to obtain consent and co-operation, and encourage participation in care**
- ensure the patient's privacy, **respecting his or her individuality**
- collect and prepare the equipment **so that everything is easily available**
- help the patient into as comfortable a position as possible, **ensuring that there is easy access to the Hickman line and entry port**
- apply sterile gloves after efficient handwashing **to reduce any risk of infection and contamination with body fluids**. If the patient performs

this procedure, he or she will usually need to use gloves; a good handwashing technique should be part of patient education prior to discharge and should be continually reinforced afterwards (Royal College of Nursing 2003)

- draw up heparinised saline solution into the syringe, *maintaining asepsis in preparation for flushing the line*
- observe the catheter site for redness, swelling or exudate, *which may indicate infection*. The patient should inform the medical practitioner and the community nurse of any change in condition of the site
- observe the catheter for any damage or cracks, *which may cause infection or an air embolus*. Report any problems immediately and clamp the line above the damage until it has been repaired or replaced
- clamp the line above the Luer lock cap if the cap needs changing. *This will ensure that air does not enter the line to cause an air embolus*
- maintaining asepsis, change the cap. *This may be necessary to ensure the continued efficiency of the valve and to reduce any risk of infection or contamination*. Refer to the health authority policy and manufacturer's instructions
- release the clamp from the line once the cap is safely in position, *to ensure that the line is safely patent again*
- swab the end of the entry port of the cap with chlorhexidine in alcohol-based solution *to prevent the transmission of infection*
- flush the line with normal saline (Royal College of Nursing 2003) (heparinised saline may be recommended by your local healthcare provider), maintaining asepsis, *to prevent a clot forming that would block the patency of the central line and prevent its continued use* (Fig. 21.9). Healthcare-provider policy will dictate the frequency of flushing with heparin. If resistance is felt, flushing should not be continued *as a clot may be dislodged*. Resistance to flushing should be reported immediately *as it may indicate a clot blocking the line*
- dress the catheter site as appropriate (*see* 'Wound care', p. 381). The site may initially be covered by a semipermeable occlusive and transparent dressing (Royal College of Nursing 2003). There may be no need for a dressing once the site is clean and healed after the stitches have been removed, usually after the first 10 days

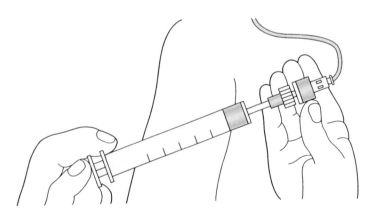

FIGURE 21.9
Care of a Hickman catheter: flushing the line with heparinised saline

- wash the site with prescribed solution and dry thoroughly with low-linting swabs *to keep the site clean and prevent any risk of infection*. Catheter care can be timed to follow a shower or bath *to prevent further any risk of infection*, but the site itself should still be cleaned separately *to prevent contamination*
- ensure that the patient is left feeling as comfortable as possible *so that he or she can resume the normal activities of living*
- dispose of equipment safely *to prevent the transmission of infection*
- document this nursing practice appropriately, monitor the after-effects and report any abnormal findings immediately *to ensure safe practice and enable prompt, appropriate medical or nursing intervention to be initiated*
- in undertaking this practice, nurses are accountable for their actions, the quality of care delivered and record-keeping according to the Code of Professional Conduct: Standards for Conduct, Performance and Ethics (Nursing and Midwifery Council 2004) and Guidelines for Records and Record Keeping (Nursing and Midwifery Council 2005).

Patient/carer education

Key points

In partnership with the patient and/or carer, ensure that they are competent to carry out any practices required. Information should be given on an appropriate point of contact for any concerns that may arise.

The reason for the particular intravenous therapy should be explained to the patient. The importance of maintaining the cannula or catheter in situ should be emphasised and the danger of disconnection explained, so that the patient does not pull the lines or dislodge the dressing.

Specific written education for care of the site and lines should be given to the patient discharged home with an intravenous infusion. This may include:
- care of the infusion site and cannula or catheter port
- changing the infusion fluid as prescribed
- flushing the line to maintain patency for intermittent intravenous therapy
- observing the site for any adverse effects.

Patients at home should know what to do if the lines become disconnected. They and their carers should be familiar with the use of a simple clamp and be able to apply a dressing with firm pressure and a tight bandage while waiting for help from the community team.

All patients should understand the importance of immediately reporting any redness, swelling or pain at the infusion site, as well as any disconnection or blockage of the lines and any other adverse symptoms. A telephone helpline gives the patient at home added confidence to be self-caring.

References

Jeanes A 2005 Infection control. A practical guide to the use of hand decontaminants. Nursing Times 101(20): 46–48

Nicol M, Bavin C, Bedford-Turner S et al 2003 Essential nursing skills, 2nd edn. Mosby, London

Nursing and Midwifery Council 2004 Code of professional conduct: standards for conduct, performance and ethics. NMC, London

Nursing and Midwifery Council 2005 Guidelines for records and record keeping. NMC, London

Pellowe CM, Pratt RJ, Loveday HP et al 2004 The epic project. Updating the evidence base for national evidence based guidelines for preventing healthcare associated infections in NHS hospitals in England: a report of recommendations. Journal of Hospital Infection 5(6): 10–16

Royal College of Nursing 2003 Standards for infusion therapy. RCN, London

Scales K 2005 Vascular access: a guide to peripheral venous cannulation. Nursing Standard 19(49): 48–52

Simcock L 2001 The use of central venous catheters for IV therapy. Nursing Times 97(18): 34–35

Websites

Royal College of Nursing: http://www.rcn.org.uk/publications/pdf/standardsinfusiontherapy.pdf

Infection Control Nurses Association: http://www.icna.co.uk

NHS Education Scotland: http://www.nes.scot.nhs.uk/docs/publications/Clinical Skillsdraft121004.doc

Self assessment

1. You are asked to assist the competent practitioner in the insertion of an intravenous cannula. List the equipment that will be required and outline the procedure as it should be undertaken.
2. Determine the differences between different administration sets and provide examples of the fluids that would be administered in each.
3. Outline the procedure for priming connecting and administering an intravenous infusion of normal saline (0.9% sodium chloride) 1 litre over 8 hours.
4. Describe how would you remove an intravenous cannula.
5. What is the rationale for a Hickman line and how is it maintained in the community setting?

Practice 22
Isolation Nursing

Historically the terms 'isolation' and 'barrier nursing' have been used by nurses to describe the physical separation of persons suspected or known to be infected with a communicable disease from those who are not. Today most patients with infective conditions can be nursed in a general hospital with modern wards and single rooms using 'Standard Precautions' (Department of Health and Hospital Infection Society 2001). However, there are certain infections that require a higher level of containment, e.g. new or 'novel' infections, or those that are extremely resistant, e.g. multi-drug resistant tuberculosis. These patients would usually be transferred to an Infectious Disease Unit where specialised accommodation and equipment would be provided according to the category of the infection.

'Protective isolation'

This is the term used to describe nursing precautions taken to keep a vulnerable patient, e.g. a person with compromised immunity, free from infection risks that might be encountered in the normal ward environment.

Different precautions may also be used to '*isolate*' non-infective patients such as those who are undergoing radiotherapy treatments that render the person a radioactive hazard to fellow patients.

This section consists of three parts:

1 **Source isolation**

2 **Protective isolation**

3 **Radioactive hazard isolation**

Learning outcomes	By the end of this section you should know how to: ▪ prevent the spread of infection while nursing a patient with a specific communicable disease (source isolation) ▪ protect a patient from infection when he or she may be at a greater risk than normal (protective isolation) ▪ prevent hazard to carers and visitors when radioactive substances are used.
Background knowledge required	Revision of the modes of transmission of infection and related microbiology Awareness of standards and legislation on infection control (Department of Health 2004) Review of health service policy in relation to the control of infection in both institutional and community settings Knowledge of the role of the infection control team in your work area

Understanding of standard infection control precautions
Review of local health service policy in relation to the handling of radioactive
substances.

Indications and rationale for nursing patients in an isolation area	The aim of this nursing practice is to create an effective barrier between an infected area and a non-infected area, to prevent the occurrence of cross-infection, or to use appropriate measures to prevent contamination from radioactive substances.

Isolation precautions are often a combination of national guidance and local experience: **always check the local policy**. In general, it is advised that all practitioners use the same general prevention strategies with all patients at all times (Department of Health 2004). The application of standard infection control precautions (*see* 'Infection prevention and control', p. 151) is the foundation for this and includes:

- an appropriate hand-hygiene technique
- the use of gloves for clinical practices
- the protection of any broken skin
- the prevention and treatment of needlestick injuries
- the use of protective clothing/equipment (aprons, gowns, eye goggles) when required
- the use and disposal of 'sharps'
- the management of spillages
- the collection and disposal of waste products.

1. SOURCE ISOLATION

In this instance, the 'infected' area is the isolation area where the infected patient is being nursed, the 'non-infected' area being that outside the isolation area.

Indications and rationale for source isolation	This is carried out **to prevent the spread of infection from patients who have or are suspected of having a specific communicable infection**, for example:

- an infection caused by methicillin-resistant *Staphylococcus aureus* (MRSA). This infection, especially if present in the bloodstream, poses the greatest problem for patients who are already at high risk, e.g. those with invasive devices or being ventilated. Guidelines for care of persons with MRSA vary between acute, community and domestic care settings. Precautions are based on an individual risk assessment and the type of healthcare setting (Working Party on MRSA 1998)
- a respiratory infection caused by untreated *Mycobacterium tuberculosis* (National Institute for Clinical Excellence 2006)
- an active enteric infection caused by *Salmonella* or *E. coli* O157 verocytotoxin (VTEC) (Scottish Infection Standards and Strategy Group 2004).

Equipment

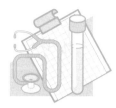

The environment and equipment required will depend on the infection, the patient's condition and the local health policies. It will usually include the following:

1. Single room with toilet facilities and sometimes an anteroom with protective clothing storage and washhand basin
2. Handwashing facilities for personnel inside and outside the isolation area
3. Alcohol-based hand gel (Ritchie et al 2005)
4. Personal protective clothing, which may include:
   — cap
   — filter-type mask or respirator
   — gown or fluid repellent clothing
   — plastic apron
   — gloves
   — protective washable shoes
   — face protection/goggles

[Many of these items are disposable and a supply of them should be kept in an adjacent area outside the isolation area]

5. Linen for the bed, and personal towels for the patient
6. Individual crockery and cutlery, which can be processed in a dishwasher should be routinely used. However, in some circumstances, disposable items may be required (please check with the local infection control policy or infection control team)
7. Facilities for the treatment, or disposal of, infected linen and rubbish
8. Equipment needed for appropriate personal and nursing care should remain within the isolation area for the duration of the isolation precautions **to prevent the transmission of infection**. All items used must be decontaminated and disinfected before reuse according to local control of infection policy
9. Thermometer, sphygmomanometer, stethoscope and watch or clock with a second hand as required for recording vital signs
10. Special containers for the collection of laboratory specimens if required
11. The patient's documentation should remain outside the isolation area and details of recordings and care be completed by 'uncontaminated' personnel **to maintain a safe environment**.

Guidelines and rationale for this nursing practice

- consult appropriate personnel **to obtain advice and guidance**. All health authorities and hospitals have a member of staff designated to be responsible for the control of infection in that area, for example an infection control nurse (Clinical Standards Board for Scotland 2001)
- carry out a risk assessment of infection (Department of Health 2004)
- plan the nursing so that everything required is carried out during one period of time in the isolation area: **personnel continually entering and leaving the area greatly increase the risk of cross-infection**
- if possible, choose personnel with known immunity to care for patients with specific infections as they will be resistant to the infection, e.g. persons who have had chickenpox or are protected against varicella, may care for patients with chickenpox or shingles
- explain the importance of the precautions to the patient **to gain consent and co-operation, and encourage participation in care**

- wash the hands and apply alcohol-gel solution before entering the isolation area *to maintain a safe environment*
- don personal protective clothing as required *to create an effective barrier against the infection*
- enter the isolation area
- perform all necessary nursing care. Two nurses may be needed for certain nursing practices for example passing equipment, the patient's meals or prescribed medication in from outside the isolation area. One nurse should remain in protective clothing within the area. The second nurse should remain at the entrance of the area and transfer articles to the nurse within the area without allowing any contamination to occur. *This prevents the transmission of infection*
- observe the patient throughout this activity *to monitor any change in condition*
- ensure that the patient is left feeling as comfortable as possible *to help to promote the healing process*
- ensure that the patient has means of local communication, such as a nurse call system, since *patients and staff can feel very isolated in this situation* (Rees et al 2000, Maunder at al 2003). If isolation precautions are to be maintained for a long period of time and the patient's general condition allows, a bedside telephone or media system may be provided
- safely dispose of any infected material according to local policy *to prevent cross-infection*
- wash the hands within the isolation area *to prevent the infection being transferred out of the area*
- remove protective clothing without touching the outside of the garments and dispose of them safely *to prevent any cross-infection and maintain a safe environment for all*
- leave the isolation area once all the nursing care has been completed
- repeat handwashing outside the isolation area and apply alcohol hand gel *to further ensure no contamination occurs*
- document the nursing practices appropriately, monitor any after-effects and report abnormal findings immediately *so that care can be evaluated and any nursing or medical interventions altered as required*
- explain the precautions to visitors, who should be restricted to close relatives and friends, to obtain their co-operation in maintaining isolation for the patient by wearing any recommended protective clothing and undertaking hand hygiene
- in undertaking this practice, nurses are accountable for their actions, the quality of care delivered and record-keeping according to the Code of Professional Conduct: Standards for Conduct, Performance and Ethics (Nursing and Midwifery Council 2004), Guidelines for Records and Record Keeping (Nursing and Midwifery Council 2005) and Healthcare Associated Infection Task Force Code of Practice (Scottish Executive Health Department 2004).

Disposal of infected material

Local guidelines should be followed regarding the disposal of contaminated waste. In an institutional setting, two nurses are required: one to remain in protective clothing within the isolation area, the second nurse to remain free from contamination outside it.

Disposal of waste

This should be put in a clinical waste disposal bag and closed as appropriate inside the isolation area by the isolation nurse before being passed out to the second ward nurse. All waste bags must be securely fastened with a permanent closure using tape and 'swan-neck' fastening (Fig. 22.1) or a self-locking tag. The bag must be marked with the ward or unit name and date to ensure that it complies with waste disposal and health and safety legislation. Bags are usually stored in locked secure containers or areas prior to uplift and consignment for processing by heat disinfection or incineration.

Disposal of linen

Infected linen should be placed in a water-soluble membrane bag or totally water-soluble bag and then the appropriate colour-coded bag designated for infected linen prior to sending to the laundry. Disposable linen may be used in an emergency situation.

Disposal of 'sharps'

The infected 'sharps' container should be safely closed by the isolation nurse and placed in a designated outer container or bag held by the second nurse, keeping the outside uncontaminated. The outer container should then be sealed, a 'danger of infection' label attached and the whole disposed of in accordance with local healthcare policy to prevent any transmission of infection.

Plastic waste bags must be sealed when no more than 0.75 full

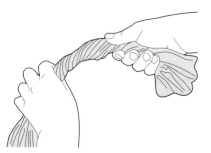

Twist firmly than double over

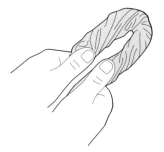

Pull together

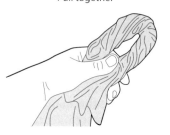

Seal firmly with tag to form a handle

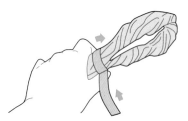

FIGURE 22.1
'Swan-neck' method for waste bag closure

Clinical Nursing Practices

Domestic cleaning

The domestic manager should be informed whenever isolation procedures are required. Arrangements for routine and terminal cleaning of the isolation area will be made in co-operation with the hospital infection control personnel to protect the patient and staff.

Decontamination of the isolation area

When a patient leaves an isolation area, the nursing staff should review and risk assess all the equipment used to nurse the infected person. The room or cubicle and its associated furniture, fixtures and fittings should be decontaminated by cleaning and disinfection as stated in the local infection control policy prior to being used again (Barker et al 2004, Rutala & Weber 2004, Scottish Executive Health Department 2004).

Specific precautions

Different precautions may be needed for specific infections.

Respiratory infections

The patient should be nursed in a single room or cubicle with the door kept closed **to reduce air-borne and/or droplet infection**. This room should ideally have an integral air circulation system with HEPA filter and failure alarm to alert staff if there is a malfunction.

- gloves should be worn during all care procedures; **to prevent contamination with body fluids**. A good handwashing technique along with gloves should give adequate protection, this **preventing contamination with body fluids**
- urine and faeces do not require special treatment, but should be disposed of immediately; the use of a separate toilet or commode helps to reduce the risk of cross-infection.

Wound infections

The patient may need to be nursed in a single room or cubicle.

- gloves should be worn, especially when performing dressings or handling potentially infected bed linen or clothing, to **prevent contamination with body fluids** as well as **preventing the transmission of infection**
- a plastic apron may be adequate protective clothing depending on the organism causing the infection. A good handwashing technique is essential **to ensure that there is no transmission of infection**.

Enteric infections

The patient should be nursed in a single room or cubicle with adequate individual toilet facilities **as enteric infections are readily transmitted** (Hospital Infection Society 2003, Department of Health 2005).

- gowns, plastic aprons and gloves should be worn, but a mask is not necessary. Crockery and cutlery should be washed in the hottest cycle of the dishwasher and not processed by hand to ensure that they are processed in a standardised manner at a set temperature
- vomitus and faeces are usually infective and should be disposed of according to local policy. In rare cases this may include covering the infected matter with disinfectant for a period of time **to destroy the causative organisms**.

Disposable bed pans and urinals are treated as infected waste **to maintain a safe environment**. Reusable bedpans, bedpan bases for disposable systems and reusable urinals should be processed on the wash and disinfection cycle of the automatic bedpan washing machine between each use and when the patient is discharged.

- before removing protective clothing, the gloved hands should be washed **to reduce contamination**, and further handwashing should be performed as in the guidelines above.

Viral blood infections

Special precautions may be required when a patient has a viral infection caused by:

- the hepatitis B or C virus
- human immunodeficiency virus (HIV), which may develop into acquired immune deficiency syndrome (AIDS).

These patients may be suffering from the disease or carrying the virus in their blood and should be treated as having infected blood and body fluids. The caring personnel are most at risk of infection in this situation. Precautions should be maintained for all patients suspected of being 'carriers' until investigations prove negative. Epidemiology and research in the last two decades have demonstrated that certain persons are at higher risk of acquiring blood-borne virus infections than others:

- intravenous drug users (via contaminated needles, syringes and equipment) **through direct blood infection**
- male homosexuals, bisexuals and heterosexual couples, especially those with numerous partners, who practise unprotected sex, **through infected blood and body fluids during sexual intercourse**
- babies born to mothers who are infected **because the virus crosses the placental barrier**
- people who have been transfused with contaminated blood or blood products **through direct blood infection**
- patients from, or those who have recently visited, countries where there is a relatively higher incidence of the disease and infection control precautions may not be adequate.

Precautions should be taken routinely to prevent healthcare personnel in contact with patients being placed at risk. It is important to remember that viruses have to enter the blood circulation via a break in the skin or through the mucosa of the non-infected individual. The degree of risk should ideally be assessed by the lead health professional and precautions planned in conjunction with the local infection control team. All proposed care plans must be explained and discussed with the patient and carers.

Low-risk situations

Precautions should be taken when handling blood and body secretions, and gloves should be worn at all times. Special care should be taken when handling and disposing of syringes and needles. Sharps containers should be treated as infected and labelled with biohazard stickers. Blood and other specimens for investigation should be labelled with special 'at risk of infection' stickers.

High-risk situations

Additional precautions may be prescribed, for example when carrying out an invasive procedure for patients known to be infected with HIV or active hepatitis B virus. Standard infection control precautions should be maintained. Protective clothing including face protection should be discretely worn by any attending personnel **to prevent any infected secretions or blood splashing the eyes or mouth of the carer**. In some areas where such patients are known to be regularly admitted, additional personal protective equipment (PPE) is routinely held available for immediate use. The local infection control and occupational health service advisors can provide more detailed advice.

Healthcare personnel should be vaccinated against hepatitis B (refer to local infection control and personnel policies).

2. PROTECTIVE ISOLATION

In this situation, the infected area is the environment of the ward and the non-infected area is the isolation area. Pathogens are prevented from entering the isolation area by the protective isolation of the patient. The principles and the guidelines are the same as above, but the procedure is reversed to protect the patient from staff and other persons.

Indications and rationale for protective isolation	This is carried out **to prevent the spread of infection to patients who have a reduced resistance to infection as a result of their disease condition or prescribed treatment, for example**:

- patients who have leukaemia, which leads to immature and defective white blood cells and decreases resistance to infection
- patients who have reduced autoimmunity as a result of cytotoxic medication used in the treatment of malignant disease, and have a reduced white blood cell count
- patients who are receiving immunosuppressive medication following transplant surgery, which also reduces the number of white blood cells.

The following precautions are emphasised. A filter-type mask may be used by personnel **to protect the prolonged neutropenic patient from droplet infection**.

The form of protective clothing depends on the patient's condition. Gowns should be worn when nursing children, but in most instances a plastic apron will be sufficient **to prevent cross-infection from the nurse's uniform**.

All personnel must be meticulous in their handwashing technique **to maintain a safe environment** (NHS Education for Scotland 2005). An alcohol hand rub should be applied frequently to the nurse's hands *to further reduce the risk of cross-infection*.

Special air flow facilities, for example a laminar flow system, may be used to prevent a flow of air from the ward area to the isolation area. This *decreases the risk of infection being transferred from the ward environment*.

Patients in protective isolation are at risk of acquiring infection from bacteria and viruses present on the surface of uncooked foods, e.g. salads and raw fruit. Sterile foods may be prescribed and supplied by the dietetics department. Preparation advice must be followed meticulously. It should be remembered that *sterile* foods may be reheated in a microwave oven but these do not kill toxins in non-sterile foods due to 'cold spots'.

The precautions should be explained to visitors, who should be limited to close relatives and friends, thus *reducing the risk of infection*. Appropriate protective clothing should be worn *to maintain a safe environment for the patient* (Clark et al 2002).

Visitors and other personnel should not be in contact with the patient if they have a cold, sore throat or other infection, however mild, *which might infect the immunosuppressed patient*. The reason for this precaution should be explained. Nursing should be planned so that only one or two staff are caring for the patient during a span of duty, *to reduce the risk of infection from ward personnel*.

3. RADIOACTIVE HAZARD ISOLATION

Patients receiving large doses of radioactive isotopes, either systemically or by implantation, are normally nursed in specially equipped units that have in-built barriers against radioactivity and are equipped with specialised screens. Radioactive isotopes are, however, being used more frequently for diagnostic purposes, and nurses may care for patients undergoing such investigations in general wards. Local policy should always be followed.

Indications and rationale for radioactive hazard isolation

This is carried out *to prevent the radioactive contamination of carers and others when radioactive substances are used*:

- to treat patients who have malignant tumours with radioactive implants or radioactive isotopes
- for diagnostic investigations using radioactive isotopes.

The isolation technique aims *to reduce the risk of radiation for other patients and caring personnel* by limiting the time spent near the patient having radioactive treatment, and enforcing a safe distance at other times. The patient should be nursed in a single room or confined to one particular area of the ward. Lead screens should be used *as a shield from radiation when radioactive implants are inserted*, according to individual requirements. Radioactive material should be transported in lead containers *to prevent any escape of radioactivity*.

Guidelines and rationale for this nursing practice	■ consult the radiation protection officer and health service policy **to ascertain the precautions appropriate for particular radioactive substances used in treatment or investigation** ■ explain the precautions and their implications to the patient **and gain consent and co-operation** ■ ensure that all staff wear radiation detection badges. This will **monitor individual doses of radiation and ensure that no one is exposed to a dangerous level** ■ plan the nursing so that no nurse is in an area of radiation for longer than necessary, and share care **so that each nurse has a reduced exposure time** ■ don protective lead aprons or use a lead board if appropriate **to block the passage of radiation** ■ wear gloves and apron for all nursing practices and when handling any bedclothes or linen that may be contaminated by radioactive excreta or body fluids, **to prevent contamination** ■ dispose of linen and waste according to health authority policy, labelling materials with special radioactive warning stickers, **in order to maintain a safe environment** ■ follow local policy when dealing with any spillage of suspected radioactive material ■ display radiation hazard notice near to the patient to alert others to the radioactive risk ■ in undertaking this practice, nurses are accountable for their actions, the quality of care delivered and record-keeping according to the Code of Professional Conduct: Standards for Conduct, Performance and Ethics (Nursing and Midwifery Council 2004).

Radioactive materials have a reducing 'half-life' so that **precautions need only be carried out for a specific, prescribed period of time**. Once the danger of radioactivity is considered negligible, the precautions may be discontinued.

It is advisable that staff who have had close contact with radioactive materials should have a shower and a change of clothing when coming off duty, **as an extra precaution**.

In radiotherapy units, special guidelines may apply, i.e. for pregnant staff, and a Geiger counter may be used to assess the radioactivity level before disposing of radioactive material.

Patient/carer education Key points 	In partnership with the patient and relative or carer, ensure that they are competent to carry out any practices required. Information should be given regarding an appropriate point of contact for any concerns that may arise. ■ the reason for the specific precautions should be explained to the patient and relatives ■ detailed patient education on the specific precautions for each individual infection will be needed throughout this nursing practice ■ the specific teaching of self-care skills such as mouth care will be needed for immunosuppressed patients and the importance of these reinforced ■ patients with a confirmed MRSA or *Clostridium difficile* infection should understand the importance of reporting that they have had these

infections when visiting the outpatient department or on readmission, as recurrence is common and certain antibiotics may be contra-indicated

- patients with blood-borne virus infections should have a good knowledge of any ongoing precautions for the prevention of cross-infection in the ward, at home, employment and community settings. Good communication skills, both verbal and non-verbal, are required to reinforce the nurse's non-judgemental attitude and to reduce any feeling of stigma on the part of the patient and family

- patients being discharged following recent investigation using radioactive isotopes should be given information sheets concerning any specific precautions. Liaison with the community team will help to reinforce any precautions needed.

References

Barker J, Vipond IB, Bloofield SF 2004 Effects of cleaning and disinfection in reducing the spread of Norovirus contamination via environmental surfaces. Journal of Hospital Infection 58: 42–49

Clark L, Smith W, Young L 2002 Protective clothing: principles and guidance. ICNA, London (Available at: http://www.icna.co.uk)

Clinical Standards Board for Scotland 2001 Standards: healthcare associated infection (HAI) infection control. CSBS, Edinburgh

Department of Health 2004 Standards for better health (Available at: http://www.dh.gov.uk/publications)

Department of Health 2005 Management, prevention and surveillance of *Clostridium difficile*: interim findings from a national survey of NHS acute trusts in England (Available at: http://www.hpa.org.uk/infections/topics_az/clostridium_difficile/InterimReport05pdf)

Department of Health and Hospital Infection Society 2001 Standard principles for preventing hospital acquired infections. Journal of Hospital Infections 47(Suppl): S21–S37 (Available at: http://www.needlestickforum.net/6bestprac/pds/EPIC-Standard-Principles-HAI.pdf)

Hospital Infection Society 2003 National *Clostridium difficile* Standards Group Report to the Department of Health. Journal of Hospital Infection (Available at: http://www.his.org.uk/_db/documents/FINAL_C_Diff_report.pdf)

Maunder R, Hunter J, Vincent L et al 2003 The immediate psychological and occupational impact of the 2003 SARS outbreak in a teaching hospital. Canadian Medical Association Journal 168(10): 1245–1251

National Institute for Clinical Excellence 2006 Revised guidance for the diagnosis, treatment and management of tuberculosis. HMSO, London

NHS Education for Scotland 2005 Promoting hand hygiene in healthcare: a short self-directed web-based learning package for healthcare workers. NES, Edinburgh (Available at: http://www.new-hai.info/)

Nursing and Midwifery Council 2004 Code of professional conduct: standards for conduct, performance and ethics. NMC, London (Available at: http://www.nmc-uk.org)

Nursing and Midwifery Council 2005 Guidelines for records and record keeping. NMC, London

Rees J, Davies H, Birchall C et al 2000 Psychological effects of source isolation nursing (2): patient satisfaction. Nursing Standard 14(29): 32–36

Ritchie K, Iqbal K, Macpherson K et al 2005 The provision of alcohol based products to improve compliance with hand hygiene, Health Technology Assessment Report. NHS QIS, Glasgow (Available at: http:// www.nhshealthquality.org)

Rutala W, Weber DJ 2004 The benefits of surface disinfection. American Journal of Infection Control 32(4): 229–231

Saint S, Higgins LA, Nallamothu BK 2003 Do physicians examine patients in contact isolation less frequently? American Journal of Infection Control 32(6): 254–256

Scottish Executive Health Department 2004 The NHS Scotland code of practice for the local management of hygiene and healthcare associated infection (HAI). SEHD Healthcare

Associated Infection Task Force, Edinburgh (Available at: http://www.scotland.gov.uk/library5/publications/hai1)

Scottish Health Facilities 2005 Infection control in the built environment. Note 30, version 2 (Available at: http://www.show.scot.nhs.uk/pef/secure/)

Scottish Infection Standards and Strategy Group 2004 Bicollegiate College of Physicians and Scottish Executive Health Department guidelines for the diagnosis and management of suspected or proven *E. coli* 0157. Journal of the Royal College of Physicians of Edinburgh 34(1): 37–40 (Available at: http://www.rcpe.ac.uk/publications/articles/vol33_4html)

Working Party on MRSA 1998 British Society for Antimicrobial Chemotherapy (BSAC), Hospital Infection Society (HIS) and the Infection Control Nurses Association (ICNA) revised guidelines for the control of methicillin-resistant *Staphylococcus aureus* infection in hospitals. Journal of Hospital Infection 39(4): 253–290 (Available at: http://www.ncbi.nlm.nih.gov/entrez/query?cmd = retrieve&db = PubMed&list_uids = 9749399&dopt = Abstract)

Websites

Department of Health: http://www.dh.gov.uk/ publications
Hospital Infection Society: http://www.his.org.uk/
Infection Control Nurses Association: http://www.icna.co.uk
Nursing and Midwifery Council: http://www.nmc-uk.org

Self assessment

1. When caring for infected patients, the emphasis is on preventing the spread of the infection. Identify three items that could be used to protect healthcare staff from enteric infection in a hospital setting and prepare a patient's care plan to include these items.

2. Protective isolation aims to maintain a safe environment for the patient at risk of infection while the treatment for the disease is underway. What information should be provided to visitors and relatives about visiting restrictions before they come to the hospital?

3. Isolation immediately affects the normal person-to-person communication process. Patients often become depressed and bored because the number of people in contact with them is greatly reduced: visitors are limited, and staff restrict the number of times they enter and leave the area (Saint et al 2003). Think of your own hospital's provision: do you have television, voice link or a local call system in isolation rooms? What other measures could be taken?

4. Isolation rooms should ideally have significant glass areas to allow the patient to see the outside environment whilst allowing occlusion for privacy and rest, and they should possess a window with an interesting view (Scottish Health Facilities 2005). What other equipment and facilities should be present in an isolation room?

5. What type of foods and supplements are recommended for patients while in protective isolation?

Practice 23
Lumbar Puncture

Learning outcomes

By the end of this section, you should know how to:
- prepare the patient for this nursing practice
- collect and prepare the equipment
- assist the medical practitioner to perform a lumbar puncture
- care for the patient following the procedure.

Background knowledge required

Revision of the anatomy and physiology of the brain and spinal cord, with special reference to the cerebrospinal fluid and meninges

Revision of the anatomy of the lumbar vertebrae

Revision of 'Aseptic technique' (*see* p. 381)

Revision of local policy on lumbar puncture.

Indications and rationale for lumbar puncture

Lumbar puncture is the insertion of a specialised needle into the lumbar subarachnoid space to gain access to the cerebrospinal fluid. This may be required:
- **to obtain a sample of cerebrospinal fluid for investigative and diagnostic purposes**, e.g.:
  — bacteriological investigation for patients suspected of having meningitis or encephalitis
  — cytological investigation for patients suspected of having a malignant tumour
- **to identify the presence of blood in the cerebrospinal fluid** following trauma or a suspected subarachnoid haemorrhage
- **to introduce radio-opaque fluid into the subarachnoid space** for radiographic investigation
- **to identify raised intraspinal/intracranial pressure and provide relief**, if appropriate, by removing some of the cerebrospinal fluid
- **to introduce intrathecal medication** such as cytotoxic agents or antibiotics (Lyndsay & Bone 2004).

The procedure may be performed on patients who are inpatients or day patients, according to their clinical status. A lumbar puncture should not be performed if raised intracranial pressure is suspected as the raised pressure might cause the brain stem tissue to herniate through the foramen magnum. This is known as 'coning' and could be fatal (Boon et al 2004).

Outline of the procedure

A lumbar puncture is performed by a medical practitioner using an aseptic technique. The patient is helped into the correct position. An area of skin above the 3rd, 4th and 5th lumbar vertebrae is prepared and cleansed with alcohol-based antiseptic solution prior to the administration of local anaesthesia. Once the local anaesthetic has taken effect, a special lumbar puncture needle is inserted between the 3rd and 4th, or 4th and 5th, lumbar vertebrae in order to gain access to the subarachnoid space below the spinal cord in the region of the cauda equina (Fig. 23.1). The needle is hollow with a stilette to ease introduction to the subarachnoid space. Once in position, the stilette of the needle is removed. A disposable manometer is attached to the end of the needle via a two-way tap, and the cerebrospinal fluid (CSF) is allowed to flow into the manometer to record the intraspinal pressure. A normal CSF pressure is 60–150 mmH$_2$O. The pressure will fluctuate with respiration and heart beat. Coughing will cause the pressure to rise (Clarke 2002).

When the pressure recording has been completed, the manometer is occluded, and 2–3 ml of cerebrospinal fluid is allowed to flow into each of the three separate sterile specimen containers as required while still maintaining asepsis. The specimen containers should be pre-labelled, numbers 1, 2 and 3 because the first specimen may contain blood as a result of the needle being introduced. The containers should collect the specimens sequentially to avoid misinterpretation of results. The medical practitioner will note the colour, consistency and opacity of the cerebrospinal fluid as well as observing the presence or absence of blood. On completion of this stage, the needle is removed, and the puncture site is covered by a small sterile dressing or plastic sealant spray. Following this procedure, according to local policy and the patient's clinical status, appropriate neurological observations, wound-site assessment and the monitoring of any localised pain or headache should be performed (Lindsay & Bone 2004).

The position of the patient

The correct position is important in order to ensure the success and safety of this procedure. Patients should lie on their side on a firm bed with one pillow, stretching their lumbar vertebrae by flexing their head and neck and drawing their knees up to the abdomen, holding them with their hands (Fig. 23.2). The nurse can assist by supporting the patient behind the knees and the neck, and helping to maintain the extension of the lumbar vertebrae, thus widening the intervertebral space. This will help to ensure that the insertion and correct placement of the lumbar puncture needle is safely achieved. Once the needle is in position, the

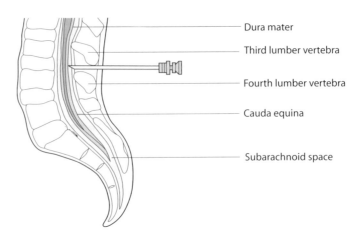

Dura mater

Third lumber vertebra

Fourth lumber vertebra

Cauda equina

Subarachnoid space

FIGURE 23.1
Lumbar puncture:
position of the needle in
relation to the vertebrae

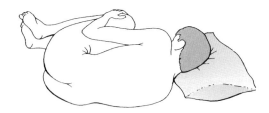

FIGURE 23.2
Lumbar puncture:
position of the patient
From Lindsay & Bone
2004, with permission

medical practitioner may ask patients to straighten their legs slowly without moving the position of their back. This will reduce the intra-abdominal pressure, which can cause an abnormal reading of intraspinal pressure.

This procedure is occasionally performed with a patient sitting straddled on a chair and facing the back of the chair with his or her head resting on folded arms. This position may be chosen by the medical practitioner when performing a lumbar puncture for an obese patient with dyspnoea who may be distressed when lying flat. Whichever position is used, it is important for the patient to remain still (Tate & Tasota 2000).

Equipment

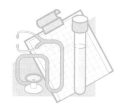

1. Trolley
2. Sterile dressings pack
3. Sterile drapes
4. Sterile surgical gloves for the medical practitioner
5. Lumbar puncture needles of appropriate size
6. Spinal manometer
7. Two-way tap
8. Alcohol-based antiseptic lotion for cleansing the skin
9. Local anaesthetic and equipment for its administration
10. Syringe and needles for administering the local anaesthetic
11. Sterile dressing, e.g. Airstrip or plastic sealant spray
12. Three sterile specimen containers appropriately labelled and numbered 1, 2 and 3, completed laboratory forms, and a plastic specimen bag for transportation. These may be required for three separate samples of cerebrospinal fluid for microbiological, biochemical and cytological investigation
13. Receptacle for disposable items
14. Sharps box.

Lumbar puncture needle

This is a rigid stainless steel needle, available between 3.8–12.7 cm in length, complete with its own sharp-pointed stilette; this helps the passage of the needle into the correct position. Once the stilette has been removed, the blunt end of the needle lies within the subarachnoid space and should cause no damage to the tissues during the procedure. Needles are usually supplied with their own metal two-way tap, but a Luer disposable tap may be used. The length and gauge of the needle will be dependent on the height and weight of the patient, the reason for the lumbar puncture and the experience of the medical practitioner undertaking the procedure. The smallest gauge needle is recommended to minimise risk of post-procedure headache (Armon & Ewans 2005).

Guidelines and rationale for this nursing practice

- help to explain the procedure to the patient **to gain consent and co-operation, and to encourage participation in care**
- ensure the patient's privacy **to respect his or her individuality and maintain self-esteem**
- help to collect and prepare the equipment **to ensure the procedure is performed efficiently**
- help the patient into the appropriate position, and remain with him or her **to maintain that position and maximise safety during the procedure**
- help to prepare the sterile field **to maintain asepsis**
- observe the patient throughout this activity **to monitor any adverse effects**
- help to expose the lumbar region of the patient's back and assist the medical practitioner, as required, **to maintain asepsis and reassure the patient**
- hold the appropriate sterile containers **to receive the flow of cerebrospinal fluid as directed, maintaining asepsis**
- once the needle has been removed, apply pressure to the site and cover with a sterile dressing or plastic sealant spray **in order to prevent leakage of the cerebrospinal fluid and maintain asepsis**
- help the patient into a comfortable position once the procedure has been completed **to promote comfort and recovery from the procedure; there is no evidence to support keeping the patient on bedrest to reduce risk of headache** (Cooper 2002)
- dispose of the equipment safely **to comply with health and safety issues and prevent transmission of infection**
- monitor the patient's conscious level **to observe for signs of possible brain stem herniation**
- monitor the patient's vital signs **to observe for abnormalities**
- document the procedure appropriately, monitor any after-effects, and report abnormal findings immediately, **ensuring safe practice and enabling prompt appropriate medical and nursing action to be initiated**
- immediately dispatch the labelled cerebrospinal fluid specimens, with their completed forms, to the laboratory **so that investigations may be initiated and decisions about appropriate treatment made as soon as possible**
- in undertaking this practice, nurses are accountable for their actions, the quality of care delivered and record-keeping according to the Code of Professional Conduct: Standards for Conduct, Performance and Ethics (Nursing and Midwifery Council 2004) and Guidelines for Records and Record Keeping (Nursing and Midwifery Council 2005).

Additional information

This is an invasive procedure that involves direct access to the spinal and brain tissue via the cerebrospinal fluid. Asepsis should therefore be maintained during and after the procedure, and an adequate handwashing technique should be practised to prevent cross-infection.

The puncture site should be observed for evidence of localised infection or leakage; accurate observations of the patient's condition will help to monitor any signs of developing infection.

Urgent medical attention must be sought if cerebrospinal fluid leakage occurs.

The patient's general and neurological condition, for example orientation, restlessness, drowsiness and nausea, should be noted. Any evidence of cerebral irritability should be observed. Fitting, twitching, spasticity or weakness of limb movements should be reported immediately and recorded. The patient's level of consciousness and vital observations should be recorded as prescribed, depending on his or her condition. Any rise in temperature that might indicate a developing infection should be reported. Neurological observations should be maintained according to local policy after this investigation (*see* 'Unconscious patient', p. 351).

The patient may complain of a headache following this procedure. Analgesic medication should be administered as prescribed. The nurse should be observant for any non-verbal communication indicating pain, and anticipate the patient's needs as appropriate. The fact that the patient might experience discomfort should be explained to him or her.

A normal diet may be ordered as the patient's condition allows. An adequate fluid intake should be maintained following the procedure. Drinks should be easily accessible to the patient and specialised cups or straws used as appropriate.

The patient should have a short period of rest and then mobilise as directed. Mobilisation should commence with the patient sitting up in bed for a period of time before progressing to further activity as the condition allows.

Patient/carer education

Key points

The reason for the investigation and the importance of a lumbar puncture for diagnostic or therapeutic purposes should be explained to the patient. This should include the fact that the investigation itself should have no long-term effects. The importance of keeping in the correct position should be carefully explained and reinforced.

Following the lumbar puncture, the patient should understand the necessity of reporting a headache or any other adverse effects to the nursing staff. Patients who have the procedure performed as an outpatient should be given written instructions with advice on taking appropriate analgesia for headache, care of the puncture site and a contact telephone number in case of any adverse effects at home.

References

Armon C, Ewans RW 2005 Smaller needle size is associated with less frequent headache. Addendum to assessment: prevention of post lumbar puncture headaches. Report of the therapeutics and technology assessment subcommittee of the American Academy of Neurologists. Neurology 65(4): 510–512

Boon JM, Abrahams PH, Meiring JH et al 2004 Lumbar puncture: review of a clinical skill. Clinical Anatomy 17: 544–553

Clarke CRA 2002 Neurological disease. In: Kumar P, Clarke M (eds) Clinical medicine, 5th edn. Elsevier Science, Edinburgh

Cooper N 2002 Evidence-based lumbar puncture: best practice to prevent headache. Hospital Medicine 63(10): 598–599

Lindsay KW, Bone I 2004 Neurology and neurosurgery illustrated, 4th edn. Churchill Livingstone, Edinburgh

Nursing and Midwifery Council 2004 Code of professional conduct: standards for conduct, performance and ethics. NMC, London

Nursing and Midwifery Council 2005 Guidelines for records and record keeping. NMC, London

Tate J, Tasota F 2000 Looking at lumbar puncture in adults. Nursing November: 91

Clinical Nursing Practices

Self assessment

1. Describe some of the indications for lumbar puncture.
2. Discuss the nurse's role in preparing the patient for lumbar puncture.
3. Why is it important to have specimen containers ready prior to the procedure?
4. Following the procedure, what observations should be made on the patient?
5. What information would a patient need when being discharged following lumbar puncture?

Practice 24
Mouth Care

Learning outcomes	**By the end of this section, you should know how to:**
	▪ prepare the patient for this nursing practice
	▪ collect and prepare the equipment
	▪ carry out mouth care according to the individual needs of the patient in both a community and an institutional setting.

Background knowledge required	Revision of the anatomy and physiology of the mouth and pharynx, with special reference to the teeth, salivary glands and oral mucosa Revision of pharmaceutical literature related to the mouthwashes and mouth-cleaning preparations in current use Revision of local policy related to mouth care.

Indications and rationale for mouth care	Mouth care is the use of a toothbrush and paste, a mouthwash or other mouth-cleaning preparation to help the patient to maintain the cleanliness of his teeth or dentures and to encourage the flow of saliva to maintain a healthy oropharyngeal mucosa. Good oral health is crucial to meeting fundamental human needs such as comfort, nutrition, communication and acceptable personal appearance (NHS Quality Improvement Scotland 2004).

This nursing practice is also known as oral hygiene and may be required:

▪ for any patient who has not eaten for a period of time or whose diet is restricted, as the reduction in mastication decreases the flow of saliva; this may occur during the preoperative or postoperative period, especially in patients who have undergone oral or abdominal surgery
▪ for patients who are dehydrated for any reason as the normal flow of saliva will be reduced
▪ for patients suffering from nausea or vomiting as they will be reluctant to eat
▪ for patients being treated with oxygen therapy, particularly using unhumidified oxygen, which has a drying effect on the oral mucosa
▪ for patients who are having radiotherapy or cytotoxic medication for malignant disease as this may adversely affect the cells of the oral mucosa (White 2000)
▪ for patients with any form of facial paralysis or muscle weakness as the inability to masticate adequately reduces the flow of saliva and may cause food debris to be retained in the mouth. This may include an unconscious patient or one in the terminal stages of illness
▪ for patients who have poor manual dexterity or cognitive impairment (White 2000)
▪ for patients with an oral infection such as candidiasis.

There is a lack of research on the frequency of mouth care, which will vary for each individual. The use of an effective oral assessment tool is strongly advised to ensure the early detection of problems within vulnerable patient groups (Roberts 2000). Intensive mouth care may be carried out every 2 hours, whereas mouthwashes may only be required two or three times a day but frequency should be based on individual assessment (Griffiths & Lewis 2002).

Equipment

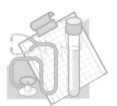

1. Suitable tray or trolley
2. Plastic gloves (non-sterile)
3. Pencil torch
4. Spatula
5. Toothbrush
6. Toothpaste
7. Container for dentures (for institutional care this should be appropriately labelled)
8. Beaker
9. Bowl or receiver
10. Towel or other protective covering
11. Mouthwash solution
12. Soft tissues for wiping the mouth
13. Receptacle for disposable items.

Additional equipment for specialised mouth care as required

Mouth-care pack or equivalent equipment
Foam sticks
Cotton buds
Prescribed medication, e.g. an antifungal agent if thrush is diagnosed
Solution for mouth cleaning
Lubrication for lips, e.g. petroleum jelly or lip balm
Suction equipment.

Toothbrush and toothpaste

The patient's own equipment may be used if it is available; otherwise, a soft, small-headed nylon brush and toothpaste can be supplied. This is usually the most appropriate equipment for this nursing practice (Clay 2000).

Foam sticks

These are ineffective in removing debris from the teeth and gums (Clay 2000), but they are useful for rinsing or refreshing the mouth (Nicol et al 2000). Care should be taken that the foam head does not become detached and obstruct the patient's airway.

Solutions to be used as mouthwashes

Various solutions are available, professional knowledge or individual prescription and patient preference influencing the choice of preparation used. All the solutions used should be clearly labelled and diluted according to their instructions. The procedure for checking the preparation is as for 'Administration of medicines' (*see* p. 13).

There remains little general consensus over the efficacy of oral-care agents (Milligan et al 2001).

Saline

This can be made up using common salt, one level teaspoon (approximately 4.5 g) in 500 ml of water, also being available in sterile sachets. This is an effective mouthwash for patients who have had oral surgery, especially dental extractions.

Thymol

This is prepared in solution and is the main component of most mouthwash tablets. It has a mild antiseptic effect and is well tolerated when diluted to suit the patient's taste.

Sodium bicarbonate

This may be made up immediately prior to use. One level teaspoon of powder in 500 ml of water is a useful mouthwash for dissolving mucus and debris. A stronger solution can be used for soaking dentures before cleaning them.

Chlorhexidene

This is the most effective chemical agent for maintaining oral hygiene and for dental plaque control (Xavier 2000). Mouthwash should not take place more than once every 12 hours (British National Formulary 2005). Stronger solutions can, however, stain the teeth, and long-term use can cause mucosal damage (British National Formulary 2005).

Water

This may be the most refreshing and appropriate mouthwash to use after brushing the teeth.

Other aids for mouth care (if permitted)

Soda water

This may be appreciated as an alternative mouthwash.

Ice cubes

These may be sucked, but the number should be limited if the patient has a restricted oral intake.

Fresh fruit

This can be sucked and then removed. Pineapple, if allowed, can be very refreshing and will stimulate the flow of saliva as it contains the enzyme ananase, which can help to clean a coated tongue (Rattenbury et al 1999).

Saliva substitutes

These are useful for the treatment of a dry mouth (NHS Quality Improvement Scotland 2004).

Soft paraffin/lip salves

These prevent the lips becoming dry and cracked.

Glycerine, with or without lemon, should not be used as it can dehydrate the oral tissue and is an ineffective cleanser. In addition, lemon is acidic and can lead to irritation and the decalcification of the teeth (Clay 2000).

Solutions for mouth cleaning

Any mouthwash solution can be used for mouth cleaning, as can solutions that actively stimulate the flow of saliva. The most efficient method of mouth cleaning remains, however, a mild toothpaste applied with a soft, small-headed toothbrush (Clay 2000). The toothbrush may be dipped in any mouthwash or mouth-cleaning solution acceptable to the patient.

Mouth-care pack

This prepared sterile pack is used when intensive mouth care is needed for patients for whom a mouthwash alone, or tooth-brushing, is not appropriate. The pack may contain:

- a plastic tray divided into compartments to hold the mouth-cleaning solution
- cotton sticks
- foam sticks
- gauze swabs.

If a pack is not available, a sterile mouth-care tray can be assembled using:

- a foil tray
- a gallipot
- gauze swabs
- foam sticks
- cotton sticks.

The mouth-care pack should be covered, labelled with the patient's name and the date, cleaned and replenished after use, and replaced every 24 hours or as required. In the patient's own home, equipment can be adapted appropriately, maintaining a safe environment.

Guidelines and rationale for this nursing practice

- explain the nursing practice to the patient **to gain consent and co-operation, and to encourage participation in care, ensuring that there is some understanding of this practice**
- collect and prepare the equipment **to ensure an efficient use of time and resources**. Some solutions are more effective if prepared immediately before use
- ensure the patient's privacy **to respect his or her individuality and maintain self-esteem**
- help the patient into a comfortable sitting position, either in bed or on a chair **to help patient co-operation and promote as much independence as possible**. It is sometimes possible for patients to sit comfortably in front of a wash basin in either their own home or an institution
- place some protective material over the patient's chest and under the chin **to protect the clothes**. The patient's own towel can be used
- observe the patient throughout this activity **to monitor any adverse effects**
- don clean plastic gloves after efficient handwashing **to prevent contamination with body fluids and to maintain a safe environment**
- it is advisable to wear gloves for all mouth care as it may involve direct contact with the oral mucosa and oral secretions

- ask or help the patient to remove his or her dentures and place them in a bowl of clean water (labelled if necessary) *to gain access and a clear view of the oral cavity*
- examine the patient's mouth and tongue using the torch and spatula, *to observe the condition of the teeth, dentures, tongue, lips, gums and mucous membrane. Note any food debris, any ulcers or sores and the condition of the lips* (Xavier 2000)
- if possible, discuss with the patient the most suitable and acceptable mouth care for his or her particular needs *to promote individualised care and aid compliance*
- help patients to clean their teeth or dentures with their toothbrush and toothpaste
- offer a suitable mouthwash, explaining that it should not be swallowed, and help to hold the equipment as necessary *to rinse the mouth until all the debris and cleaning paste have been removed*
- offer tissues *for drying the mouth*
- help to apply lubrication to the lips as required *to maintain the integrity of the skin of the lips*. This can be done by placing the lubricant on a gloved finger and applying it directly, or patients may apply it themselves, *encouraging independence*
- return the patient's clean dentures in a bowl of clean water and encourage the patient to wear them *to maintain the shape of the oral cavity*
- ensure that the patient is left feeling as comfortable as possible. A period of rest should ideally be encouraged after this nursing practice
- dispose of equipment safely *to maintain a safe environment*
- document the nursing practice appropriately and immediately report any deterioration or improvement in the condition of the mouth, as well as abnormal findings. *This enables changes in practice to be implemented to maintain optimum mouth care for each patient*
- in undertaking this practice, nurses are accountable for their actions, the quality of care delivered and record-keeping according to the Code of Professional Conduct: Standards for Conduct, Performance and Ethics (Nursing and Midwifery Council 2004a), Guidelines for the Administration of Medicines (Nursing and Midwifery Council 2004b) and Guidelines for Records and Record Keeping (Nursing and Midwifery Council 2005).

Intensive mouth care for dependent patients

- explain the nursing practice *to gain the patient's consent and co-operation if possible*
- ensure the patient's privacy *to respect individuality*
- help the patient into a comfortable position *so that he or she tolerates the practice*
- collect and prepare the equipment, including the mouth-cleaning pack or tray
- don clean plastic gloves *to prevent contamination with body fluids*
- remove dentures if present *to gain access and a clear view of the oral cavity*
- examine the patient's mouth as before
- clean all round the mouth, gums and tongue with the mouth-cleaning solution, using a soft toothbrush if possible. *This will help to dislodge debris and remove plaque* (Pearson & Hutton 2002)

- help the patient to use a mouthwash if possible, or rinse the mouth with a gauze swab soaked in mouthwash solution, allowing the patient to suck it. For patients with a wired mandible following oral surgery, a syringe of mouthwash in conjunction with suction may be used. This will require good co-operation from the patient and an adequate swallowing reflex **to prevent inhalation of the rinsing fluid**
- help the patient to clean the dentures, or clean them for him or her, using a toothbrush and toothpaste, under a running tap if possible, **to retain a healthy oral mucosa**
- proceed with the nursing practice as before.

Mouth care for an unconscious patient

Mouth-care guidelines are as for a dependent patient, with the following exceptions:
- position the patient on his or her side, with no pillow, and the head supported **so that no secretion or mouth-cleaning solution can flow into the trachea and be inhaled** (Major 2005)
- place waterproof material on the bed before placing tissues under the lower side of the face **to absorb solution and saliva draining from the mouth**
- check that suction equipment is at hand and in working order, and, if required, perform oral suction before commencing and during the nursing practice **to prevent any danger of fluid being inhaled**.

The dentures should have been removed, cleaned, appropriately labelled and stored with the patient's belongings on admission (*see* 'Unconscious patient', p. 351).

Patient/carer education
Key points

In partnership with the patient and/or carer, ensure that they are competent to carry out any practices required. Information should be given on an appropriate point of contact for any concerns that may arise.

Health promotion with regard to mouth care should be multidisciplinary from childhood to old age: the public health nurse, school nurse, practice nurse and district nurse, as well as the dentist and dental hygienist, may be involved. The correct use of dental floss can be included when discussing dental hygiene (Fig. 24.1). General oral hygiene advice should include:
- the importance of good care of the mouth, teeth and gums related to general health
- good tooth-cleaning technique and care of the dentures
- nutritional advice about the relationship of the incidence of dental caries to food and drink with a high sugar content
- the importance of removing debris from the teeth and fornices of the mouth after meals
- the influence of fluoride in the development of teeth
- the correct method of brushing and flossing the teeth.

Patients with a suppressed immune system should be taught oral hygiene procedures to prevent mucosal infection.

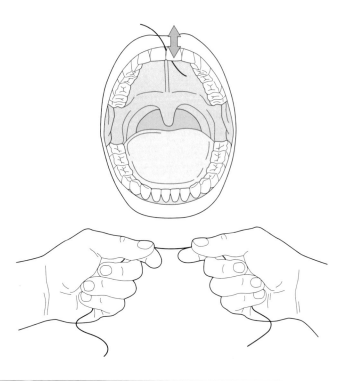

FIGURE 24.1
**Mouth care: use of
dental floss**

References

British National Formulary 2005 Mouthwashes, gargles and dentrifrices. Section 12.3.4: 556. BMJ Publishing Group, London

Clay M 2000 Oral health in older people. Nursing Older People 12(7): 21–26

Griffiths J, Lewis, D 2002 Guidelines for oral care of patients who are dependent, dysphagic or critically ill. Journal of Disability and Oral Health 3(1): 30–33

Major C 2005 Meeting hygiene needs. In: Baillie L (ed) Developing practical nursing skills, 2nd edn. Arnold, London

Milligan S, McGill M, Sweeney M et al 2001 Oral care for people with advanced cancer: an evidence-based protocol. International Journal of Palliative Nursing 7(9): 418–426

NHS Quality Improvement Scotland 2004 Working with dependent older people to achieve good oral care. NHS/QIS, Edinburgh

Nicol M, Bavin C, Bedford-Turner S et al 2000 Essential nursing skills. Mosby, London

Nursing and Midwifery Council 2004a Code of conduct: standards for conduct, performance and ethics. NMC, London

Nursing and Midwifery Council 2004b Guidelines for the administration of medicines. NMC, London

Nursing and Midwifery Council 2005 Guidelines for records and record keeping. NMC, London

Pearson LS, Hutton JL 2002 A controlled trial to compare the ability of foam swabs and toothbrushes to remove dental plaque. Journal of Advanced Nursing 39(5): 480–489

Rattenbury N, Mooney G, Bowen J 1999 Oral assessment and care for patients. Nursing Times 95(49): 52–53

Roberts J 2000 Developing an oral assessment and intervention tool for older people, 3. British Journal of Nursing 9(19): 2073–2078

White R 2000 Nurse assessment of oral health: a review of practice and education. British Journal of Nursing 9(5): 260–266

Xavier G 2000 The importance of mouth care in preventing infection. Nursing Standard 14(18): 47–51

Website
The British Dental Association: http://www.bda.org/smile/
Provides advice on oral health across different age spans

Self assessment

1. When may a patient require oral hygiene?
2. What is the most appropriate equipment to carry out mouth care?
3. What other aids may be used for mouth care?

Practice 25
Moving and Handling

Learning outcomes

By the end of this section you will:

- understand the relevance and use of moving and handling legislation
- identify the four areas of risk assessment
- have a knowledge of the ethical and legal issues relating to moving and handling
- relate the principles of evidence-based practice, ergonomics, balance and stability in relation to practice.

Background knowledge required

Sickness and absence related to moving and handling costs the NHS approximately £300 million per year and is responsible for approximately 40% of all sickness and absence in the NHS (National Health Service 2002). The reasons for this include lack of education, inadequate staffing, cumulative loads, poor postures, illness, stress and poor work practice (Retsas & Pinikahana 2000, Royal College of Nursing 2005).

Before this can be addressed the nurse needs to understand why the practice of safe handling is so important. Therefore you should review the following:

Manual Handling Operations Regulations (MHOR 1992), which came into force on the 1 January 1993

The RCN Code of Practice for Patient Handling (Royal College of Nursing 2002)

The EEC Directive 90/269/EEC (Commission of European Communities 1990)

The Health and Safety at Work Act (HSMO 1974), the lifting equipment regulations (LOLER; Health and Safety Executive 1998b) and provision and use of work equipment regulations (PUWER; Health and Safety Executive 1998c)

You should also review the anatomy and physiology of the spinal column and main joints and muscles of the body. Your focus should be on the curves of the spine and the make-up of vertebrae and discs as well as the inherent problems relating to 'slipped' discs and their presentation

Review your local policy on safer moving and handling as well as the current theories on safe and efficient moving and handling practices. The Guide to the Handling of People (Smith 2005) is a good place to start

You should also revise the Guidelines for Safer Handling during Resuscitation in Hospital (Resuscitation Council 2001)

Review incidence and demographics of manual handling injuries on the Health and Safety website (http://www.hse.gov.uk)

Review what is meant by unsafe moves such as drag lift, cradle lift, shoulder lift or Australian lift, pivot transfers, and moves where the handler is directly in front of the patient.

Clinical Nursing Practices

Indications and rationale for moving and handling	Moving and handling should be considered as: ▪ any transporting or supporting of a load – including the lifting, putting down, pushing, pulling, carrying, throwing and moving by hand or bodily force (Health and Safety Executive 1998a, p. 6). With this definition in mind, as a nurse, moving and handling encompasses all of our work practices and in order to practise safely all nursing tasks should be underpinned by the principles presented in this chapter. It is not solely about moving patients/clients who are unable to move themselves but it includes walking, moving equipment and furniture and even carrying small loads and it impacts on all aspects of our lives.
Outline of the procedure	Before starting any moving and handling task you should first ask the question, 'Do I need to do this task?' Following this you should undertake a risk assessment. By undertaking a risk assessment you should be made aware of any potential problems and how big they might be. In assessing the risk you should not only consider what you are moving but also yourself, the environment and the task. An easy way to remember this is to use the acronyms LITE or TILE. These letters stand for: L = Load (the patient, package, piece of equipment, etc.) I = Individual (you the nurse) T = Task (what it is you need to do) E = Environment. These four areas of assessment are not independent of each other but should be assessed together. The implications of how they impact on each other should be considered. This is not an easy thing to do as in a survey of D and E grade nurses 82 variables were generated for the load alone (Cook & Nendick 1999). When assessing the load, consider the size, shape and weight of it. If it is a patient/client ask yourself whether they can move themselves. All nurses have struggled at some point to move a patient only to discover them wandering up the corridor independently later. The stability of the load also needs consideration. If it is likely to behave unpredictably this puts you at the highest level of risk. Once you have assessed the load you should assess yourself. Consider your state of health, because when we are 'under the weather' we do not work to our full capacity. Reflect on whether you fully understand what you are being asked to do and if you really know what is involved. If you intend using a piece of equipment ensure that you know what the weight limits are for it and how it operates. When considering the task, i.e. what it is you want to do, identify whether it involves distances, variations in height, and/or use of equipment. Your assessment of the environment should involve the type of floor, height and movability of furniture, the amount of space around the area and the visibility of the area. Once this assessment has been completed it should be recorded in the patient's handling record and only after all this has been completed are you ready to consider the move. When starting the move you should ensure that taking an ergonomic approach means that the task is prepared to suit you and that does not mean you adapting

to the task. This may mean ensuring that you have room to move, that beds/chairs that are height adjustable are altered to suit you. Next you need to think about your positioning and movement pattern (Box 25.1). Start by moving in close to your patient before finding your centre of gravity. By being close to your load you will make the load feel lighter. If you hold the load away from your body it will affect your centre of gravity and stability and make the load feel heavier and less stable. You can test this by holding a heavy folder at arms' length for a minute. You will experience how heavy it begins to feel. If you then hold it close to your chest for the same length of time you will discover that the folder feels much lighter.

In adults the imaginary 'centre of gravity' point lies near the base of the spine and should always be anchored within the pelvic girdle. If suspended from this point the body would, in theory, balance (Fig. 25.1). The feet form what is called the 'base' and if the centre of gravity moves out beyond the 'base', the body will become unbalanced and fall unless all the major muscles of the trunk and legs tense to hold the body upright. A prolonged period of imbalance can lead to stress and strain of these muscles and ultimately injury and pain (Fig. 25.2). Widening the 'base' to keep the centre of gravity within the baseline will help to avoid this and lead to more safe and efficient movement. However, too wide a base will also unbalance you. Your feet should be between shoulder and hip width apart and your knees should be soft not locked or bent.

BOX 25.1
Positioning and movement pattern

Once you have found your base:
- Offset your feet so that you are ready to move in the direction in which you want to go
- Lower your bottom and tuck it under as this ensures your centre of gravity is centred
- Gently relax your shoulders before taking a hold of your load using a flat palm. Hand holds will need to be adjusted to suit the size and height of your load but the important thing is to avoid grasping
- Once you have a hold of your load bob down slightly and lead with your head into the move. This gives your rise more momentum and makes the move more efficient.

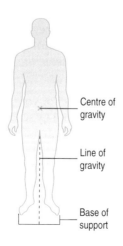

Centre of
gravity

Line of
gravity

Base of
support

FIGURE 25.1
Centre of gravity

Clinical Nursing Practices

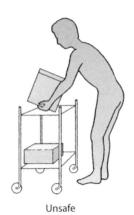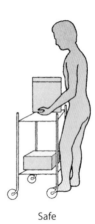

Unsafe   Safe

FIGURE 25.2
Examples of safe and unsafe lifting

Equipment

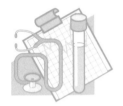

1. As decided on the risk assessment form.

Health and Safety Regulations, i.e. The Operations and Lifting Equipment Regulations (Health and Safety Executive 1998b) and the Provision and Use of Work Equipment Regulations (Health and Safety Executive 1998c) apply to all items of patient moving and handling equipment including the maintenance of slings and hoists.

Nurses are accountable for their actions and prior to using any lifting aid they should ensure that the manufacturer's instructions for use are available and are complied with. In their study published in 2003, Swain et al identified that lack of available equipment meant nurses moved patients manually, which contravened the first duty of Manual Handling Operations Regulations (1992), i.e. to avoid manual handling whenever possible. However, Brown (2004) found that as well as a lack of availability of equipment, the suitability of the equipment needed to be taken into account, particularly manually operated hoists and wheelchairs. Student nurses in Brown's survey identified that using certain pieces of equipment had caused some damage to the arm and shoulder girdle and had strained the lower back.

Slings should be cleaned in line with manufacture guidelines and checked for any wear prior to each use.

Hoists should display the most recent mechanical check by the manufacturer. These checks should be carried out at six-monthly intervals. Any problems should be reported to the maintenance department immediately and the hoist should be withdrawn from use.

Guidelines and rationale for this nursing practice

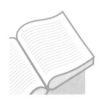

You are responsible for your own health and safety and also that of others who may be affected by what you do or fail to do (HMSO 1974). All employers must provide adequate moving and handling training and information to all employees. Written safety policies should also be provided. It is the duty of each nurse to ensure attendance at all moving and handling induction and update sessions. The NMC Code of Professional Conduct (2004) states that not only are you accountable for your own actions but that it is your responsibility to keep your knowledge and skills up to date. If an area of practice, e.g. safe moving and handling, is outside your level of competency you must obtain help and appropriate supervision. This responsibility extends to all other colleagues encountered in the workplace. If you have reason to believe their practice is unsafe or puts the patient at risk you must protect your patient and report your colleague to a senior person.

The NHS Quality Improvement Scotland (NHS QIS) Standards for Clinical Governance and Risk Management came into effect in November 2005. These standards, as applied to moving and handling, should ensure that organisations are accountable for monitoring and improving the quality of their services. Additionally, there should be a systematic identification and evaluation of risk. All staff should be fully supported and adequately trained in safe moving and handling to enable them to contribute to safe effective patient-focused care.

- in undertaking this practice, nurses are accountable for their actions, the quality of care delivered and record-keeping according to the Code of Professional Conduct: Standards for Conduct, Performance and Ethics (Nursing and Midwifery Council 2004) and Guidelines for Records and Record Keeping (Nursing and Midwifery Council 2005).

Patient/carer education
Key points

There has been some recent academic debate (Griffith & Stevens 2004), which has highlighted that the dignity and distress of the patient must be considered when they are asked to comply with a move that they are unwilling to undertake, i.e. be moved by a mechanical hoist. It is important, therefore, that nurses ensure that they consider the wishes of their patient and use effective communication skills to negotiate a solution with the patient with regard to safe moving and handling.

In order to provide patient-centred care, power and authority must be transferred from the nurse to the patient (Russell 2003). Professionals often assume that patients do not comply with what they are asked to do because they do not understand the evidence presented to them. More time should be taken to listen to the patient's point of view and to discuss the safest way to move them. This may involve demonstrating and explaining the benefits of lifting equipment. The more dynamic the relationship between the nurse and patient the easier it should be for the nurse to understand the patient's point of view and for them to arrive at a solution that is agreeable to both. According to Russell (2003) to increase patient compliance acceptance of the patient's point of view is necessary, not education or coercion.

Many patients in the community depend on relatives or friends to help them move. Healthcare professionals must ensure that a risk assessment has been carried out and that the carers have been taught to take an ergonomic approach to moving and handling. It must also be ensured that they are competent in using any necessary moving aids.

References

Brown AM 2004 A descriptive survey of the moving and handling experiences of student nurses in one school of nursing and midwifery and their thoughts on the teaching they received. Unpublished dissertation, RCN, London

Commission of European Communities (CEC) 1990 Council Directives of 29th May 1990 (90/269/EEC) on the minimum health and safety requirements for the manual handling of loads where there is a risk particularly of back injury to workers. Fourth Individual Directive within the meaning of Article 16 (1) of Directive 89/391/EEC. Official Journal of the European Communities, NO L 156/9–13, Brussels

Cook G, Nendick C 1999 Manual handling: what patient factors do nurses assess? Journal of Clinical Nursing 8(4): 422–430

Griffith R, Stevens M 2004 Manual handling and the lawfulness of no lifting policies. Nursing Standard 18(21): 39–43

Health and Safety Executive 1998a Guidance on manual handling regulations. HMSO, Norwich

Health and Safety Executive 1998b Lifting operations and lifting equipment regulations (LOLER). HMSO, London

Health and Safety Executive 1998c Provision and use of work equipment regulations. HMSO, London

HMSO 1974 Health and Safety at Work Act. HMSO, London

MHOR 1992 Manual Handling Operations Regulations 1992. UK Government Statutory Instrument No 2392. HMSO, London

National Health Service 2002 Back in work back pack. Department of Health, London

NHS Quality Improvement Scotland 2005 Standards for clinical governance and risk management. Scottish Executive, Edinburgh

Nursing and Midwifery Council 2004 Code of professional conduct: standards for conduct, performance and ethics. NMC, London

Nursing and Midwifery Council 2005 Guidelines for records and record keeping. NMC, London

Resuscitation Council 2001 Guidance for safer handling during resuscitation in hospital. Resuscitation Council (UK), London

Retsas A, Pinikahana J 2000 Manual handling activities and injuries among nurses: an Australian hospital study. Journal of Advanced Nursing 31(4): 875–883

Royal College of Nursing 2002 Code of practice for patient handling. RCN, London

Royal College of Nursing 2005 The guide to the handling of people, 5th edn. National Back Pain Association, Teddington, UK

Russell S 2003 Nurses and 'difficult' patients: negotiating non compliance. Journal of Advanced Nursing 43(3): 281–287

Smith J (ed) 2005 The guide to the handling of people, 5th edn. National Back Pain Association (BackCare)/Royal College of Nursing, Teddington, UK

Swain J, Pufahl E, Williamson G 2003 Do they practice what we teach? A survey of manual handling practice amongst student nurses. Journal of Clinical Nursing 12(2): 297–306

Website

UK Government health and safety website: http://www.hse.gov.uk

Self assessment

1. In what year did the Manual Handling Operations Regulations come into force?
2. Name the four main factors to be considered when undertaking a moving and handling assessment.
3. Identify two manual lifts that are considered unsafe.
4. What does ergonomic mean?
5. Identify the stages of positioning oneself prior to any moving and handling task.

Practice 26
Nebuliser Therapy

Learning outcomes	**By the end of this section, you should know how to:** ▪ prepare the patient for this nursing practice ▪ collect and prepare the equipment ▪ administer drugs via a nebuliser, either in the community or in an institutional setting ▪ maintain equipment safely before and after nebulisation ▪ document drug administration (Nursing and Midwifery Council 2004b).
Background knowledge required	Revision of anatomy and physiology of the respiratory system Revision of 'Oxygen therapy' (*see* p. 245) Revision of 'Administration of medicines' (*see* p. 13). Revision of local policy on nebuliser therapy.
Indications and rationale for using nebuliser therapy	Nebulisers allow drugs to be administered directly into the lower respiratory tract. Drugs are usually available in solution, in single use containers called nebules. A nebuliser attached to a flow of air or oxygen converts the solution of a drug into an aerosol for therapeutic inhalation (British Thoracic Society 2004). The nebuliser will convert the drug into respirable particles that are small enough (2–5 microns in diameter) to reach the bronchioles. Lung deposition of the drug will be dependent upon the particle and droplet size, the type of nebuliser chamber, the volume of fluid, the flow rate of gas driving the nebuliser as well as the patient's respiratory pattern. Treatment with nebulisers aims to deliver a therapeutic dose of a drug within a reasonably short period of time, i.e. between 5 and 10 minutes (British Thoracic Society 2004). Nebulisers can be useful when a large dose of a drug is required, or if a patient is unable to use any other device to inhale a drug, often in an acute situation. Nebulised drugs can be used without the need for the patient to co-ordinate breathing with inhalation, unlike using inhalers. Occasionally drugs for inhalation are unavailable in other forms of inhalers. Nebulised drugs are used for patients with primary respiratory diseases such as asthma (Rees & Kanabar 2006) and also for patients with other diseases with respiratory symptoms, such as cancer or heart failure. Thus, the nebuliser can be used in acute, emergency situations such as acute asthma or chronic obstructive pulmonary disease (COPD), in primary health care or institutional settings. Equally, routine use for chronic disease management or palliative care can also occur in different care settings. Common reasons for using nebulisers are: ▪ ***to administer bronchodilators,*** e.g. —asthma —COPD

- **to administer nebulised sodium chloride 0.9%** to aid expectoration, e.g.
  —palliative care
- **to administer an antibiotic** (British Thoracic Society 2003, 2004, Rees & Kanabar 2006), e.g.
  —cystic fibrosis
  —HIV.

The drug and driving gas for the nebuliser is prescribed by a medical practitioner and is often administered by the nurse. Sometimes treatment will be co-ordinated with chest physiotherapy. Compressed air is the most common driving gas used although high-flow oxygen may be used during an acute asthmatic event. A flow rate of 6–8 L min^{-1} is required for either air or oxygen to ensure the drug particle size is small enough to allow lung deposition and drug effectiveness. For patients who have acute severe asthma, it is recommended that the driving gas is oxygen, to prevent desaturation of oxygen during nebulisation. For patients who have COPD, it is recommended that the driving gas is air to prevent diminishing the hypoxic drive leading to hypercapnia.

If long-term domiciliary nebuliser treatment is needed, the patient may become efficient in his or her own self-care using nebuliser treatment at home, with access to a local nebuliser service for ongoing support and education as well as maintenance of equipment.

There are currently three main types of nebuliser with research ongoing to create ones that have improved efficiency of drug delivery (Esmond 2001):
- **jet**: is most commonly used
- **ultrasonic**: is a more expensive system
- **adaptive aerosol delivery**: provides more precise drug delivery.

The decision to use a mask or mouthpiece depends upon the individual patient and the drug being administered. Some patients may be unable to hold a mouthpiece and so a mask would be more suitable. Some drugs have side effects and it is recommended that they are used in conjunction with either a mask or mouthpiece. For example, anticholinergic drugs (e.g. Ipratropium Bromide) can cause eye problems (glaucoma) and are better suited to a mouthpiece (British Thoracic Society 2004). It is important to follow the manufacturer's instructions to ensure the most appropriate delivery devices and equipment are used to maximise drug delivery and minimise side effects to the patient.

For some patients requiring nebulisation, it is important to measure Peak Expiratory Flow Rate (PEFR) before and after nebulisation to measure the effectiveness of drug administration. It is commonly required in patients with asthma (Rees & Kanabar 2006).

Equipment

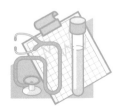

1. Prescribed air supply: most commonly an electric or battery-operated air compressor
2. Prescribed oxygen supply, either piped or in cylinders
3. Oxygen tubing
4. Nebuliser (Fig. 26.1)
5. Mouthpiece or appropriate oxygen mask (Fig. 26.1)
6. Prescribed drugs

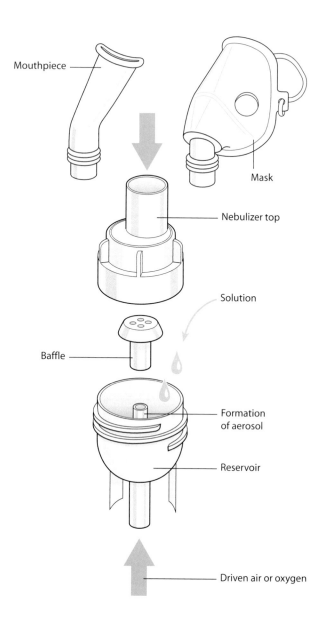

Mouthpiece

Mask

Nebulizer top

Solution

Baffle

Formation of aerosol

Reservoir

Driven air or oxygen

FIGURE 26.1
Jet nebuliser
From Brooker & Nicol
2003, with permission

7. Sputum carton as required
8. 'No Smoking' signs as appropriate (*see* 'Oxygen therapy', p. 245)
9. Receptacle for soiled disposable items.

For peak flow measurement

1. Peak flow meter (Fig. 26.2)
2. Disposable mouthpiece
3. Specific chart for documenting the results.

1. Fit disposable mouthpiece to peak flow meter

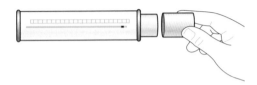

2. Ensure patient stands up or sits upright and holds peak flow meter horizontally without restricting movement of the marker. Ensure the marker is at the bottom of the scale

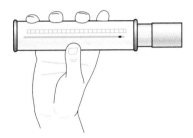

3. Ask patient to breathe in deeply, seal lips around mouthpiece and breathe out as quickly as possible

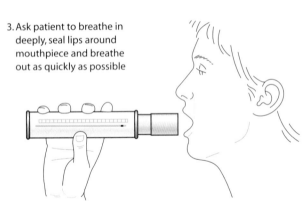

4. Repeat steps 2 and 3 twice more. Choose and record the highest of the three readings

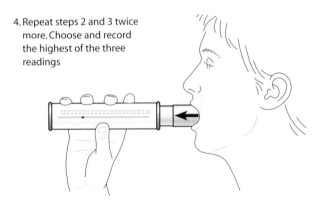

FIGURE 26.2
Measuring peak expiratory flow rate (PEFR)
From Brooker & Nicol 2003, with permission

Guidelines and rationale for this nursing practice

- explain the nursing practice to the patient *to gain consent and co-operation, to encourage participation in care and reduce anxiety*
- explain to the patient that they should breath normally during nebulisation *to enhance drug deposition*
- explain to the patient they should avoid talking during nebulisation *to enhance drug deposition*
- ensure the patient's privacy *to respect individuality and maintain self-esteem*
- prepare and assemble the equipment *to ensure efficient administration of the drug*
- if oxygen is the driving gas for nebulisation, explain the dangers of smoking to the patient and his or her family/carers, positioning the 'No Smoking' signs as appropriate, thus *making sure that they understand that there is an increased risk of fire when oxygen is being administered*
- if indicated, help the patient to measure their PEFR by recording the best of three results on the peak flow meter before commencing nebuliser therapy *to help to evaluate the effects of the treatment*
- help the patient into a comfortable position, upright if possible, *so that he or she will tolerate the therapy without distress*
- prepare the patient for the noise of the nebuliser *to minimise anxiety and encourage concordance*
- identify and check the drug administration prescription (*see* 'Administration of medicines', p. 13). to ensure safe administration of the drug and to fulfil *professional requirements for drug administration*
- if more than one drug is prescribed, follow manufacturer's instructions *to ensure correct equipment is used as some drugs cannot be mixed and some drugs require particular nebuliser chambers*
- fill the nebuliser chamber with the prepared medication, *keeping the nebuliser chamber upright to avoid spillage of the drug* (Fig. 26.3)

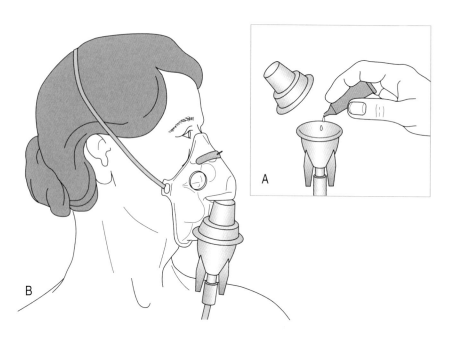

FIGURE 26.3
Adding the nebuliser solution
From Nicol et al 2003, with permission

- connect the equipment together *to ensure efficient drug delivery*
- turn on the air compressor or oxygen source *to ensure the drug will be converted into an aerosol*
- observe the fine spray from the nebuliser *to check that the equipment is working*
- encourage the patient to breathe the nebulised aerosol through the mouthpiece or mask *for maximum effect*
- observe the patient closely during nebulisation *to monitor the effects and watch for side effects such as tremor or tachycardia*
- time the nebulisation *as nebulisation should take no more than 10 minutes*. There may still be solution in the nebuliser chamber after this time, however when the noise of the nebuliser changes from a hissing to a spluttering of the solution turn off the nebuliser
- encourage the patient to expectorate *if the medication has been prescribed to loosen the bronchial secretions*
- offer the patient oral hygiene *as some drugs can cause huskiness and oral candidiasis*
- ensure that the patient is left feeling as comfortable as possible
- measure and record the patient's PEFR if indicated *to monitor the effect of treatment*
- wash and dry the nebuliser, tubing and mask or mouthpiece according to manufacturer's instructions and local policy *to minimise the risk of infection and ensure equipment remains functional*
- follow the manufacturer's instructions and local policy for safe storage of the equipment *to comply with health and safety needs regarding infection control*
- monitor the patient's respiratory rate and pulse according to instructions *to provide ongoing information of their clinical status*
- document the nursing practice appropriately, monitor after-effects and report any abnormal findings immediately *to ensure safe practice and enable prompt, appropriate medical and nursing intervention to be initiated*
- in undertaking this practice, nurses are accountable for their actions, the quality of care delivered and record keeping according to the Code of Professional Conduct: Standards for Conduct, Performance and Ethics (Nursing and Midwifery Council 2004a), Guidelines for the Administration of Medicines (Nursing and Midwifery Council 2004b) and Guidelines for Records and Record Keeping (Nursing and Midwifery Council 2005).

Additional information　　If oxygen is used, all precautions to prevent the risk of fire should be maintained, as with 'Oxygen therapy' (*see* p. 245).

This is not a sterile procedure, but adequate standards of cleanliness should be maintained. The nurse should wash his or her hands before commencing and on completing this nursing practice. The equipment for each patient should be kept clean and dry when not in use. It should be changed according to manufacturer's instructions to prevent infection.

Regular maintenance checks of all equipment should be carried out as per local policy.

During the nursing practice itself, the patient will not be encouraged to speak.

The solution is normally administered over a period of up to 10 minutes, which can be explained to the patient.

Monitor the respiration rate and depth and type of respiration, taking readings as frequently as required. The patient should take deep regular breaths through the mouthpiece of the nebuliser to ensure that the medication reaches the mucosa of the bronchi and bronchioles rather than just the oropharynx. Patients will often experience less dyspnoea after this procedure, and there may be a dramatic relief of bronchospasm for patients with asthma. This can be monitored by peak flow recording over a period of time.

Observe and record the amount, colour and type of any sputum.

A healthy mouth and oropharyngeal mucosa is essential for maximum absorption of the medication. Frequent oral hygiene should therefore be performed as appropriate. A mouthwash after expectorating may be appreciated and should be available if desired.

Patient/carer education Key points 	In partnership with the patient and/or carer, ensure that they understand the goals of treatment. The reason for the nebuliser therapy should be carefully explained to the patient and his or her family so that concordance is continued and the patient feels empowered. If oxygen is used for nebulisation, information about fire risks and the precautions needed should be explained (*see* 'Oxygen therapy', p. 245). If the patient is self-caring, instructions about preparing the medication and using the equipment should be given, and the nurse should ensure that these continue to be followed correctly. At home, the nurse should ensure that the patient and carers keep the equipment clean and separate from other household equipment, in order to maintain a safe environment. In the home, patient and family should have written instructions regarding the care and maintenance of the equipment. Contact with the provider of the nebuliser should be made available to encourage regular servicing of the equipment to ensure its effectiveness. A telephone contact for an appropriate member of the healthcare team should be provided. The patient should understand the importance of immediately reporting any changes in respiratory function, such as increased dyspnoea, cough or sputum, or any general feeling of distress (National Institute for Clinical Excellence 2004).

References

British Thoracic Society 2003 British guideline on the management of asthma: a national clinical guideline. BTS, London

British Thoracic Society 2004 British guideline on the management of chronic obstructive airways disease: a national clinical guideline. BTS, London

Brooker C, Nicol M 2003 Nursing adults: the practice of caring. Mosby, Edinburgh

Esmond G 2001 Respiratory nursing. Ballière Tindall, Edinburgh

National Institute for Clinical Excellence 2004 Chronic obstructive pulmonary disease: management of chronic obstructive pulmonary disease in adults in primary and secondary care. NICE, London

Nicol M, Bavin C, Bedford-Turner S et al 2003 Essential nursing skills, 2nd edn. Mosby, London

Nursing and Midwifery Council 2004a Code of professional conduct: standards for conduct, performance and ethics. NMC, London

Nursing and Midwifery Council 2004b Guidelines for the administration of medicines. NMC, London

Nursing and Midwifery Council 2005 Guidelines for records and record keeping. NMC, London

Rees J, Kanabar D 2006 The ABC of asthma, 5th edn. Blackwell, Oxford

Websites
British Thoracic Society: http://www.brit-thoracic.org.uk
Scottish Intercollegiate Guidelines Network: http://www.sign.ac.uk

Self assessment

1. What are the benefits of administering drugs via a nebuliser?
2. What information would the patient need to be given before nebulisation?
3. Consider any patient you have seen using a nebuliser and think about why it was appropriate for the patient.
4. How can peak flow measurement (PEFR) help to measure the response to treatment with nebulised bronchodilators?
5. What information would a carer need to support a patient on domiciliary nebuliser therapy?

Practice 27
Neurological Examination

Learning outcomes	**By the end of this section, you should know how to:** ▪ prepare and support the patient for a neurological examination ▪ collect and prepare the equipment ▪ if required, assist the medical practitioner during the neurological examination.
Background knowledge required	Revision of the anatomy and physiology of the nervous system Revision of 'Care of the unconscious patient' (*see* p. 351).
Indications and rationale for neurological examination	Neurological examination is a method of obtaining some objective data on the functioning of a patient's nervous system (Hickey 2003). This may be required: ▪ ***to aid in the diagnosis of a neurological disease*** ▪ ***to monitor the effect of a neurological disease*** ▪ ***to aid in the assessment of treatment during the course of a neurological disease***.
Outline of the procedure	This procedure is carried out by a medical or skilled nurse practitioner, usually in conjunction with an examination of the motor and sensory function of the patient's trunk and limbs. The ophthalmoscope and pen torch are used to assess the function of the optic, oculomotor, trochlear and ophthalmic branch of the trigeminal cranial nerves. The auriscope and tuning fork are used to examine the ears and assess the function of the vestibulocochlear cranial nerve respectively. An assessment of the patient's sensation to pain, touch and temperature is made using a sterile needle, a cotton-wool ball and test tubes of hot and cold water. The olfactory cranial nerve is assessed when the patient is asked to identify the odours of various strong-smelling substances. The tendon hammer is used by the medical practitioner when testing a spinal reflex such as the knee jerk. Assessment for an upper motor neurone lesion will also require the use of a tendon hammer for stroking the lateral aspect of the sole of the patient's foot. The function of the facial cranial nerve is assessed by asking the patient to identify various substances, i.e. salt, sugar, vinegar and lemon juice. To prevent inaccurate results, the patient will be asked to use a mouth rinse after each substance has been tasted.
Equipment 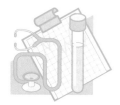	1. Ophthalmoscope 2. Pen torch 3. Auriscope 4. Tuning fork 5. Sterile injection needle

6. Non-sterile cotton-wool balls
7. Test tubes filled with hot and cold water
8. Small containers of various strong-smelling substances, e.g. peppermint and oil of cloves
9. Tendon hammer
10. Small samples of salt, sugar, lemon juice and vinegar
11. Glass of water for rinsing the patient's mouth
12. Trolley or tray for equipment
13. Receptacle for used mouth rinse
14. Receptacle for soiled disposable items.

Guidelines and rationale for this nursing practice

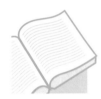

- help to explain the procedure to the patient **to gain consent and co-operation**
- wash the hands **to reduce cross-infection**
- prepare the equipment **to ensure that all the equipment is available and ready for use**
- ensure the patient's privacy **to reduce anxiety**
- observe the patient throughout this activity **to note any signs of distress**
- help the patient into a comfortable position **to allow the patient to maintain the position and to provide easy access for the practitioner**
- assist the medical practitioner during the examination **to enhance the overall quality of the procedure**
- ensure that the patient is left feeling as comfortable as possible, thus **maintaining the quality of this nursing practice**
- dispose of the equipment safely **to reduce any health hazard**
- document the nursing practice appropriately, monitor the after-effects and report any abnormal findings immediately, **providing a written record and assisting in the implementation of any action should an abnormality or adverse reaction to the practice be noted**
- in undertaking this practice, nurses are accountable for their actions, the quality of care delivered and record-keeping according to the Code of Professional Conduct: Standards for Conduct, Performance and Ethics (Nursing and Midwifery Council 2004) and Guidelines for Records and Record Keeping (Nursing and Midwifery Council 2005).

Patient/carer education
Key points

In partnership with the patient and/or carer, ensure that they are competent to carry out any practices required. Information should be given on an appropriate point of contact for any concerns that may arise.

The patient should be given an initial explanation of the procedure by the medical practitioner, but the nurse may need to repeat this. The patient should have the initial results of the examination explained and discussed (Hickey 2003).

References

Hickey J 2003 Neurological assessment. In: Hickey J (ed) The clinical practice of neurological and neurosurgical nursing, 5th edn. Lippinicott Williams & Wilkins, Philadelphia, PA
Nursing and Midwifery Council 2004 Code of professional conduct: standards for conduct, performance and ethics. NMC, London

Nursing and Midwifery Council 2005 Guidelines for records and record keeping. NMC, London

Websites

Multiple Sclerosis Society: http://www.mssociety.org.uk

The Stroke Association: http://www.stroke.org.uk

Self assessment

1. What equipment is used to assess the function of the optic, oculomotor, trochlear and ophthalmic branch of the trigeminal nerves?
2. How can the patient's responses to pain, touch and temperature be assessed?

Practice 28
Nutrition

There are three parts to this section:

1 Feeding a dependent patient

2 Enteral feeding

3 Parenteral nutrition

1. FEEDING A DEPENDENT PATIENT

Learning outcomes

By the end of this section, you should know how to:
- prepare the patient for this nursing practice
- collect and prepare the equipment
- carry out the feeding of a dependent patient.

Background knowledge required

Revision of the anatomy and physiology of the mouth and oesophagus, with special reference to the physical acts of mastication and swallowing.

Indications and rationale for the feeding of a dependent patient

The nurse may be required to feed a dependent patient **to maintain adequate nutrition in**:
- a patient who is unable to use his or her upper limbs because of paralysis or serious illness
- a patient who has lost upper limb co-ordination because of a physical or mental disease
- a patient who has recently lost his or her eyesight
- a patient who has an injury around the mouth.

Equipment

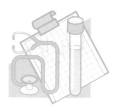

1. Feeding utensils such as a fork, knife, spoon, drinking cup with a spout or cup with an angled straw
2. A cloth, disposable napkin or paper towel
3. Diet, as ordered by the patient
4. Trolley or tray for equipment
5. Receptacle for soiled disposable items.

Clinical Nursing Practices

Guidelines and rationale for this nursing practice

In hospital or at home, this practice may be undertaken by the patient's relatives or carers.

- explain the nursing practice to the patient **to gain consent and co-operation**
- collect and prepare the equipment **to ensure that all the equipment is available and ready for use**
- help the patient into a comfortable position **to allow easy access to the patient by the nurse and also allow the patient to maintain his or her position during the practice**
- observe the patient throughout this activity **to note any signs of distress**
- wash the hands and put on an apron **for general hygiene purposes and to reduce the risk of cross-infection**
- **for patient satisfaction and enjoyment**, keep the food not being eaten at a suitable temperature
- remind the patient of his or her ordered menu **to permit psychological preparation for the food**
- when possible, the nurse should sit down while feeding the patient **so that this is made an enjoyable social occasion**
- ask the patient which food he or she wishes to eat first, thereby **giving the patient some control over the activity**
- offer the food to patients at a rate set by them **as hurrying them while they are eating may induce nausea or vomiting**
- **to prevent gagging or choking**, place the spoon or fork accurately into the patient's mouth
- offer sips of fluid during the meal **to aid in the mastication and swallowing of the food**
- discontinue feeding when asked by the patient in order **to prevent a feeling of distension and excessive fullness**
- assist the patient with mouth care following the meal **as this will promote dental health and may reduce the incidence of dental caries**
- ensure that the patient is left feeling as comfortable as possible, thus **maintaining the quality of this nursing practice**
- dispose of equipment safely **to reduce any health hazard**
- document the nursing practice appropriately, monitor the after-effects and report any abnormal findings immediately, **thus providing a written record and assisting in the implementation of any action should an abnormality or adverse reaction to the practice be noted**
- in undertaking this practice, nurses are accountable for their actions, the quality of care delivered and record-keeping according to the Code of Professional Conduct: Standards for Conduct, Performance and Ethics (Nursing and Midwifery Council 2004) and Guidelines for Records and Record Keeping (Nursing and Midwifery Council 2005).

Patient/carer education

Key points

Advice on a healthy dietary intake and the benefits of such a diet should be given by the nurse to both the patient and the carers. The nurse should provide information and education on the constituents of any special diet that is required by the patient.

Information regarding the maintenance of oral health should also be given by the nurse.

2. ENTERAL FEEDING

There are two parts to this section:

A Enteral feeding via a nasogastric tube as an intermittent bolus or continuous enteral feed

B Enteral feeding via a gastrostomy/jejunostomy tube.

Learning outcomes

By the end of this section, you should know how to:
- prepare the patient for this nursing practice
- collect and prepare the equipment
- describe the principles of enteral feeding
- outline some of the problems of enteral feeding.

Background knowledge required

Revision of the anatomy and physiology of the gastrointestinal tract
Revision of the nutritional requirements of the human body.

Indications and rationale for enteral feeding

Enteral feeding is the introduction of the daily nutritional requirements, in liquid form, directly into a patient's stomach or small intestine by means of a tube. The tube may be inserted through the nostril and passed down into the stomach, or introduced directly into the stomach or small intestine via a surgical incision made in the abdominal wall.

Enteral feeding may be performed **to maintain adequate nutrition** in the following circumstances:
- obstruction of the oesophagus, e.g. by a neoplasm
- loss of the swallowing reflex
- oesophageal fistula
- preoperative preparation of malnourished patients
- during radiotherapy treatment
- postoperatively for patients who have had some types of oral surgery, or oesophageal surgery
- some unconscious patients
- patients who have severe burns.

Enteral feeding can be administered in several ways. It may be given through a fine tube with its own administration set and container for the feed, or it can be channelled through a pump. Enteral feeds may also be introduced via a self-retaining tube such as a Foley's catheter or percutaneous endoscopic gastrostomy (PEG) tube via a surgical opening in the abdominal wall into the stomach, duodenum or jejunum. The liquid feed is usually purchased ready prepared, which can greatly reduce the potential of health care-associated infection (National Institute for Clinical Excellence 2003).

2A. ENTERAL FEEDING VIA A NASOGASTRIC TUBE AS AN INTERMITTENT BOLUS OR CONTINUOUS ENTERAL FEED

Equipment

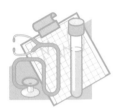

1. Enteral feeding tube and introducer
2. Lubricant, e.g. iced water or jelly
3. Hypoallergenic tape
4. Container with prepared feed
5. Enteral feed administration set
6. Intravenous infusion stand
7. Gravity or volumetric pump if required
8. Water
9. Syringe (50 ml)
10. Gallipot, syringe and pH indicator strips
11. Stethoscope
12. Receptacle for soiled disposable items.

The second syringe should be a 10 ml size if a fine-bore tube is being used or a 50 ml catheter-tip syringe for a Ryles-type tube.

Guidelines and rationale for this nursing practice

- explain the nursing practice to the patient *to gain consent and co-operation*
- collect and prepare the equipment *for efficiency of practice*
- help the patient into a comfortable position, ideally sitting upright (Smith et al 1999) but otherwise at an angle of 30–45° (Murray 2000)
- observe the patient throughout this activity *to detect any signs of discomfort or distress*
- insert the enteral feeding tube as described in 'Gastric aspiration' (*see* p. 147) and then remove the introducer or assist the qualified practitioner as requested
- before commencing the feed, an X-ray is necessary *to confirm the position of the tube* as the lumen is too narrow to allow the usual tests to be carried out and it is necessary to ascertain that the tube has been correctly positioned. If a Ryles-type tube has been used the correct positioning of the tube can be checked by flushing the tube with 20 ml of air to ensure that it is clear (Dougherty & Lister 2004). A small amount of stomach contents is then

aspirated and placed in the gallipot. The pH-sensitive paper can then be dipped into it. A pH of 3 or less indicates stomach contents

- attach the prepared feed in the container to the infusion stand
- join the administration set to the container using a non-touch technique (Smith et al 1999) and allow the feed to run through to the end of the set before it is connected to the feeding tube *so that as little air as possible is introduced into the patient's stomach*
- adjust the flow rate as required or connect to the appropriate pump and ensure the rate of flow is as prescribed *so that the patient's stomach does not become over-distended and produce feelings of nausea*
- when intermittent bolus feeding is the method of choice, run some water through at the end of the feed *to clear the tube*
- ensure that the patient is left feeling as comfortable as possible, thus *maintaining the quality of this practice*
- record appropriately the time of commencement of feeding and the amount and type of feed given, monitor the after-effects and report any abnormal findings immediately, *providing a written record and assisting in the implementation of any action should an abnormality or adverse reaction to the practice be noted*
- in undertaking this practice, nurses are accountable for their actions, the quality of care delivered and record-keeping according to the Code of Professional Conduct: Standards for Conduct, Performance and Ethics (Nursing and Midwifery Council 2004) and Guidelines for Records and Record Keeping (Nursing and Midwifery Council 2005).

Narrow-bore tubes for continuous enteral feeding are made of silicone or polyurethane, with a diameter ranging from 1 to 3 mm. They are more comfortable for the patient than the wide-bore tube and less likely to cause ulceration, inflammation, stricture, haemorrhage and erosion of the mucosa (Woods 1998). They do, however, become blocked more easily, and it is almost impossible to clear them by aspiration.

2B. ENTERAL FEEDING VIA A GASTROSTOMY/JEJUNOSTOMY TUBE (FIG. 28.1)

Equipment

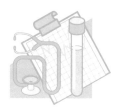

1. Water
2. Syringe
3. Prepared feed in its container
4. Enteral feed administration set
5. Enteral feed pump if required
6. Intravenous infusion stand if required
7. Receptacle for soiled disposable items.

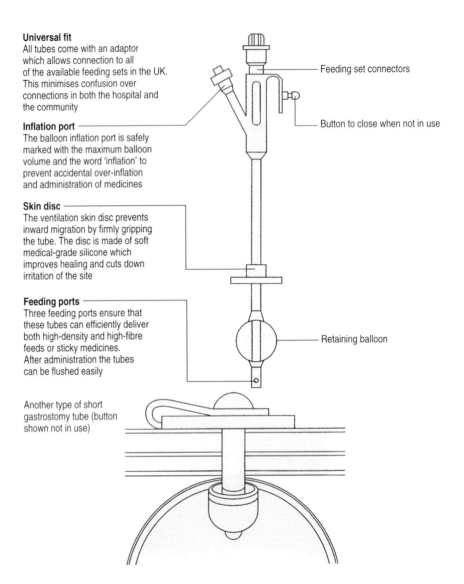

Universal fit
All tubes come with an adaptor which allows connection to all of the available feeding sets in the UK. This minimises confusion over connections in both the hospital and the community

Feeding set connectors

Inflation port
The balloon inflation port is safely marked with the maximum balloon volume and the word 'inflation' to prevent accidental over-inflation and administration of medicines

Button to close when not in use

Skin disc
The ventilation skin disc prevents inward migration by firmly gripping the tube. The disc is made of soft medical-grade silicone which improves healing and cuts down irritation of the site

Feeding ports
Three feeding ports ensure that these tubes can efficiently deliver both high-density and high-fibre feeds or sticky medicines. After administration the tubes can be flushed easily

Retaining balloon

Another type of short gastrostomy tube (button shown not in use)

FIGURE 28.1
Enteral feeding: examples of gastrostomy tubes

Guidelines and rationale for this nursing practice

- explain the nursing practice to the patient **to gain consent and co-operation**. Patients should be encouraged to be active partners in care
- assist the patient into a suitable position, for example semi-recumbent, **to allow easy access to the gastrostomy site and to lessen the risk of a kink in the tube**. The patient should ideally not lie flat as this increases the risk of reflux and aspiration
- observe the patient throughout this activity **to detect any signs of discomfort or distress**
- collect and prepare the equipment **for efficiency of practice**
- insert the administration set into the feed bottle in an aseptic manner **to prevent infection**
- allow the feed to run through the set in order to expel all the air **as unnecessary air introduced into the stomach can cause pain and distension**

- the plastic cap at the end of the administration set should remain in place at this time **to prevent infection**
- flush the tube with about 10–50 ml of water via a syringe **to ensure that the tube is patent**
- insert the administration set into the tube (via the pump if used)
- start the flow by switching on the pump or adjusting the administration set
- disconnect the administration set when all the feed has been delivered
- flush the tube through with water **to clear the tube**
- ensure that the patient is left feeling as comfortable as possible, thus **maintaining the quality of this practice**
- dispose of the equipment safely **to reduce any health hazard**
- record appropriately the time and amount and type of feed administered, monitor the after-effects and report any abnormal findings immediately, **providing a written record and assisting in the implementation of any action should an abnormality or adverse reaction to the practice be noted**
- in undertaking this practice, nurses are accountable for their actions, the quality of care delivered and record-keeping according to the Code of Professional Conduct: Standards for Conduct, Performance and Ethics (Nursing and Midwifery Council 2004) and Guidelines for Records and Record Keeping (Nursing and Midwifery Council 2005).

Patient/carer education
Key points

A clear explanation of the necessity of this form of feeding will help to gain the patient's co-operation. If the patient is self-administering feeds, the importance of hygiene needs to be stressed (National Institute for Clinical Excellence 2003). The feeding pattern also needs to be agreed with the patient.

3. PARENTERAL NUTRITION

Learning outcomes

By the end of this section, you should know how to:
- prepare and support the patient for this nursing practice
- collect and prepare the equipment
- assist the medical practitioner with the insertion of a central venous catheter
- maintain an infusion of parenteral nutrition for a period of time in an institutional or community setting.

Background knowledge required

Revision of the anatomy and physiology of the cardiopulmonary system, with special reference to the circulation of the blood, and the veins of the neck and upper thorax
Revision of the nutritional needs required to maintain health

Revision of 'Intravenous therapy' (*see* p. 169) and 'Care of a Hickman catheter' (*see* p. 181)

Revision of 'Aseptic technique' (*see* p. 341)

Revision of the 'Principles of infection prevention and control' (*see* p. 341)

Review of health authority policy regarding parenteral nutrition in both community and institutional care.

Indications and rationale for parenteral nutrition	Parenteral nutrition is the intravenous infusion of essential nutrients into patients who are unable to maintain an adequate nutritional intake by the oral or nasogastric route (Burnham 1999, Dougherty & Lister 2004). ***It may be indicated for anyone who is unable to ingest, digest or absorb sufficient oral or enteral feeding***, for example:

- patients who have had surgery involving major resection of the intestine as they will have a reduced ability to digest food
- patients who have extensive inflammatory disease of the alimentary system as inflammation of the gut reduces the efficiency of the digestive process
- patients who have malabsorption problems because, despite a reasonable intake, an inadequate amount of nutrients will be absorbed and be available for the cells
- patients who have severe nausea and vomiting, e.g. following chemotherapy for malignant disease. The appetite is reduced, and food will not remain in the stomach long enough for digestion to occur.

'Parenteral nutrition' (PN) is the term used when all the patient's nutritional requirements are given by a central venous catheter. However, it has been demonstrated that some parenteral nutrition solutions can be infused for a short time using a peripheral vein access route. Parenteral nutrition may also be given as a supplement to nasogastric or oral feeding (Zainal 1994).

Outline of the procedure	This procedure should be performed ideally in the operating theatre. If it is performed in the ward, it should take place in the treatment room.

The insertion of the intravenous catheter for the infusion of parenteral nutrition is usually performed by a medical practitioner using an aseptic technique, however some specifically educated and trained nurses are now undertaking this practice in specialised units (Benton & Marsden 2002). A cap and theatre mask are worn. Having washed his or her hands, the medical practitioner dons a theatre gown and gloves, and prepares the sterile equipment on the trolley, maintaining asepsis. When the patient is in the correct position, sterile drapes are placed round the area of the access site. A local anaesthetic may be administered. The skin area of the access site is cleansed prior to the insertion of an intravenous catheter through the subclavian or internal jugular vein to allow the tip of the catheter to lie in the superior vena cava. A flow of prescribed infusion fluid is established, and the distal end of the catheter is stitched in position. The access site is covered with a sterile dressing.

A catheter will occasionally be tunnelled subcutaneously so that the entry site to the vein is separated from the skin entry site; this will reduce the risk of infection. It is performed when long-term parenteral nutrition is envisaged (Benton & Marsden 2002).

The concentration of the nutrients is irritant to peripheral vessels and could cause damage to peripheral veins. The infusion fluid enters the circulation at the superior vena cava, is rapidly diluted by the volume of blood entering the heart and is quickly distributed by the circulation, thus reducing any problems of irritation of the vessels involved.

The position of the patient is important during this procedure and depends on the choice of entry site for catheterisation. There are three main entry sites.

The subclavian vein

The patient lies supine with no pillow, the neck being extended. The head of the bed is lowered by 10°.

The internal jugular vein

The patient lies supine with no pillow, and the neck is extended. The head is rotated away from the site of entry and is well supported in position. The head of the bed is lowered by 10°. This position is important to prevent the development of an air embolus.

The median cephalic vein

The patient lies supine. The chosen arm is extended with the palm upwards and the elbow supported. Peripherally inserted central catheters, introduced via the cephalic or basilic vein, are increasingly being used as technology advances.

Equipment

As for intravenous infusion (*see* p. 169).

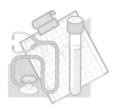

Additional equipment

1. Theatre cap and mask
2. Sterile gown
3. Sterile gloves
4. Sterile minor operation pack or sterile drape and towels
5. Waterproof protection for the bed
6. Alcohol-based lotion for cleansing the skin
7. Prescribed infusion fluid for parenteral nutrition
8. An appropriate sterile catheter depending on the site of entry used, e.g. a Hickman catheter or double- or triple-lumen catheter
9. Sterile needles and black silk sutures
10. ECG monitoring equipment if required
11. Volumetric infusion pump
12. Cassette for priming the infusion pump or a specialised infusion set
13. Dark bag for excluding light from the prepared infusion fluid.

Infusion fluid for parenteral nutrition

This will be prescribed by the medical practitioner for each 24-hour period as to the patient's nutritional needs and related blood chemistry. A combination of nutrients will be used to give a balanced intake, and vitamins and trace elements will be included in the prescription (Green and Jackson 2006).

The infusion bags will either be purchased ready prepared from pharmaceutical companies or prepared by a hospital pharmacy service with the required equipment such as a laminar flow to ensure the sterility of the infusion fluid. Everything for parenteral nutrition, including vitamins and trace elements, may be added individually. This reduces the risk of infection that might occur when an infusion of several different fluids in separate containers is prescribed; a series of taps, or Y-connectors, are thus needed for the infusion.

A combination of the following intravenous fluids may be prescribed. All are usually available in 500 ml containers (see the current pharmaceutical literature and British National Formulary 2006):
- carbohydrates, e.g. dextrose
- fats, e.g. Intralipid
- proteins, e.g. Aminoplex, Vamin.

Many products are available, the choice depending on the patient's needs and the pharmaceutical contractual arrangements within each health authority. A medical practitioner may have also have a preference for specific products. A number of commercial pharmaceutical companies provide ready prepared combined parenteral infusion bags for a 24-hour period.

The following may also be added:
- vitamins. Some vitamins are destroyed by sunlight so if these are added to a 24-hour parenteral infusion, the container must be covered by a dark bag to exclude light
- electrolytes, e.g. potassium and phosphates
- trace elements, e.g. zinc and magnesium.

Hickman catheter

A Hickman intravenous catheter may be chosen by the medical practitioner for a parenteral infusion that is needed over a period of weeks. This radio-opaque silastic catheter has a small sponge-like Dacron cuff at its distal end. The line is tunnelled subcutaneously, the cuff helping to retain the line in position as fibrous tissue forms round it. Patients may go home with this catheter in situ and become proficient in self-care under the supervision of the primary healthcare team (Corbett et al 1993). Patients will require extensive training in the care and maintenance of parenteral nutrition, the British Association for Enteral and Parenteral Nutrition (1994a) suggesting that this should be provided only in specialised centres where a co-ordinated multidisciplinary service is available (British Association for Enteral and Parenteral Nutrition 1994b).

The Hickman catheter is also used for infusions of intravenous cytotoxic medication that are prescribed over a long period and are not suitable for a peripheral infusion because of their irritant properties.

Volumetric infusion pumps

Parenteral nutrition should be infused using a continuous volumetric infusion pump. This ensures that a steady flow of prescribed nutrients is infused at a rate suitable for the patient's metabolism. If a pump is unavailable, a burette administration set should be used. Infusion pumps are primed with a special cassette and introduced into the infusion circuit between the administration set from the infusion fluid and the infusion catheter. There are clear manufacturer's instructions for all infusion pumps, which should be followed when setting up infusions.

Infusion pumps can normally be set to give an hourly flow rate of between 1 and 999 ml per hour. All pumps are fitted with alarm systems that monitor for any occlusion of the lines, air bubbles and completion of the available fluid. Recent equipment has a digital readout of details of the infusion and the alarm system. New equipment for the controlled administration of intravenous infusion is continually being developed. There are different types of infusion pump and gravity-feed infusion set on the market, and the choice of use may depend on health authority policy.

Guidelines and rationale for this nursing practice

- help to explain the procedure to the patient ***to gain consent and co-operation, and to encourage participation in care*** (Hamilton 1993)
- ensure the patient's privacy, respecting ***individuality and maintaining self-esteem***
- collect and prepare the equipment ***for efficiency of practice***
- check the prescribed intravenous fluid for parenteral nutrition (*see* 'Administration of medicines', p. 13)
- wash hands ***to reduce cross-infection*** (Jeanes 2005)
- prime the equipment (*see* 'Intravenous infusion', p. 171)
- help the patient into the appropriate position, depending on the site of entry used for the insertion of the central venous catheter, ***so that optimum safety is maintained for the patient***
- observe the patient throughout this activity ***to monitor any adverse effects***. The central line enters the large veins adjacent to the heart and may occasionally cause arrhythmias so monitoring the patient's ECG may be helpful
- adjust the tilt of the bed to lower the patient's head if necessary in order ***to minimise the risk of an air embolus***
- remain with the patient and help to maintain his or her position. Reassurance will be needed ***as the patient may find this part frightening***
- assist the medical practitioner as required ***to ensure a safe outcome for this practice***
- commence the infusion of parenteral nutrition at the prescribed rate once the catheter is in position and the sterile dressing has been applied to the access site
- if required cover the infusion with a dark bag ***to protect any vitamins from light, which may cause their deterioration***
- ensure that the patient is left feeling as comfortable as possible. The patient should ideally have a period of rest after this nursing practice ***to reduce anxiety and stress***
- if using an infusion pump, set as per the manufacturer's instructions ***to maintain the infusion as prescribed***
- dispose of the equipment safely ***to maintain a safe environment***

- document the nursing practice appropriately, monitor the after-effects and report any abnormal findings immediately. ***This ensures safe practice and enables prompt and appropriate medical and nursing intervention to be initiated***
- in undertaking this practice, nurses are accountable for their actions, the quality of care delivered and record-keeping according to the Code of Professional Conduct: Standards for Conduct, Performance and Ethics (Nursing and Midwifery Council 2004) and Guidelines for Records and Record Keeping (Nursing and Midwifery Council 2005).

Patient/carer education

Key points

In partnership with the patient and/or carer, ensure that they are competent to carry out any practices required. Information should be given on an appropriate point of contact for any concerns that may arise.

Explanations given before, during and after the line has been inserted, as well as the rationale for continuing parenteral nutrition, will help the patient to understand and interpret the condition and its treatment. The nurse should be sensitive to the timing and relevance of the information for each stage of this practice.

The community team will help to encourage the independence of the person receiving PN at home. This will include teaching the relevant aspects of:
- aseptic technique
- care of the central venous catheter
- observation of the site
- preparation of the intravenous feed
- use of the volumetric infusion pump
- mouth care.

Patients requiring long-term care should understand the importance of reporting redness, swelling or pain at the catheter site or any feeling of being generally unwell. Their independence may be increased if they are taught the principles of blood glucose monitoring.

Patient education should be part of the discharge planning and should commence well before the patient goes home. It is helpful to have a liaison nurse working between the community and the institution, written information in the form of an education leaflet reinforcing the patient's and carer's knowledge and confidence.

A contact telephone number to use as a 'helpline' will improve the patient's confidence and independence.

References

Benton S, Marsden C 2002 Training nurses to place tunnelled central venous catheters. Professional Nurse 17(9): 531–535

British Association for Parenteral and Enteral Nutrition 1994a Enteral and parenteral nutrition in the community. BAPEN, Maidenhead, UK

British Association for Parenteral and Enteral Nutrition 1994b Organisation of nutritional support in hospitals. BAPEN, Maidenhead, UK

British National Formulary 2006 BNF. British Medical Association and Royal Pharmaceutical Society of Great Britain, London

Burnham W 1999 Parenteral nutrition. In: Dougherty L, Lamb J (eds) Intravenous therapy in nursing practice. Churchill Livingstone, Edinburgh

Corbett K, Meehan L, Sackey V 1993 A strategy to enhance skills. Developing intravenous skills for community nursing. Professional Nurse 9(1): 60–63

Dougherty L, Lister S (eds) 2004 Royal Marsden manual of clinical nursing procedures, 6th edn. Blackwell Science, Oxford

Green S, Jackson P 2006 Nutrition. In: Alexander M, Fawcett J, Runciman P (eds) Nursing practice – hospital and home: the adult 3rd edn. Churchill Livingstone, Edinburgh

Hamilton H 1993 Care improves, while costs reduce. The clinical nurse specialist in total parenteral nutrition. Professional Nurse 8(9): 592–596

Jeanes A 2005 Infection control. A practical guide to the use of hand decontaminants. Nursing Times 101(20): 46–48

Murray A 2000 Enteral tube feeding: helping to provide nutritional support. Community Nurse (May): 13–17

National Institute for Clinical Excellence 2003 Care during enteral feeding. Infection control – prevention of health care associated infection in primary and community care: Clinical guideline 2. NICE, London

Nursing and Midwifery Council 2004 Code of professional conduct: standards for conduct, performance and ethics. NMC, London

Nursing and Midwifery Council 2005 Guidelines for records and record keeping. NMC, London

Smith L, Baker F, Stead L et al 1999 Feeding via a nasogastric tube. Nursing Times 95(8 Suppl): 1–2

Woods S 1998 Use of enteral and parenteral feeding. Professional Nurse 14(1): 44–46

Zainal G 1994 Nutrition of critically ill people. Intensive and Critical Care Nursing 10(3): 165–169

Websites

Nursing and Midwifery Council: http://www.nmc-uk.org

Royal College of Nursing: http://www.rcn.org.uk

Self assessment

1. When is it necessary to feed a patient?
2. Outline the procedure for feeding a patient.
3. Under what circumstances is it considered necessary to commence enteral feeding?
4. In what ways is enteral feeding administered?
5. When is parenteral nutrition used?

Practice 29
Oxygen Therapy

Learning outcomes	**By the end of this section, you should know how to:** ■ prepare the patient for this nursing practice ■ collect and prepare the equipment ■ administer oxygen therapy at home or in an institutional setting.
Background knowledge required	Revision of the anatomy and physiology of the cardiopulmonary system, with special reference to the exchange of gases and the mechanism of respiration Revision of the dangers of the use of oxygen Review of local policies and procedures regarding fire precautions and oxygen therapy, in both institutional and community care.
Indications and rationale for oxygen therapy	Oxygen therapy is the introduction of increased oxygen to the air available for respiration to prevent hypoxia, a condition in which insufficient oxygen is available for the cells of the body, especially those in the brain and vital organs. Hypoxia may occur in the following circumstances: ■ respiratory disease in which the area available for respiration is reduced by, for example: — infection — chronic conditions such as chronic obstructive pulmonary disease (COPD) and carcinoma — pulmonary infarction or embolus — asthma ■ chest injuries following trauma, when the mechanism of respiration may be impaired ■ heart disease, when the cardiac output is reduced by, for example: — myocardial infarction — congestive cardiac failure ■ haemorrhage, reducing the oxygen-carrying capacity of the blood ■ preoperatively and postoperatively when analgesic drugs, e.g. morphine (an opiate), may have an effect on respiratory function ■ in emergency situations, e.g. cardiac or respiratory arrest and hypovolaemic, septic or cardiogenic shock, as the cardiac output will fall, reducing the amount of oxygenated blood available to the vital organs ■ head or spinal injuries. Except in emergency situations, oxygen therapy will be prescribed by a medical practitioner, who will specify both the percentage of oxygen and the method of administration. The administration of oxygen is one of the specific medical treatments: patients will have individually assessed requirements related to their particular medical problem (British National Formulary 2006).

Oxygen therapy can be administered in the patient's own home under the care of the community nurse or in an institutional setting, but the principles underlying this nursing practice remain the same wherever it takes place. At home, the oxygen cylinder and its associated equipment will be delivered regularly to the patient's home from a central supply, depending on the policy of the individual health board, as prescribed and ordered by the general practitioner. Alternatively, oxygen may be administered via an oxygen concentrator, which is an effective and economical way to deliver therapy to a patient who requires long-term intervention (British National Formulary 2006). Guidelines on the monitoring of patients outside institutional settings is provided by the Royal College of Physicians (1999) and NICE in the COPD national guideline (National Institute for Clinical Excellence 2004).

Equipment

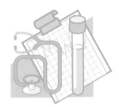

1. Oxygen supply, e.g. piped oxygen or oxygen cylinder
2. Oxygen concentrator (for use in the community)
3. Reduction gauge as required
4. Flow meter
5. Oxygen mask or nasal cannulae as appropriate
6. Oxygen tubing
7. Humidifier as appropriate
8. 'No Smoking' signs
9. Receptacle for soiled disposable items.

Oxygen masks

Oxygen masks (Fig. 29.1) are designed to provide an accurate percentage of oxygen by entraining an appropriate amount of air for a specific flow rate of oxygen (Francis 2006). Instructions are available for each type of mask and these should be used accordingly (Francis 2006).

They can be classified according to their performance, which can be fixed or variable. Fixed-performance masks provide a concentration of oxygen that does not vary with the patient's rate and depth of breathing. An example of these is the Venturi masks (Fig. 29.2), which, through the addition of a colour-coded attachment to the jets, can provide a variety of oxygen concentrations from 24 to 60%. Venturi masks are suitable for use with patients who have chronic obstructive pulmonary disease (COPD).

Variable performance masks, such as the Hudson, can be attached to a reservoir bag. Used alone they provide an oxygen concentration, depending on oxygen flow rate and the patient's respiratory rate and depth, of 30–60%. If the mask is

FIGURE 29.1
Oxygen therapy: mask in position

Specific adaptor for prescribed oxygen percentage

attached to a reservoir bag, which does not permit rebreathing, and oxygen at 12 L min^{-1}, oxygen concentrations of 95% can be delivered (Boumphrey et al 2003, Francis 2006) The performance of nasal cannulae is also variable with respiratory effort. These are light plastic tubes inserted into each nostril and shaped to fit over the ears to maintain their position (Fig. 29.3). Patients find them more comfortable and less claustrophobic than a conventional mask. However, they are not suitable for all patients as they should only be used with an oxygen flow rate of 4 L min^{-1} or less and deliver oxygen concentrations of between 22 and 35% (Francis 2006).

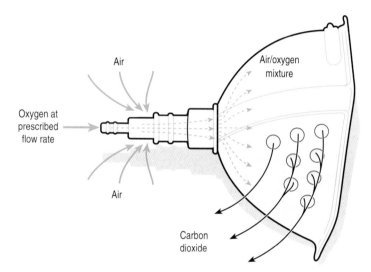

Air

Air/oxygen mixture

Oxygen at prescribed flow rate

Air

Carbon dioxide

FIGURE 29.2
Venturi fixed-performance oxygen mask
From Brooker & Nicol 2003, with permission

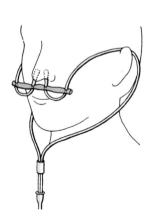

FIGURE 29 3
Oxygen therapy: nasal cannulae in position

T-piece

Oxygen may be delivered directly into an endotracheal tube or tracheostomy tube via wide corrugated tubing and a T-piece. Adequate humidification is essential here.

Oxygen tents

These are used mainly in paediatrics, when babies and young children would not tolerate masks. The danger of fire is increased further using this method, because of the larger area of concentrated oxygen within the oxygen tent, and the difficulty of confining the gas to a small area when nursing the patient.

Emergency situations

For emergency resuscitation procedures, oxygen may be administered via an Ambu bag and resuscitation mask for a higher percentage of oxygen to be given with assisted ventilation (*see* 'Cardiopulmonary resuscitation', p. 71).

Humidifiers

It is important that the oxygen administered is adequately humidified to prevent drying of the mucosa of the respiratory tract. The inspiration of the, usually, cold, dry gas can interfere with ciliary action and increase mucous viscosity. This will lead to the production of secretions that are difficult to expectorate, lead to alveolar collapse and infection. Gas exchange may also be impaired. In order to prevent these complications a humidifier may be added to the oxygen delivery system (Fig. 29.4). Various humidifiers that use hot or cold water or heat moisture exchange membranes are available. Heat moisture exchangers are used predominantly in the critical care setting for patients who are breathing with the aid of a mechanical ventilator. Hot or cold water systems involve the attachment of the oxygen delivery tubing to the humidifier. Moisture is gathered by the gas as it passes either through or over the water, nebulised and delivered to the patient.

Humidifier bottles should be changed according to local policy or manufacturer's instructions (Pilkington 2004, Francis 2006).

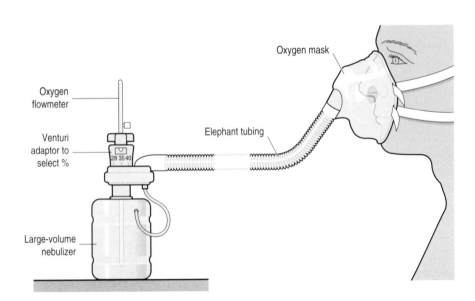

FIGURE 29.4
Humidification of oxygen
From Brooker & Nicol
2003, with permission

Oxygen mask

Oxygen flowmeter

Venturi adaptor to select %

Elephant tubing

Large-volume nebulizer

Guidelines and rationale for this nursing practice

- identify and check the prescription for oxygen therapy **to ensure that the correct percentage is administered**
- explain the nursing practice to the patient **to gain consent and co-operation, and encourage participation in care**. Oxygen masks can be a barrier to communication by making it more difficult for the patient to speak and be heard, so there is a risk of misunderstanding. This may cause the patient to remove the mask so the nurse needs good communication skills to help the patient tolerate the procedure while it is necessary. The use of closed (direct) questions, to which only a 'yes' or 'no' answer is needed, may be of help
- explain the dangers of smoking to the patient, family and friends, and display appropriate 'No Smoking' signs, **making sure that all understand the increased risk of fire when oxygen is administered**. Oxygen is a gas that readily supports combustion, so in areas where it is used, the risk of fire is greatly increased. Every precaution to prevent fire should be taken. The patient should, if possible, be aware of the problem and help in maintaining a safe environment. Health authority policy on fire precautions should be familiar to all staff and carers
- alcohol-based solutions, oils and grease should not be used in areas where oxygen is being administered **as these volatile substances are readily flammable and the presence of oxygen increases the risk of fire**. All such precautions should also be part of patient education when therapy is being administered in a community setting, involving all the family and the associated carers as well
- at home, hang the 'No Smoking' sign on the oxygen cylinder, **as a reminder for all the family and visitors**
- collect and assemble the equipment as required **so that everything is at hand**
- help the patient into a comfortable position **so that he or she will tolerate the oxygen therapy without distress**. A need for oxygen therapy usually indicates that the patient has some difficulty with breathing. This dyspnoea may be relieved by helping the patient into an appropriate and comfortable position as the condition allows, for example sitting upright, leaning over a bed table supported on a pillow, or sitting in a chair
- observe the patient's vital signs, including type and depth of respirations, throughout this activity **to monitor any adverse effects as well as any improvement in respiratory function**. The patient's general condition should be observed to identify any deterioration or improvement in the hypoxic state, for example degree of drowsiness, level of orientation or level of consciousness. The colour and condition of the patient's skin should be observed for cyanosis, clamminess or sweating
- fill the humidifier with sterile water to the correct level **so that there is efficient humidification of the inspired oxygen**
- adjust the flow rate of oxygen as prescribed **so that the correct percentage is administered**. Patients who have COPD have permanently altered respiratory physiology. The respiratory drive or stimulus for respiration responds only to a low arterial blood level of oxygen so only low percentages of oxygen, for example 24–28% should be prescribed and administered. Raising the arterial blood oxygen level too high in these patients could cause respiratory arrest. It is important that the patient and family understand the importance of not

altering the prescribed flow rate and the danger of increasing the amount of oxygen administered

- observe the flow of oxygen and water vapour through the mask or cannulae before administration **to check that the equipment is working efficiently**
- place the mask in the correct position, and adjust it to fit firmly and comfortably over the patient's nose and mouth (*see* Fig. 29.1 above) **so that all the oxygen prescribed is administered and as little as possible escapes from the mask**
- remain with the patient as necessary **and help him or her to keep the equipment in position**
- top up the level of water in the humidifier as required **to maintain humidification**
- check the oxygen tubing regularly for any build up of condensation, **which may reduce the flow**
- assist the medical practitioner with the estimation of arterial blood gases as required **to evaluate the efficiency of the treatment**
- monitor the saturation levels using pulse oximetry if required **to evaluate the effect of the oxygen administered**
- ensure that the patient is left feeling as comfortable as possible **so that he or she will continue to tolerate the oxygen therapy**. The removal of the mask for drinking should be supervised by the nurse and will depend on the patient's condition. It may be possible to change to nasal cannulae at mealtimes, using a mask at other times to maintain the accuracy of the oxygen percentage being administered
- oxygen, even when adequately humidified, causes the mouth and nasal passages to become dry. Frequent oral and nasal hygiene will therefore be required **for the patient's comfort and to maintain a healthy oropharyngeal mucosa**. Oral fluids should be encouraged to counteract the drying effect on the mucosa
- the inside of the oxygen mask may become wet with condensation so the patient's face can be washed and the inside of the mask dried as appropriate. **This will greatly increase the patient's comfort and tolerance of this nursing practice**
- dispose of the equipment safely to prevent any transmission of infection
- document the nursing practice appropriately, monitor the after-effects and report any abnormal findings immediately, **ensuring safe practice and enabling prompt appropriate medical and nursing intervention to be initiated as soon as possible**
- in undertaking this practice, nurses are accountable for their actions, the quality of care delivered and record-keeping according to the Code of Professional Conduct: Standards for Conduct, Performance and Ethics (Nursing and Midwifery Council 2004) and Guidelines for Records and Record Keeping (Nursing and Midwifery Council 2005).

Pulse oximetry

It is possible to measure the oxygen saturation level (Sa_{O_2}) by a non-invasive technique. An electronic device called a pulse oximeter measures the absorption of red and infrared light passing through living tissue. The equipment is normally a specialised, sensitive electronic clip that fits comfortably on a finger, a toe or an earlobe (Fig. 29.5), the result being recorded on the patient's electronic monitor. The oximeter reading responds closely to the arterial blood gas level (Sao_2), so fewer blood samples are needed for monitoring the arterial blood oxygen level. The fact that a continuous readout of the level can be observed helps to evaluate the effect of oxygen therapy and, being non-invasive, aids maintaining a safe environment for both patient and staff. Pulse oximetry is used to monitor oxygen status to determine oxygen requirements, during general anaesthesia or through periods where the patient may be sedated. It is also used to assess the severity of the patient's condition. However, pulse oximetry does not detect respiratory rate and depth so should not replace these vital-sign observations. In addition there are a number of contraindications for its use when an inaccurate and misleading reading may be obtained. For example:

- reduced pulsatile flow during periods of cold, hypotension, cardiac arrhythmias
- anaemia
- shivering or movement of the limbs
- direct light sources that are shining on the probe
- nail varnish.

Arterial blood gas estimation

In intensive care areas and accident and emergency units, and during perioperative care, the effectiveness of oxygen therapy may be monitored by assessing the arterial blood gases. The results are recorded in relation to the percentage of oxygen administered, changes in the percentage of oxygen or method of administration being made accordingly. Samples of arterial blood are usually obtained from the radial artery, either from an indwelling arterial cannula or by individual sampling. The nurse should maintain observations of the arterial puncture site for bleeding.

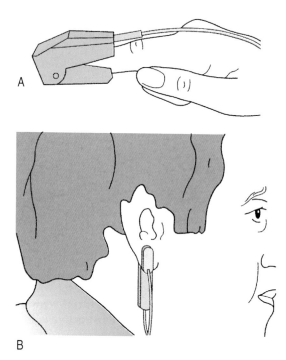

FIGURE 29.5
Oxygen therapy: pulse oximeter
A Hand sensor
B Earlobe sensor

Patient/carer education

Key points

In partnership with the patient and/or carer, ensure that they are competent to carry out any practices required. Information should be given on an appropriate point of contact for any concerns that may arise.

The reason for the administration of oxygen therapy should be explained to the patient and the family and carers involved. They should understand that it is a specific part of the treatment.

At home, the patient and carers should be shown how to adjust the flow rate to the prescribed rate only, how to fill the humidifier, maintaining a safe environment, and how to connect the mask and tubing. The procedure for changing oxygen cylinders or using an oxygen concentrator, and the personnel involved, will depend on health authority policy; carers may in some instances be instructed in this.

The increased risk of fire should be explained and simple instructions about fire precautions given. The danger of smoking when oxygen is used should be continually reinforced: patient and family co-operation is needed for this. They can choose where 'No Smoking' signs should be displayed.

For patients with COPD, everyone should understand the importance of never increasing the prescribed flow of oxygen delivered to the patient. This may need reinforcing if there is a change of carer in the community setting. The reason for this should be part of patient education.

The patient should understand the importance of immediately reporting any changes in respiratory function such as increased dyspnoea, cough, sputum or a general feeling of distress.

References

Boumphrey SM, Morris EAJ, Kinsella SM 2003 100% Inspired oxygen from a Hudson mask – a realistic goal? Resuscitation 57: 69–73

British National Formulary 2006 Oxygen. British Medical Association and the Royal Pharmaceutical Society of Great Britain, London

Brooker C, Nicol M 2003 Nursing adults: the practice of caring. Mosby, Edinburgh

Francis C 2006 Respiratory care. Blackwell Publishing, Oxford

National Institute for Clinical Excellence 2004 Chronic obstructive pulmonary disease. Management of chronic obstructive pulmonary disease in adults in primary and secondary care. Clinical guideline 12. NICE, London

Nursing and Midwifery Council 2004 Code of professional conduct: standards for conduct, performance and ethics. NMC, London

Nursing and Midwifery Council 2005 Guidelines for records and record keeping. NMC, London

Pilkington F 2004 Humidification for oxygen therapy in non-ventilated patients. British Journal of Nursing 13(2): 111–115

Royal College of Physicians 1999 Domiciliary oxygen therapy services: clinical guidelines and advice for prescribers. Royal College of Physicians, London

Websites

British Lung Foundation: http://www.lunguk.org/

British Thoracic Society: http://www.brit-thoracic.org.uk/

Living with Chronic Obstructive Pulmonary Disease: http://www.livingwithcopd.co.uk/

Self assessment

1. What type of oxygen mask would be used for a patient who has chronic obstructive pulmonary disease?
2. What safety precautions should be taken while caring for a patient receiving oxygen therapy either at home or in hospital?
3. What are the contraindications for the use of pulse oximetry?

Practice 30
Paracentesis: Abdominal

Learning outcomes	**By the end of this section, you should know how to:**
	▪ prepare the patient for this procedure
	▪ collect and prepare the equipment
	▪ assist the medical practitioner with abdominal paracentesis as required.

Background knowledge required

Revision of the anatomy and physiology of the abdominal organs, with special reference to the peritoneum

Revision of 'Aseptic technique' (*see* p. 381)

Revision of 'Infection prevention and control' (*see* p. 151).

Indications and rationale for abdominal paracentesis

Abdominal paracentesis is the removal of fluid from the peritoneal cavity through a sterile cannula or needle (Campbell 2001). Medication is sometimes introduced into the peritoneal cavity by the same route. The procedure may be performed for the following reasons:

▪ **to obtain a specimen of abdominal fluid for diagnostic purposes**

▪ **to relieve intra-abdominal pressure** caused by increased fluid within the abdominal cavity. This is called ascites and may occur in association with several conditions:
   — congestive cardiac failure involving dysfunction of the right side of the heart
   — chronic hepatic disease
   — malignant disease with metastases in the liver

▪ **to introduce medication into the peritoneal cavity**, e.g. cytotoxic therapy for malignant disease.

Outline of the procedure

Abdominal paracentesis is carried out by a medical practitioner using an aseptic technique. A mask and sterile gown, as well as sterile gloves, should be worn.

The site of insertion is midway between the umbilicus and the symphysis pubis along the midline. The skin is cleansed with antiseptic lotion and a local anaesthetic is administered, the area round the site being covered with sterile towels. A small skin incision is made with a sterile blade, and a trocar and cannula or a catheter and introducer are inserted into the peritoneal cavity. The trocar/introducer is removed, allowing fluid to flow through the cannula. The specimens of abdominal fluid required for investigation are collected at this stage by holding the appropriately labelled sterile containers under the flow of fluid, maintaining asepsis. The cannula may be removed and a sterile dressing applied, or it may be stitched in position and attached to sterile tubing and a closed drainage bag if drainage is to be maintained. A suitable sterile dressing should be applied around the cannula.

The flow of drainage fluid is regulated with a gate clamp or roller clamp to prevent too rapid a reduction of intra-abdominal pressure. Initially, only 1 L of fluid should be allowed to drain, before regulating the flow to 100 ml per hour or as prescribed by the medical practitioner. This should prevent the patient developing symptoms of shock because of the sudden lessening of pressure in the abdominal cavity.

In palliative care settings having a drainage catheter in situ may be considered, to reduce the discomfort associated with ascites (McNamara 2000). Some patients may be managed at home (Moorsom 2001).

Equipment

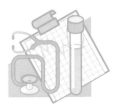

1. Trolley
2. Theatre mask
3. Sterile gown
4. Sterile gloves
5. Sterile dressings pack
6. Sterile towels
7. Sterile bowl
8. Sterile specimen containers, appropriately labelled, completed laboratory forms and a plastic specimen bag for transportation
9. Antiseptic lotion
10. Sterile abdominal paracentesis set containing:
    — a specialised trocar and cannula or catheter and introducer
    — forceps
    — a blade and holder
    — tubing
11. Local anaesthetic and equipment for its administration
12. Sterile sutures and a needle for stitching the cannula in position
13. Sterile drainage bag
14. Gate clip or roller clamp
15. Disposable tape measure
16. Measuring jug
17. Receptacle for soiled disposable items.

Guidelines and rationale for this nursing practice

- help to explain the procedure to the patient **to gain consent and co-operation, and encourage participation in care**
- ask the patient to empty his or her bladder immediately prior to the procedure. This will ensure that the bladder remains within the pelvis, thus **preventing any risk of perforation when the trocar is inserted**
- ensure the patient's privacy, **respecting individuality and maintaining self-esteem**
- wash hands **to prevent cross-infection** (Jeanes 2005)
- measure and record the patient's abdominal girth before commencing the procedure **to compare with measurements taken after abdominal paracentesis**
- wash hands **to prevent cross-infection** (Jeanes 2005)
- help to collect and prepare the equipment, **making good use of time and resources**
- help the patient into a suitable, comfortable position. He or she may sit upright with the back well supported. If possible the legs should be lowered **to**

allow easier access to the insertion site and to increase the patient's comfort. A bed that can be adjusted to allow only the lower limbs to be lowered is the most suitable. In some instances, the medical practitioner may prefer the patient to lie flat. The position chosen depends on the reason for the abdominal paracentesis

- help to adjust the patient's clothing *to expose the site of insertion*
- wash hands to prevent cross-infection (Jeanes 2005)
- observe the patient throughout this activity *to monitor any adverse effects*
- help to prepare the sterile field as required *to maintain asepsis*
- assist the medical practitioner as required during the procedure
- measure the amount of drainage and adjust the flow of drainage fluid as required *to ensure that the volume drawn does not cause a sudden reduction in intra-abdominal pressure*. Initially only 1 L of fluid should be removed, then regulating the flow to 50–150 ml per hour as prescribed
- ensure that the patient is left feeling as comfortable as possible in a sitting position *so that drainage is encouraged*
- dispose of equipment safely *to prevent the transmission of infection*
- dispatch labelled specimens of abdominal fluid to the appropriate laboratory with their completed forms immediately *so that investigations can be commenced as soon as possible*
- document the procedure appropriately, monitor the after-effects and report any abnormal findings immediately *to ensure safe practice and enable prompt, appropriate medical and nursing intervention to be initiated*
- in undertaking this practice, nurses are accountable for their actions, the quality of care delivered and record-keeping according to the Code of Professional Conduct: Standards for Conduct, Performance and Ethics (Nursing and Midwifery Council 2004) and Guidelines for Records and Record Keeping (Nursing and Midwifery Council 2005).

Patient/carer education
Key points

In partnership with the patient and/or carer, ensure that they are competent to carry out any practices required. Information should be given on an appropriate point of contact for any concerns that may arise.

Explain the reason for the procedure and the importance of the patient's position during the insertion of the catheter. Reassure the patient that he or she should feel more comfortable once some of the abdominal fluid has drained away.

If the catheter is to remain in situ for some time, explain how the patient can cope with toileting, personal cleansing and dressing, and outline the help he or she will be given with this.

The patient should understand the importance of reporting redness, swelling, pain or discomfort at the access site, even after the catheter has been removed.

References

Campbell C 2001 Controlling malignant ascites. European Journal of Palliative Care 8(5): 187–190

Jeanes A 2005 Infection control. A practical guide to the use of hand decontaminants. Nursing Times 101(20): 46–48

McNamara P 2000 Paracentesis – an effective method of symptom control in the palliative care setting? Palliative Medicine 14: 62–64

Moorsom D 2001 Paracentesis in the home care setting. Palliative Medicine 15: 169–170

Nursing and Midwifery Council 2004 Code of professional conduct: standards of conduct, performance and ethics. NMC, London

Nursing and Midwifery Council 2005 Guidelines for records and record keeping. NMC, London

Self assessment

1. Why may a patient need to have an abdominal paracentesis?
2. Identify three potential complications during or following an abdominal paracentesis.

Practice 31
Personal Hygiene

There are three parts to this section:

1 **Bed bath, immersion bath and showering**

2 **Facial shave**

3 **Hair washing**

Due to the volume of material on personal hygiene, guidelines for mouth care and skin care are given in separate sections.

Learning outcomes	**By the end of this section, you should know how to:** ▪ prepare the patient for this nursing practice ▪ collect the equipment ▪ carry out a bed bath ▪ help the patient with an immersion bath or shower ▪ carry out a facial shave ▪ wash the hair of a bed fast or ambulant patient.
Background knowledge required	Revision of the anatomy and physiology of the skin tissue Revision of 'Skin care' (*see* p. 297) and 'Mouth care' (*see* p. 205) Review of local policy on pre- and postoperative skin care Revision of infection control policy in respect of skin care, hair infestation and cleaning of equipment Review of local policy on moving and handling Review of local policy on these practices.
Indications and rationale for personal hygiene	A patient may require personal hygiene care: ▪ to clean the skin prior to surgery ▪ postoperatively following major surgery when mobility is restricted ▪ following an acute illness, e.g. myocardial infarction ▪ while in an unconscious state ▪ following trauma, e.g. a patient in traction ▪ when extremely weak and debilitated as a result of the prolonged effects of a disease, trauma or a treatment being administered.

For infection control purposes personal hygiene equipment should be for single-patient use or should be cleaned according to local policy. The nurse should cleanse their hands before and after each practice according to local policy and wear a disposable plastic apron.

1. BED BATH, IMMERSION BATH AND SHOWERING

Equipment

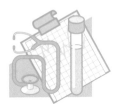

1. Soap, or prescribed antibacterial preparation/aqueous cream/emulsifying lotion
2. Patient's toiletries such as deodorant and talcum powder
3. Bath towels
4. Two face cloths/sponges or disposable wipes
5. Disposable paper towel or similar
6. Patient's brush and comb
7. Nail scissors and nail file if required
8. Clean nightdress, pyjamas or clothing
9. Clean bed linen
10. Plastic apron and disposable gloves
11. Continence products if required
12. Equipment for catheter care (*see* p. 91) if required
13. Equipment for skin care (*see* p. 297)
14. Equipment for mouth care (*see* p. 205)
15. Receptacle for the patient's soiled clothing
16. Receptacle for soiled bed linen
17. Receptacle for soiled disposable items.

Additional equipment

1. Basin of hot water at 35–40°C (bed bath)
2. Trolley or adequate surface (bed bath)
3. Bath thermometer (immersion bath)
4. Chair or shower stool (immersion bath and shower)
5. Disposable floor mat (immersion bath and shower)
6. Bathing/showering equipment aids as appropriate (immersion bath and shower).

Guidelines and rationale for this nursing practice

Bed bath

- explain the nursing practice to the patient *to gain consent and co-operation*
- collect and prepare the equipment *to ensure that all equipment is available and ready for use*
- ensure the patient's privacy *to reduce anxiety*
- observe the patient throughout this activity *to note any signs of distress*
- check that the bed brakes are in use *to prevent the patient or nurse sustaining an injury from a sudden uncontrolled movement of the bed*
- adjust the bed height *to ensure safe moving and handling practice*
- help the patient into a comfortable position *permitting the nurse easy and comfortable access to the patient*

- arrange the furniture around the patient's bed space **to allow easy access to equipment on the trolley or surface**
- remove any excess bed linen and bed appliances if in use, **allowing easy access to the patient**, but leaving the patient covered with a bed sheet **to maintain modesty**
- help the patient to remove their pyjamas or gown and anti-embolic stockings if required **to reduce exertion as this can be a strenuous activity for a person who is in a weakened state**
- check the temperature of the basin of water, **ensuring that the water is neither too hot nor too cold**
- check with the patient whether he or she uses soap on his or her face, **ensuring individualised care**
- wash, rinse and dry the patient's face, ears and neck; when possible, assist patients to do this for themselves **to encourage independence**
- if the face cloth is not going to be laundered after the procedure, the second face cloth should be used to wash the rest of the body **in order to reduce the risk of cross-infection**
- expose only the part of the patient's body being washed in order **to maintain the patient's modesty and self-esteem**
- change the water as it cools or becomes dirty, and immediately after washing the patient's pubic area, **preventing the cooling of the patient and reducing the risk of cross-infection, respectively**
- wash, rinse and thoroughly dry the patient's body in an appropriate order, such as the upper limbs, chest and abdomen, back and lower limbs, **preventing excessive exertion on the part of the patient**
- change the water immediately after perineal hygiene or leave this action until last, **reducing the risk of cross-infection from the normal skin flora of the perineal region to the rest of the skin**
- when washing the patient's limbs, first wash the limb furthest away from you. **This will allow the assistant to dry that limb as the other limb is being washed, thus reducing the time during which the patient's body is exposed to the cooling effect of the environment**. When possible, assist the patient to immerse the feet and hands in the basin of water (Fig. 31.1)
- as each part of the patient's body is washed, observe the skin for any blemishes, redness or discoloration, **which will alert the nurse to the potential problem of pressure sore development** (*see* 'Skin care', p. 297)
- apply body deodorants and/or other toiletries as desired by the patient, **ensuring individualised care**
- assist the patient to wash, rinse and dry the pubic area using the disposable wipes, washing from the front of the perineal area to the back **to prevent cross-infection from the anal region**
- carry out catheter care or use appropriate continence products if required
- help the patient to dress in clean pyjamas or gown and replace anti-embolic stockings if required to **reduce exertion on the part of the patient**
- **to prevent injury, reduce the risk of cross-infection and promote self-esteem**, assist the patient to cut and clean the fingernails and toenails if required and unless otherwise instructed
- **to promote patient comfort**, remove any soiled or damp bed linen and remake the patient's bed

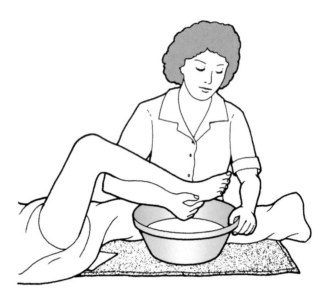

FIGURE 31.1
Foot immersion: the patient's foot and leg should be supported. The upper limbs can be supported in a similar way

- assist the patient with mouth care (*see* p. 205) *to promote a positive body image*
- assist the patient to brush or comb the hair into its usual style, *promoting independence and self-esteem*
- ensure that the patient is left feeling as comfortable as possible while *maintaining the quality of this nursing practice*
- rearrange the furniture as wished by the patient *so that any articles needed are within easy reach and the patient is given control of the environment*
- dispose of the equipment safely *to reduce any health hazard*.

Immersion bath

- discuss the arrangements for the bath with the patient *to gain consent and co-operation and encourage participation in care*. In the community, the patient should have an assessment carried out; *this will assess the need for the use of equipment available from occupational therapy and whether help with bathing and showering should be given by social-care staff*
- help the patient to collect and prepare the equipment *so that everything is ready for use*
- help the patient to the bathroom; this may include the use of mechanical lifting aids or a wheelchair *if the patient has any difficulty with mobilising*
- ensure the patient's privacy as far as possible, *to respect individuality and maintain self-esteem*

- prepare the water in the bath, maintaining a safe temperature, and gain the patient's approval *as bathing is a very personal activity*
- help the patient to undress *if he or she needs help, giving encouragement for the patient to be as independent as possible*
- observe the patient throughout this activity *to observe any adverse effects*
- help the patient into the bath. For some patients, mechanical aids may be used as appropriate according to the manufacturer's instructions
- help the patient to wash himself or herself, commencing with the face and neck *so that clean water is used first on these areas*
- help to wash the patient's hair *if required* (*see* 'Hair washing', p. 265)
- help the patient out of the bath. The patient may sit on a chair that is protected with a towel *to prevent any unsteadiness and danger of falling*
- help the patient to dry *as required and encourage independence*
- help the patient to dress as required. *To promote patients' self-esteem and independence*, they should choose what they want to wear
- allow the patient time to clean his or her teeth or dentures at the basin, *to promote oral hygiene*, giving help as required
- help to brush or comb the patient's hair *to help self-esteem*
- help the patient to a chair or bed, whichever is chosen, or as the condition allows, *for a period of rest after the exercise of bathing*
- ensure that the patient is left feeling as comfortable as possible *to promote relaxation*
- clean the bath according to local policy *to promote a safe environment*
- dispose of equipment safely *to prevent any transmission of infection*.

Showering

Many clinical areas now have open shower units where patients can be assisted to a fixed seat or can be transferred in a mobile shower chair (Fig. 31.2).

- discuss the arrangements for the shower with the patient *to gain consent and co-operation*
- help to collect and prepare the equipment *so that everything is ready for use*
- help the patient to the shower room. This may include the use of mechanical lifting aids or a wheelchair *if the patient has any difficulty with mobilising*
- help the patient to undress as required, *maintaining privacy to respect individuality*
- help the patient to sit on the shower chair or stool *so that there is no danger of falling*
- adjust the flow of water from the shower *to maintain a safe water temperature and gain the patient's approval*
- help the patient to wash while showering as required *so that he or she may have an enjoyable body wash*
- help the patient to wash his or her hair if required (see 'Hair washing', p. 265) *to promote self-esteem*
- help the patient to dry
- proceed as in the guidelines for immersion bathing, above.

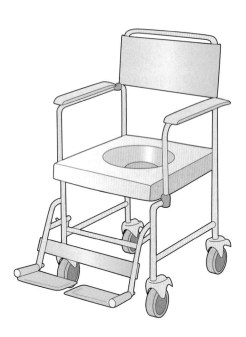

FIGURE 31.2
Mobile shower chair

2. FACIAL SHAVE

Equipment

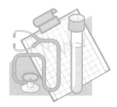

1. Bowl of hand-hot water
2. Patient's own razor or disposable safety razor or single-patient use electric shaver
3. Shaving soap and brush or shaving foam/gel
4. Face cloth or disposable wipe
5. Towel
6. Receptacles for used razor and soiled disposable items
7. Aftershave (if requested by patient)
8. Plastic apron.

Guidelines and rationale for this nursing practice

Facial wet shave

- protect the patient's upper body with a towel *to avoid patient's clothing becoming damp*
- note any skin blemishes *so that tissue damage can be avoided during shaving*
- wet the patient's face with warm water
- use shaving brush to produce a good lather from the shaving soap or use shaving foam/gel as per manufacturer's instructions and apply over face and neck *to ease shaving procedure and prevent unnecessary skin trauma*
- hold skin taut with one hand and with the other use short strokes on the skin, moving the razor in the direction of the hair growth *to ensure a close shave*
- after each stroke rinse the razor in warm water *to prevent blockage of the blades with hair*
- on completion rinse the skin *to remove all traces of soap*
- apply aftershave if requested by the patient.

Facial dry shave

This is often the preferred method especially if the patient is on anticoagulant therapy that will increase the risk of bleeding if the skin is cut with a razor. Electric shavers should not be shared among patients as this presents a cross-infection risk.

- ensure the skin is clean and dry
- hold skin taut with one hand, with the other hand place the shaver head against the skin, and use short circular movements to remove hair growth
- apply aftershave if requested by the patient
- on completion clean the shaver as per manufacturer's instructions.

3. HAIR WASHING

Equipment

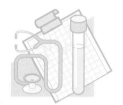

1. Small jug or hair spray tap attachment
2. Towels
3. Plastic sheeting
4. Patient's shampoo/conditioner
5. Patient's own brush and/or comb
6. Flannel or disposable cloth
7. Plastic apron
8. Hair dryer
9. Trolley or adequate surface for equipment
10. Receptacle for soiled disposable items.

Additional equipment for bedfast patient

1. Basin
2. Large container of warm water
3. Container for used water, or a bedfast rinser.

Guidelines and rationale for this nursing practice

If hair is being treated for a hair infestation then local guidelines should be followed according to current effective treatments. Infection control policies should be adhered to in order to prevent spread to family members, other patients and staff.

Washing hair of the bedfast patient

- remove the back frame of the bed
- help the patient into a comfortable position, e.g. with the shoulders supported by a pillow and the head overhanging the edge of the bed or on the bedfast rinser (Baker et al 1999). If the patient is unable to lie flat then they can sit upright supported by pillows with head bent forward over a basin on the bed trolley **to promote comfort and allow the patient to maintain the position during the practice**
- protect the patient's clothing, pillows and bedclothes using the plastic sheeting **to reduce water penetration**

- place a towel around the patient's shoulders **to absorb any water spillage**
- if the patient is able to lie flat then position the basin under the patient's head or place the basin on a chair at the top of the bed **to catch the water as it drains from the scalp**
- one person should support the patient's neck and head during this practice **to minimise discomfort**
- protect the patient's eyes with the flannel or disposable cloth, **preventing irritation from the shampoo**
- using the basin to catch the water, wet the hair, and apply the shampoo **to commence washing the patient's hair**
- rinse off the lather **to remove the shampoo and leave the patient's hair clean**. Repeat if the patient wishes
- apply the patient's hair conditioner if used, and leave for the manufacturer's recommended time before rinsing. **This helps to detangle the hair and may improve the hair's overall condition**
- towel the hair dry, **removing excess moisture**
- assist the patient to comb his or her hair into its usual style and dry using the hair dryer **to allow a positive body image to be reinstated**
- ensure that the patient is left feeling as comfortable as possible, **confirming the quality of care delivered**
- dispose of the equipment safely **to reduce any health hazard**.

Hair washing of the ambulant patient

This procedure can be carried out at the wash basin, or as part of a shower or immersion bath using a hair spray tap attachment.

- help the patient to the bathroom and ensure that he or she is sitting comfortably, **to promote comfort and allow the patient to maintain the position during the practice**
- if the patient is having their hair washed at the basin then protect the clothing using plastic sheeting **to reduce water penetration** and drape a towel around the shoulders **to absorb any water spillage**
- protect the patient's eyes with the flannel or disposable cloth, **preventing irritation from the shampoo**
- using the small jug or the hair spray tap attachment, wet the hair, and apply the shampoo **to commence washing the patient's hair**
- rinse off the lather **to remove the shampoo and leave the patient's hair clean**. Repeat if the patient wishes
- apply the patient's hair conditioner, if used, and leave for the manufacturer's recommended time before rinsing. **This helps to detangle the hair and may improve the hair's overall condition**
- towel the hair dry, **removing excess moisture**
- assist the patient to comb his or her hair into its usual style and dry using the hair dryer, **to allow a positive body image to be reinstated**
- ensure that the patient is left feeling as comfortable as possible, **confirming the quality of care delivered**.

For all practices associated with personal hygiene

- document the nursing practice appropriately, monitor any after-effects and report abnormal findings immediately, **providing a written record and** *assisting in the implementation of any action should an abnormality or adverse reaction to the practice be noted*

- in undertaking these practices, nurses are accountable for their actions, the quality of care delivered and record-keeping according to Code of Professional Conduct: Standards for Conduct, Performance and Ethics (Nursing and Midwifery Council 2004a), Guidelines for the Administration of Medicines (Nursing and Midwifery Council 2004b), and Guidelines for Records and Record Keeping (Nursing and Midwifery Council 2005).

Additional information

In many societies, feeling fresh and clean is known to create a positive body image and maintain self-esteem. The nurse should be sensitive to the beliefs of different cultures regarding the practice of bathing and personal care. Cultural, ethnic and religious preferences should therefore be observed in respect of personal hygiene (Holland et al 2003).

It is necessary to wash the skin at regular intervals to keep the natural flora of micro-organisms within manageable limits. When a patient is confined to bed, a bed bath is one of the nursing practices used to reduce the potential problem of cross-infection or self-infection during the period of vulnerability caused by illness (Roper et al 2000).

All equipment used should be clean or disposable, and all precautions must be taken to prevent cross-infection. Equipment should be cleaned and dried thoroughly according to local policy. Both at home and in hospital, it is preferable that the patient has a personal wash basin during the period of confinement to bed.

In general, bathing at home is no longer the responsibility of the community nursing service but has become the task of social-care workers. However, it is important that guidance is provided by nurses with regards to skin products especially for patients with urinary or faecal incontinence – see below. If the bed bath is part of an overall package of care, such as for a terminally ill patient, the community nurse will be involved in the management of the delivery of care.

The patient should be offered the facilities to empty his or her bladder prior to commencing a bed bath, immersion bath or shower.

Skin is easily damaged through contact with urine and faeces. The patient with incontinence is at risk of developing continence dermatitis (Ronda & Falce 2002). Burr & Penzer (2005) advise the following management regime for these patients:

- full continence assessment
- use of appropriate continence products
- introduction of a skin-care plan to reduce damage to skin
- avoidance of soaps that can dehydrate the skin. Instead use prescribed aqueous or emollient products. These products should be for single-patient use to prevent cross-infection
- care should be taken in the selection of barrier creams because some include chemicals that can further irritate the skin.

Patient movement during a bed bath should be kept to a minimum, especially when a patient suffers from dyspnoea; changing the bottom sheet should, for example, be planned to minimise movement and effort if the patient is acutely ill. When oxygen therapy is being administered, the mask or cannula can be removed for facial cleansing, hair care and mouth care at separate times during the bed bath.

The nurse and patient should talk to each other during personal hygiene care, but this may have to be kept to a minimum when the patient is acutely ill. For acutely ill or unconscious patients, non-verbal cues can be used as a method of communication, and touch will become of increased importance.

The nurse should check that the patient who is suffering pain has had recent pain relief before starting personal hygiene as the movement during bathing and hair washing may exacerbate the pain.

A patient who does not wash on a regular basis may require some assistance and education from the nurse on the benefit of this practice during his or her period of incapacity. Assisting a patient who has a pyrexia with personal hygiene can be comforting in terms of removing excess perspiration and providing clean, fresh clothing.

In hospital, it is usual to have disposable toiletries available in ward areas for patients who may have been admitted as an emergency, until their own personal equipment is brought from home. When possible, patients should be dressed in their own bed clothing for their comfort and to help maintain their individuality.

A patient who has the power, movement or sensation of a limb altered either temporarily or permanently, such as by the position of an intravenous infusion or following a cerebral vascular accident, will require some assistance and education on how to dress and undress during a bed bath. The weak or affected limb is undressed last and dressed first.

Soap should be used with caution as it has a drying effect on the skin (Burr & Penzer 2002). A patient who has dry skin may have an aqueous cream or emollient prescribed, some preparations can be added to the water for washing. The patient's skin must be rinsed well and thoroughly dried during the bed bath to reduce the potential problem of skin irritation. The nurse should carry out skin care (*see* p. 297) during personal hygiene.

Patients should be assisted to keep their fingernails and toenails clean and manicured. A podiatry service may not be available for all patients but should be used when special care has to be taken of a patient's nails, for example with a diabetic patient or a patient suffering from peripheral vascular disease, to prevent injury to the nail or nailbed. The nurse may assist the patient to apply nail polish if clinically appropriate and desired.

When patients are confined to bed, the friction between their heads and the pillow can cause their hair to become tangled and matted. A patient's hair should therefore be brushed and combed into its usual style during personal hygiene and at regular intervals throughout the day to prevent tangling and discomfort to the patient.

The patient can have his or her hair washed while in bed to maintain its cleanliness. Should a patient be confined to bed over a prolonged period, a hairdresser or barber may be required to cut and style the hair to improve morale.

Before starting personal hygiene care, the nurse should check that the environment around the patient's bed space is at a comfortable temperature and that no draughts are evident. During the procedure, the nurse should ensure that the patient is kept warm as an excessive loss of body heat can lead to hypothermia.

A patient confined to bed will not only feel more comfortable, but will also benefit psychologically from assisted personal care. The provision of privacy during this nursing practice is very important in the maintenance of the patient's self-esteem and individuality.

When possible, help patients to maintain their individuality and independence by allowing them to wash and dry any part of their body they wish, such as their face, hands and pubic area. As the patients have no choice of the method used for cleansing, instead allow them to make decisions in other areas, such as which clothing they wish to wear. The use of body deodorant, perfume and make-up is determined by personal preference, and the nurse should be guided by patients in their application.

An alternative to the traditional bed bath procedure is a commercial pack that provides disposable single-use products. The commercial BagBath® product is described by Collins & Hampton (2003) as a 'quick-drying, one-step product' that has been shown to provide a patient-friendly, cost-effective, soap-free alternative.

Before and after bathing and showering a chair should be available so that the patient can sit to dry or dress themselves without any danger of falling.

The water temperature of an immersion bath should be checked to ensure that there is no danger of scalding; the maximum temperature should be 43°C. The ability to judge temperature may be impaired in elderly patients or those with diabetic neuropathy, so the water temperature should always be checked by a nurse or a responsible adult. The use of a bath thermometer will help with this.

The bath, shower area and bath hoist, if used, should be cleaned after each use. Bath hoists in particular may harbour harmful organisms (Boden 1999). If the nurse is not confident that this has been done, the bath should be cleaned as per local policy before preparing it for the patient in order to prevent any cross-infection.

Mechanical lifting aids should be used appropriately, according to the manufacturer's instructions, to help the patient in and out of the bath or shower. In the community, this will be in accordance with the individualised community bathing assessment.

The patient's manual handling plan should be followed in order to prevent injury to the patient and the staff. For safety, it is advised that a frail, disabled or elderly person should always enter and leave a bath while sitting rather than by climbing over the side of the bath. Variable height or adjustable baths may be used.

To prevent the patient or staff slipping, the spillage of water onto the floor should be avoided; any spills that do occur should be dried immediately.

Patient/carer education

Key points

In partnership with the patient and/or carer, ensure that they are competent to carry out any practices required. Information should be given on an appropriate point of contact for any concerns that may arise.

The carer may be taught how to perform this nursing practice. Preventing infection because of the maintenance of personal hygiene should be explained to the patient and carers. Advice on the direction of washing to reduce the risk of cross-infection from the anal region to the rest of the perineal area should be given to the patient and carer.

The importance of a safe water temperature for bathing and showering should be explained, and the height of the controls or taps may need to be adapted for safe use.

The use of aids, both simple and mechanical, should be explained to the patient. This helps to maintain a safe environment by preventing accidental falls and also ensures safe moving and handling techniques for nurses and carers. Advice and teaching on the availability of aids and the adaptation of the patient's home should be part of the responsibility of the community nursing team and the occupational therapist.

The patient should understand the importance of reporting any redness, swelling or breakdown of the skin to the nurse or medical practitioner so that any further deterioration in the condition of the skin can be prevented.

It is important for carers to understand how to protect skin from urinal and faecal fluid damage.

References

Baker F, Smith L, Stead L 1999 Washing a patient's hair in bed. Nursing Times 95(5 Suppl): 1–2

Boden M 1999 Contamination of moving and handling equipment. Professional Nurse 7: 484–487

Burr S, Penzer R 2005 Promoting skin health. Nursing Standard 19(36): 57–65

Collins F, Hampton S 2003 The cost-effective use of BagBath: a new concept in patient hygiene. British Journal of Nursing 12(16): 984–990

Holland K, Jenkins J, Solomon J et al 2003 Applying the Roper–Logan–Tierney model in practice. Churchill Livingstone, Edinburgh

Nursing and Midwifery Council 2004a Code of professional conduct: standards for conduct, performance and ethics. NMC, London

Nursing and Midwifery Council 2004b Guidelines for the administration of medicines. NMC, London

Nursing and Midwifery Council 2005 Guidelines for records and record keeping. NMC, London

Ronda L, Falce C 2002 Skin care principles in treating older people. Primary Health Care 12(7): 51–57

Roper N, Logan W, Tierney A 2000 The Roper–Logan–Tierney model of nursing. Churchill Livingstone, Edinburgh

Self assessment

1. Under what circumstances would a patient require personal hygiene?
2. How can the skin be protected from urine and faecal damage?
3. What precautions should be taken to ensure the patient is not at risk during this practice?
4. What alternative product could be used instead of soap?

Practice 32
Preoperative Nursing Care

The guidelines in this nursing practice apply to both patients experiencing day surgery and those undergoing surgery that requires a longer stay in hospital.

Learning outcomes

By the end of this section, you should know how to:
- explain the standard preoperative preparation of a patient who is scheduled for surgery
- describe the nurse's role in looking after a patient prior to surgery.

Background knowledge required

Revision of the cardiopulmonary system
Review of health authority policy on the preoperative preparation of patients
Review of health authority policy on preoperative deep vein prophylaxis.

Indications and rationale for preoperative care

Preoperative nursing care is required to promote the optimum physical and psychological condition of patients undergoing surgical procedures (National Association of Theatre Nurses 2004a, Royal College of Nursing 2005).

Guidelines and rationale for this nursing practice

- explain the pre- and postoperative routines to the patient and answer any questions appropriately; the discussion of any fears or anxieties that the patient may have should be encouraged. Studies have demonstrated that patients' *anxiety levels are reduced by receiving information and explanation. Preoperative reduction of anxiety may affect postoperative analgesia use, wound healing and length of hospital stay* (Boore 1975, Hayward 1978, Fyffe 1999)
- record the temperature, pulse, respiration rate, blood pressure and urinalysis results, if required, *to give baseline findings with which to compare postoperative observations and detect abnormalities. Any abnormalities should be discussed with the nurse in charge and medical staff*
- carry out an evacuation of the patient's bowel using suppositories or the specific bowel preparation requested by the surgeon. This is usually requested if the surgical procedure involves the bowel *as evacuation helps to reduce the risk of contamination of the wound by intestinal organisms.* Intravenous fluids may be required during this time to ensure patient hydration prior to surgery
- offer the sedative that was ordered by medical staff the night before surgery *in order to help the patient sleep well*
- fast healthy adult patients of oral clear fluids 2 hours prior to induction of anaesthesia *to reduce the risk of aspiration pneumonitis.* Healthy adults are

defined as healthy patients without gastrointestinal disease or disorders (Royal College of Nursing 2005). Clear fluids include tea and coffee (without milk)

- solid foods, including milk, should be withheld for six hours prior to induction of anaesthesia *in order to avoid the risk of regurgitation and the inhalation of gastric contents while under the anaesthetic* (National Association of Theatre Nurses 2004a)

- prepare the skin according to health authority policy. This may involve the removal of an area of body hair by shaving or depilatory cream, showering or bathing using an antiseptic soap and putting on a theatre gown and perhaps socks and paper pants. These actions *may reduce the risk of a postoperative infection*. However, research into the removal of body hair and the use of antiseptic preparations in baths and showers has, however, produced contradictory findings (Brown 2002)

- ensure that all underwear has been removed, although paper pants may be worn on some occasions. Nail varnish should be removed from fingernails and toenails and make-up removed *so that these sites can be used by the anaesthetist to assess for signs of hypoxia*. Dentures must be removed *because of the danger of inhaling them, causing asphyxiation*.
  Health authority policies on the removal of spectacles, hair grips, contact lenses, hearing aids and other prostheses, e.g. wigs and artificial eyes or limbs, vary

- tape the wedding ring to the patient's finger. All other jewellery and valuables that the patient has brought into hospital should be recorded, put into an envelope, labelled appropriately and placed in a valuables box or safe. Pay special attention to any body piercing that patients may have. It may not be possible to remove some piercings, so these should be taped. If these are within the mouth area discuss with anaesthetist. Metal jewellery may be accidentally lost or may be a cause of harm to the patient, e.g. a diathermy burn (National Association of Theatre Nurses 2004b)

- document on the preoperative assessment chart any body piercing, whether taped or untaped, *to highlight to all staff who will be involved in the patient's care*

- check the patient's identification verbally and from the identification band, and confirm that the form of consent for the operation has been signed. Confirm the side of the operation if appropriate. This is done *to comply with legal requirements and hospital policy*

- after the patient has had the opportunity to micturate, administer the premedication ordered by the anaesthetist. Premedication can *help to relax the patient and may dry up any secretions*. All normal medications should be administered or withheld according to the anaesthetist's instruction

- help the patient to put on anti-embolic stockings if these have been recommended. This is *to reduce the risk of deep vein thrombosis* (Scottish Intercollegiate Guidelines Network 2002)

- leave the patient to rest quietly when the premedication has been given, but observe him or her for any reaction to the drugs. Request that the patient does not get out of bed unsupervised after the administration of premedication *to reduce the risk of falls when a sedative drug has been given*.
  Rest may also *encourage relaxation and maximise the effect of the*

premedication. In day surgery units, premedication is often only offered to patients who appear to have a high anxiety level

- when the porter from the theatre reception area arrives to collect the patient, accompany them to the theatre reception area and hand the patient over to the care of a theatre nurse. There is a checklist that the ward nurse and theatre nurse complete, the content of which will be determined by health authority policy. The patient may travel to theatre on a hospital bed or a theatre trolley, according to health authority policy. Ensure that all the relevant documentation, e.g. case notes, medicine prescription chart, X-rays, ECG tracings and reports, accompanies the patient to theatre. Research studies have demonstrated that a known person accompanying the patient **helps to reduce anxiety**

- appropriate relevant information should have been given to the relatives beforehand so that they can, with the patient's permission, telephone to check progress **to help reduce the relatives' anxiety**

- in undertaking this practice, nurses are accountable for their actions, the quality of care delivered and record-keeping according to the Code of Professional Conduct: Standards for Conduct, Performance and Ethics (Nursing and Midwifery Council 2004) and Guidelines for Records and Record Keeping (Nursing and Midwifery Council 2005).

Patient/carer education

Key points

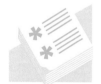

In partnership with the patient and/or carer, ensure that they are competent to carry out any practices required. Information should be given on an appropriate point of contact for any concerns that may arise.

It is important that patients undergoing day surgery should have obtained beforehand all the information and knowledge necessary for them to undergo their surgery successfully. This will probably involve nurses at the outpatient clinic, in the community and in the day surgery unit. Written material should be provided to reinforce the verbal information given. Patients will need to carry out at home many of the preoperative preparations, such as bowel preparation, skin preparation and fasting.

References

Boore J 1975 Prescription for recovery. RCN, London

Brown A 2002 The patient undergoing surgery. In: Walsh M (ed) Watson's clinical nursing and related sciences, 6th edn, Chapter 10. Baillière Tindall, London

Fyffe A 1999 Anxiety and the perioperative patient. British Journal of Theatre Nursing 3(4): 12–14

Hayward J 1978 Information: a prescription against pain. RCN, London

National Association of Theatre Nurses 2004a Standards and recommendations for perioperative practice. NATN, Harrogate, UK

National Association of Theatre Nurses 2004b Electrosurgery: managing the risks. NATN, Harrogate (Available at: http://www.afpp.org.uk/document_downloads/position_statements/Electrosurgery%20Guidance%202004.pdf [accessed 30 March 2006])

Nursing and Midwifery Council 2004 Code of professional conduct: standards for conduct, performance and ethics. NMC, London

Nursing and Midwifery Council 2005 Guidelines for records and record keeping. NMC, London

Royal College of Nursing 2005 Perioperative fasting in adults and children. RCN, London

Scottish Intercollegiate Guidelines Network 2002 Guidelines prophylaxis of venous thromboembolism No 62. SIGN, Edinburgh

Websites

Association for Perioperative Practice, incorporating National Association of
    Theatre Nurses: http://www.afpp.org.uk
Royal College of Nursing: http://www.rcn.org.uk
Scottish Intercollegiate Guidelines Network: http://www.sign.ac.uk

Self assessment

1. Why is it important to ensure patients' anxiety is reduced preoperatively?
2. What is the preoperative fasting requirement for healthy patients?
3. Describe the current guidelines for prophylaxis of deep vein thrombosis?

Practice 33
Postoperative Nursing Care

In the case of day surgery, many of the guidelines described here will be carried out by the community nurse, the patient or the carers at home.

Learning outcomes

By the end of this section, you should know how to:
- explain the general postoperative care of a patient
- describe the nurse's role in carrying out general postoperative care.

Background knowledge required

Revision of airway management
Revision of the signs and symptoms of hypoxia
Revision of the signs of difficulty with breathing – respiratory rate changes, stridor, colour, use of accessory muscles
Revision of the signs and symptoms of haemorrhage
Revision of the strengths and weaknesses of pulse oximetry
Revision of the effects of postoperative hypothermia
Revision of the clinical features of shock
Revision of the physiology of wound healing
Review of health authority policy on postoperative care.

Indications and rationale for postoperative care

Postoperative nursing care is required to monitor the patient's condition *in order to prevent and identify any problems that may occur after a surgical procedure*.

Guidelines and rationale for this nursing practice

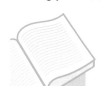

When receiving the patient back into the ward

- read the patient's theatre notes to confirm the surgical procedure that has been carried out and ascertain any instructions from the surgeon or anaesthetist, e.g. the positioning of the patient or any oxygen therapy required
- check that the airway is patent and that the patient is breathing adequately. The patient is usually conscious before leaving the recovery room, but check the level of consciousness on the return to the ward. If he or she is heavily sedated, *the tongue may slip back and obstruct the airway*. If this happens, first perform the head tilt, chin lift manoeuvre and call for assistance if required. The use of an adjunct airway may be required to secure a patent airway. If the patient is nauseated it may be safer to nurse them in the recovery position if possible.
- monitor the respiratory rate and rhythm and look for any signs of breathing distress
- monitor oxygen saturation *to ensure adequate perfusion. Check the colour of the patient – nail beds, lips for signs of cyanosis*

- on initial return to the ward 15 minute observations should be performed; *this may vary from patient to patient*. Record the temperature, pulse (feel the radial pulse for rate and rhythm), blood pressure, and urine output and compare the results with the patient's preoperative and intraoperative recordings. This will give some indication of the stability of the patient's condition and allow for prompt recognition of deterioration and improvements in the patient's condition (NHS Quality Improvement Scotland 2004). The use of a Modified Early Warning Scoring (MEWS) system has been shown to help with prompt recognition of patients at risk of deterioration (Parissopoulos & Kotzabassakis, 2005)

- observe the wound, note any staining of the dressing. Observe any drains, e.g. a Redivac free drainage, suction, or corrugated drain, that may be present, monitor patency, amount of drainage and type of fluid *to ensure prompt recognition if there are problems such as haemorrhage or blockage*

- monitor the patient's pain score (resting and moving) and administer analgesics as required by the patient and as prescribed by the medical staff *to relieve pain and anxiety* (NHS Quality Improvement Scotland 2004). Check the intraoperative and recovery record for type and last dose of painkiller *to ensure over-dosage of analgesia is avoided*. Several research studies have demonstrated that patients rate being in pain as the most anxiety-provoking issue when undergoing surgery (Nendick 2000)

- if an intravenous infusion is present, check that it is functioning according to medical staff instructions

- ensure that the patient is lying in as comfortable a position as possible and that the limbs are positioned in a manner that will not endanger muscle and nerve tissue. These measures can *help to control the level of pain*

- if a problem occurs with the patient's condition alert the nurse in charge and the doctor caring for the patient. It may be necessary to increase the frequency of observations, catheterise the patient and record hourly urine volumes and increase oxygen. It may also be necessary to move the patient to a high-dependency unit (NHS Quality Improvement Scotland 2004).

Continuing postoperative nursing

- record blood pressure, pulse and respiration rate until these are within the normal range and stable. *This usually indicates the reduction of physiological stress induced by the surgery*

- assist the patient to wash and change into his or her own nightwear and offer a mouthwash, *to aid comfort and the recovery of a sense of individuality*. If the patient has been wearing anti-embolic stockings, the continued benefit of these is to be emphasised

- encourage the patient to sit up in bed well supported by pillows (unless contraindicated) and move around as much as possible, helping him or her out of bed when the blood pressure recordings are satisfactory. These measures *help to minimise the risk of complications such as skin breakdown and deep venous thrombosis and postoperative chest infection* (Scottish Intercollegiate Guidelines Network 2004)

- unless contraindicated (e.g. by the presence of a nasogastric tube), allow a graduated amount of fluid; then gradually introduce solid food if there is no vomiting and if bowel sounds are present, *in order to rehydrate the patient and to help restore the blood glucose level to within the normal range*

- observe the wound regularly for leakage, bleeding or haematoma
- record the amount and time when the patient passes urine and has a first bowel movement *as constipation is a common postoperative problem because of immobility, dehydration and the use of narcotic analgesics*
- arrange an ongoing pain control assessment *to reduce unnecessary distress to the patient*
- ensure that the patient has adequate periods of rest *as this will aid recovery*
- give encouragement and support to the patient and any explanation or information that may be requested
- the breathing exercises described on page 27 should be encouraged *to help avoid the problems mentioned above*
- in undertaking this practice, nurses are accountable for their actions, the quality of care delivered and record-keeping according to the Code of Professional Conduct: Standards for Conduct, Performance and Ethics (Nursing and Midwifery Council 2004) and Guidelines for Records and Record Keeping (Nursing and Midwifery Council 2005).

Patient/carer education

Key points

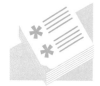

In partnership with the patient and/or carer, ensure that they are competent to carry out any practices required. Information should be given on an appropriate point of contact for any concerns that may arise.

Depending on the surgical procedure performed, the hospital patient may require a planned education programme delivered by an appropriately experienced nurse. All patients should be informed of ways of reducing the risk of occurrence of the common postoperative complications.

Day surgery patients and their carers assume a large degree of responsibility for postoperative care, and staff must ensure that they are able to cope with this before allowing the patient to be discharged. Close liaison should be maintained with the community nursing service (*see* 'Transfer of patients between care settings', p. 343).

Discharge medications should be clearly explained, especially if they are new to the patient. Involvement of the family and carers can help to ensure compliance. Ensure the patient and carer are fully aware of the risks of deep venous thrombosis in the early recuperation period and clearly explain the need for continued mobilisation and wearing of anti-embolic stockings where necessary (Scottish Intercollegiate Guidelines Network 2004).

References

Nendick M 2000 Patient satisfaction with postoperative analgesia. Nursing Standard 14(22): 32–37

NHS Quality Improvement Scotland 2004 best practice statement: postoperative pain management. HMSO, Edinburgh

Nursing and Midwifery Council 2004 Code of professional conduct: standards for conduct, performance and ethics. NMC, London

Nursing and Midwifery Council 2005 Guidelines for records and record keeping. NMC, London

Parissopoulos S, Kotzabassakis S 2005 Critical care outreach and the use of early warning scoring systems: a literature review. ICUS Nursing Web Journal 1–13 (Available at: http://www.nursing.gr/WARNING.pdf)

Scottish Intercollegiate Guidelines Network 2004 Postoperative management in adults: a practical guide to postoperative care for clinical staff. SIGN, Edinburgh

Websites
Scottish Intercollegiate Guidelines Network: http://www.sign.ac.uk/
NHS Quality Improvement Scotland: http://www.nhshealthquality.org

Self assessment

1. What are the signs and symptoms of respiratory distress?
2. How would you maintain a patient's airway?
3. What are the signs and symptoms of hypovolaemia?
4. If using a MEWS system, when would you call for senior help?

Practice 34
Pulse

This section has two parts:

1 Pulse

2 Apical–radial pulses

Learning outcomes	**By the end of this section, you should be able to:**

- provide an understanding and rationale for this practice
- prepare the patient for this nursing practice
- locate, assess, measure and record the radial pulse
- locate the major pulse points of the body
- locate, assess, measure and record the apical–radial pulses.

Background knowledge

To help you to palpate the pulse and interpret the results, it is necessary to have some knowledge of the structure, function and pathology of the cardiovascular system, particularly the heart, the conduction system and the arteries

For the practice of apical–radial pulse you should demonstrate competence in measuring and recording a radial pulse and in the correct use of a stethoscope.

1. PULSE

Indications and rationale for assessing the radial pulse

A pulse is the rhythmic expansion and recoil of the elastic arteries caused by the ejection of blood from the left ventricle. It can be palpated where an artery near the body surface can be pressed against a firm structure such as bone. Three aspects are usually noted when a pulse is being palpated – its rate, rhythm and strength.

The pulse may be assessed for the following reasons:

- on admission *to ascertain the patient's pulse and assess whether or not it falls within the normal range for the person's age*
- preoperatively *to ascertain the patient's baseline pulse rate, rhythm and quality so that comparisons can be made with postoperative assessments*

- postoperatively **to monitor the rate, rhythm and quality as indicators of the patient's cardiovascular stability and to compare the findings with the preoperative baseline data**
- **to help to estimate, in general terms, the degree of fluid loss when the level of body fluids is lowered**, e.g. after excessive vomiting, excessive diarrhoea or haemorrhage. In the event of a large fluid loss from the body, the pulse is thready and rapid. Severe electrolyte imbalance causes impaired cell function and cardiac arrhythmias
- **to compare with baseline admission assessments to help to evaluate the effect of treatment on patients who have cardiovascular or pulmonary disease**. The majority of patients with these problems will have pulse irregularities that should stabilise with treatment
- **to monitor the patient who is receiving a blood or blood product intravenous infusion**. Elevated pulse and temperature are among the first signs of reaction to the infusion.

The following terms are used to describe the differing ranges of pulse **rate**:
— normal resting heart rate for adults and adolescents 60–100 beats per minute
— a pulse rate over 100 beats per minute is known as **tachycardia**
— a pulse rate below 60 beats per minute is known as **bradycardia**

Tachycardia (a rapid pulse rate) can be the result of pain, anger, fear or anxiety, all of which stimulate the sympathetic nervous system and cause the release of adrenaline (epinephrine). It can also occur in some heart diseases, anaemia and fever, and during exercise, all of which require a greater amount of oxygen and thus increase the cardiac output (Alexander et al 2006). **Bradycardia** (a slow pulse rate) occurs in any condition, for example raised intracranial pressure, which stimulates the parasympathetic nervous system. Specific heart conditions such as damage to the conducting mechanism after a myocardial infarction can also cause bradycardia. It also occurs in fit athletes, who develop a very efficient heart muscle action.

Rhythm

The rhythm should be regular; any irregularities should be noted. It should be observed whether the irregularities occur at regular or irregular intervals. A normal regular irregularity may occur, particularly in younger people, in conjunction with inspiration and expiration.

Strength

The pulse pressure is the difference between the systolic and the diastolic pressure. The force is a reflection of the pulse strength. The pulse is usually recorded as being normal, bounding, weak and thready, or absent (Goodall 2000).

Elasticity

The elastic recoil of the artery wall should be noted. The artery of a healthy young adult feels flexible and non-tortuous, quite different from that of an elderly patient suffering from a condition such as arteriosclerosis, whose artery will feel hard and cord-like.

The pulse rate is much higher in babies and young children than adults because they have a higher metabolic rate. A pacemaker occasionally 'fires' before the sinoatrial node; the resulting decrease in filling time of the heart chambers causes a pause in the rhythm, which can be detected when assessing the pulse.

Remember you are not solely assessing the pulse rate. You are also assessing the pulse for rhythm and strength. As pulse forms one part of the observation of your patient's cardiovascular or respiratory status, it should be remembered that assessment of the colour of the lips, skin, nail beds and breathing pattern should also be noted.

Outline of the procedure

The pulse can be felt by placing two fingers over any artery lying close to the skin's surface. The radial artery is the most commonly used site for assessing rate and rhythm. If the pulse is irregular, an apical–radial pulse should be performed (*see* Section 2).

Equipment

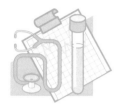

1. Watch with a second hand
2. Observation chart
3. Black pen.

Guidelines and rationale for this nursing practice

- explain the nursing practice to the patient **to obtain consent and co-operation**. Patients should be encouraged to be active partners in their care
- wash your hands **to prevent cross-infection between patients** (Jeanes 2005)
- ensure that the patient is in a position that is as comfortable and relaxed as possible. **This will help the nurse to obtain a true baseline measurement**
- observe the patient throughout this activity for any signs of discomfort or distress. **This should allow the nurse to intervene immediately in the event of an adverse reaction**
- locate the radial artery, place the first and second fingers along it and press gently (Fig. 34.1). Sufficient pressure should be applied to allow the artery to be against an underlying bone **so that the pulse of blood passing through the artery can be felt**, but care must be taken not to press too hard or the artery may be occluded
- count the pulse for 60 seconds **to allow sufficient time to detect any irregularities or other defects**
- document the findings appropriately, comparing past recordings, and report any abnormal findings immediately **to enable early intervention to improve the problem**
- wash hands after taking the pulse (Jeanes 2005)
- in undertaking this practice, nurses are accountable for their actions, the quality of care delivered and record-keeping according to the Code of Professional Conduct: Standards for Conduct, Performance and Ethics (Nursing and Midwifery Council 2004) and Guidelines for Records and Record Keeping (Nursing and Midwifery Council 2005).

It should be noted that although some research suggests that the pulse can be measured over 15 or 30 seconds and then multiplied by 4 or 2 respectively to give

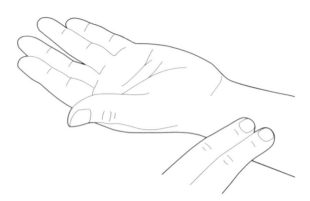

FIGURE 34.1

Taking a radial pulse
From Trim 2005. Copyright
Emap Public Sector Ltd
2005. Reproduced by
permission of Nursing
Times

the beats per minute (Hwu & Coates 2000), the student or novice nurse should palpate the pulse for a full 60 seconds to assess regularity and strength. Although electronic devices exist that have the capability to measure the pulse rate these do not have the ability to assess for irregularities or arterial insufficiency. Additionally, poor understanding of equipment and a lack of competence in its correct use can result in inaccurate recording and subsequent poor outcomes for your patient (Davidson & Barber 2004).

Sites of major pulse points of the body

Although the pulse assessment is usually made using the radial artery, there are other sites where an artery near the body surface can be pressed against an underlying bone or other firm body structure. The major pulses (Fig. 34.2) are the:
- temporal
- carotid – assessing strength of the pulse
- brachial – when measuring blood pressure
- radial – assessing rate and rhythm
- femoral – assessing the characteristics of the pulse
- popliteal – assessing for peripheral vascular disease (PVD)
- posterior tibial – assessing for PVD
- dorsalis pedis – assessing for PVD.

2. APICAL–RADIAL PULSES

Indications and rationale

The rate at the apex of the heart and a peripheral pulse rate, usually the radial pulse, are counted simultaneously and compared to ascertain whether there is a discrepancy in the rate. It may be assessed **to estimate the degree of dysfunction on admission and the effect of treatment on**:
- patients, who have cardiac impairment, for example frequent ventricular ectopic beats, atrial fibrillation or atrial flutter. This is because in such cases each ventricular contraction may not be sufficiently strong to transmit an arterial pulse (Jevon et al 2000). Apex and radial pulse measurement represents an important component in your patient's care if they have been diagnosed with atrial fibrillation

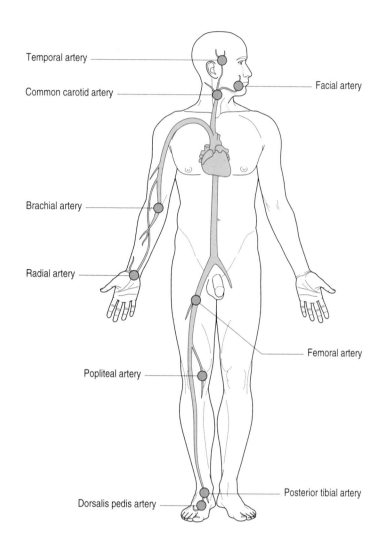

Temporal artery

Common carotid artery

Facial artery

Brachial artery

Radial artery

Femoral artery

Popliteal artery

Posterior tibial artery

Dorsalis pedis artery

FIGURE 34.2
Locating the pulse
From Trim 2005. Copyright
Emap Public Sector Ltd
2005. Reproduced by
permission of Nursing
Times

■ patients who are receiving medication to improve heart action, e.g. digoxin
■ patients who have peripheral arterial disease.

The assessment elicits a pulse–apex deficit and helps in decisions on the necessity for treatment (Alexander et al 2006). The wider the deficit, the less efficient the cardiac contraction.

Equipment

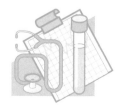

1. Watch with a second hand
2. Stethoscope
3. Observation chart
4. Red pen
5. Black pen.

Guidelines and rationale for this nursing practice

- measurement is carried out by two nurses simultaneously over 1 minute **to allow accuracy in recording an irregular rate**
- explain the nursing practice to the patient, including the reasons for the procedure and the manner in which it will be carried out **to gain consent and co-operation. Patients should be encouraged to be active, informed partners in their care**
- the patient should rest for at least 15 minutes prior to the procedure **as this will give an indication of the ventricular rate at rest**
- ensure the patient's privacy **to maintain dignity and a sense of self**
- collect the equipment for efficiency of practice and to reduce any unnecessary stress for the patient (Fig. 34.3)
- wash hands **to prevent cross-infection**
- assist the patient to a comfortable position, inclined slightly forward if possible so that there is easy access to the chest wall and gravity will move the heart to the front of the thoracic cage. Patient comfort will also prevent an artificial elevation of the pulse rate
- observe the patient throughout this activity **to detect any signs of discomfort**
- place the diaphragm of the stethoscope over the apex of the heart (nurse 1) (Figs 34.4 & 34.5). This is usually located at the 5th intercostal space and 12 cm left of the midline
- locate the peripheral, usually radial, pulse (nurse 2) (Fig. 34.6)
- ensure that the watch is visible to both nurses, who begin counting the rates simultaneously for 1 minute (Fig. 34.7)
- at the end of 1 minute, the nurses compare results and document them appropriately, **compare these with past recordings and report any abnormal findings immediately**. The apex rate is recorded in red ink and the peripheral in black ink **to distinguish the two recordings**

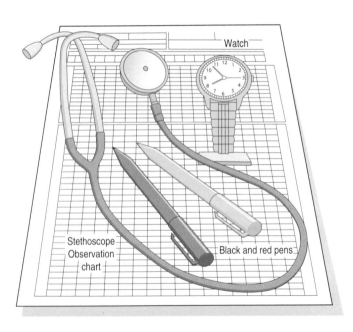

FIGURE 34.3

Assemble equipment
From Jevon et al 2000. Copyright Emap Public Sector Ltd 2000. Reproduced by permission of Nursing Times

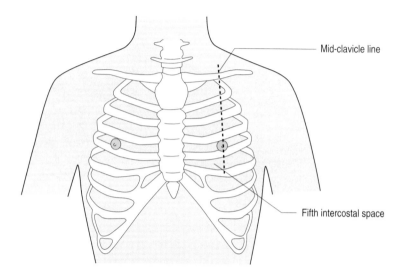

Mid-clavicle line

Fifth intercostal space

FIGURE 34.4
Locate the apex beat (a)
From Jevon et al
2000. Copyright Emap
Public Sector Ltd
2000. Reproduced by
permission of Nursing
Times

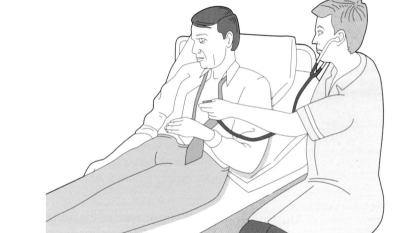

FIGURE 34.5
Locate the apex beat (b)
From Jevon et al
2000. Copyright Emap
Public Sector Ltd
2000. Reproduced by
permission of Nursing
Times

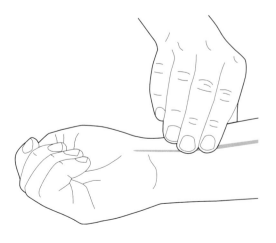

FIGURE 34.6
Locate the radial pulse
From Jevon et al
2000. Copyright Emap
Public Sector Ltd
2000. Reproduced by
permission of Nursing
Times

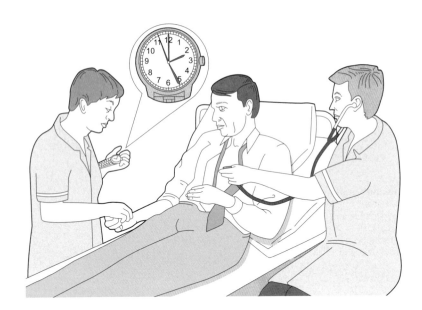

FIGURE 34.7
Count the pulse
From Jevon et al
2000. Copyright Emap
Public Sector Ltd
2000. Reproduced by
permission of Nursing
Times

- if the apex rate is too quick to be recording accurately you should consider using cardiac monitoring
- the patient's clothing should be repositioned if appropriate and the patient made comfortable *to maintain comfort and dignity*
- wash hands and clean the stethoscope *to prevent cross-infection*
- in undertaking this practice, nurses are accountable for their actions, the quality of care delivered and record-keeping according to the Code of Professional Conduct: Standards for Conduct, Performance and Ethics (Nursing and Midwifery Council 2004) and Guidelines for Records and Record Keeping (Nursing and Midwifery Council 2005).

**Patient/carer
education**
Key points

The patient and carer must receive meaningful explanations regarding their care and the rationale for this nursing practice. In addition patients and their carers should be given relevant information and support in relation to the health problem.

It is helpful to explain to patients that their pulse rate will increase with exercise. If they wish to palpate their own pulse, they should be shown the correct way to do this, staff monitoring the results until the patient has been shown to be competent.

References

Alexander M, Fawcett J, Runciman P 2006 Nursing care – hospital and home: the adult, 3rd edn. Churchill Livingstone, Edinburgh
Davidson K, Barber V 2004 Electronic monitoring of patients in general wards. Nursing Standard 18(49): 42–46
Goodall S 2000 Peripheral vascular disease. Nursing Standard 14(25): 48–52
Hwu JY, Coates V 2000 A study of the effectiveness of different measuring times and counting methods of human radial pulses. Journal of Clinical Nursing 9(1): 146–152
Jeanes A 2005 Infection control. A practical guide to the use of hand decontaminants. Nursing Times 101(20): 46–48

Jevon P, Ewens B, Lowe R 2000 Measuring apex and radial pulse. Nursing Times 96(50): 43–44

Nursing and Midwifery Council 2004 Code of professional conduct: standards for conduct, performance and ethics. NMC, London

Nursing and Midwifery Council 2005 Guidelines for records and record keeping. NMC, London

Trim J 2005 Monitoring pulse. Nursing Times 101(21): 30–31

Self assessment

1. What do you understand by the terms rhythm and strength in relation to pulse assessment?
2. You are admitting a patient to hospital. How would you assess their radial pulse? Write down the steps you would perform.
3. Name three sites for pulse measurement other than radial and identify their location on the human body.
4. List two reasons why your patient may require apex–radial pulse assessment.
5. Where should you place the diaphragm of the stethoscope to measure apical heart rate?
6. How would you maintain patient dignity throughout this practice?

Practice 35
Rectal Examination

Learning outcomes	**By the end of this section, you should know how to:** ▪ prepare the patient for this procedure ▪ collect and prepare the equipment ▪ assist the practitioner performing this procedure as requested.
Background knowledge required	Revision of the anatomy and physiology of the sigmoid colon, rectum and anus A basic understanding of the potential complications for spinal injury patients in relation to bowel care.
Indications and rationale for rectal examination	Rectal examination is used as a diagnostic aid when there is: ▪ *rectal bleeding* ▪ *severe constipation* ▪ *severe diarrhoea* ▪ *pain in the anal or rectal area* ▪ *a suspected enlarged prostate gland* ▪ *a suspected rectocele*. An experienced nurse who has undergone appropriate training may perform a digital rectal examination as part of the assessment process for severe constipation (Royal College of Nursing 2000). This procedure assists the nurse practitioner in the decision-making process when choosing an appropriate laxative or enema (*see* 'Enemas', p. 129, and 'Suppositories', p. 321 for further information). The nurse practitioner may also use this procedure to remove faeces present in the lower rectum if appropriate.
Outline of the procedure	The medical or nursing practitioner will put a disposable glove on the dominant hand and apply some lubricant to the fingertips. He or she will then insert one or two fingers into the patient's rectum and perform the examination. On completing the examination, the practitioner will remove the glove by turning it inside out as he or she takes it off. A lubricated rectal speculum may be inserted by a medical practitioner and, using the light source, a visual examination carried out. An anal or rectal swab may also be taken for laboratory examination. Digital rectal examinations (DREs) must be performed with caution on patients with a spinal injury at T6 or above. A DRE can stimulate the vasal nerve, causing the heart beat to slow and blood pressure to fall. The patient may demonstrate a flush over the upper body and experience a sense of impending doom. This is known as 'autonomic dysreflexia' and requires prompt medical attention. It is important to note that this is an invasive and embarrassing procedure for the patient. Care and consideration should be taken by the practitioner at all stages

of this procedure, remaining alert to potential issues that could arise, e.g. previous radiotherapy to this area, detection of a previously undiagnosed rectal carcinoma or a past history of abuse.

Equipment

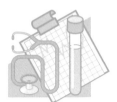

1. Tray/flat surface
2. Disposable gloves
3. Apron
4. Sterile rectal speculum (Fig. 35.1), if required
5. Water-soluble lubricant
6. Protective covering for the bed
7. Receptacle for soiled disposable items
8. Swabs
9. Sterile laboratory swab in a container, if required
10. Light source.

Guidelines and rationale for this nursing practice

- help to explain the procedure to the patient **to gain consent and co-operation**
- collect and prepare the equipment **for efficiency of practice**
- assist the patient into the position requested by the medical practitioner, ensuring privacy. This is usually the left lateral position
- obtain a baseline pulse **to allow for quick identification of any complications related to stimulating the vasal nerve during the procedure**
- observe the patient throughout this activity **to detect any signs of discomfort or distress**
- assist the medical practitioner as requested
- ensure that the patient is left feeling as comfortable as possible. If any bleeding is likely as a result of the examination, ensure that the patient's underwear is protected
- dispose of the equipment safely **for the protection of others**
- document the examination in the patient's records, monitor the after-effects and report any abnormal findings immediately **to provide a written record and assist in the implementation of any action should an abnormality or adverse reaction to the practice be noted**
- in undertaking this practice, nurses are accountable for their actions, the quality of care delivered and record-keeping according to the Code of Professional Conduct: Standards for Conduct, Performance and Ethics (Nursing and Midwifery Council 2004) and Guidelines for Records and Record Keeping (Nursing and Midwifery Council 2005).

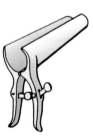

FIGURE 35.1
Rectal speculum

Patient/carer education

Key points

In partnership with the patient and/or carer, ensure that they are competent to carry out any practices required. Information should be given on an appropriate point of contact for any concerns that may arise.

A careful explanation should help to gain the patient's co-operation and aid relaxation, which will in turn reduce the discomfort of the examination.

The patient should be informed who to contact if severe pain, discharge or bleeding is experienced after the examination. Contact numbers for appropriate counselling services should be available in the event of distress caused by issues in relation to abuse experienced by the patient.

References

Nursing and Midwifery Council 2004 Code of professional conduct: standards for conduct, performance and ethics. NMC, London

Nursing and Midwifery Council 2005 Guidelines for records and record keeping. NMC, London

Royal College of Nursing 2000 Digital rectal examination and manual removal of faeces. RCN, London

Website

NHS Scotland (SHOW): http:// www.show.scot.nhs.uk/spinalunit/ Spinal%20Documents/AUTDYS.pdf

Self assessment

1. Describe the complications associated with performing a DRE on a patient with a spinal injury.
2. Describe and justify the correct position to place a patient prior to a rectal examination.
3. Explain why a patient may be apprehensive prior to undergoing a rectal examination.

Practice 36
Respiration

Learning outcomes	**By the end of this section, you should know how to:** ▪ prepare the patient for this nursing practice ▪ assess, measure and record the respirations ▪ recognise any abnormalities.
Background knowledge required	To help you to assess, record and interpret respiration, it is necessary to have some knowledge of the respiratory system, particularly the physiology of the bronchi, bronchioles and alveoli.
Indications and rationale for assessing respiration	The basic activity of the respiratory system is to supply sufficient oxygen for the body's metabolic needs and remove carbon dioxide. This is achieved through inspiration and expiration. One respiration consists of an inspiration and an expiration. Respiration may be assessed for the following reasons: ▪ to obtain a baseline measurement **so that any alteration in the patient's breathing pattern can be promptly noticed** ▪ to monitor a patient who has breathing problems **to help in diagnosis** ▪ to compare against baseline measurements **to help evaluate the effect of treatment on patients who have pulmonary disease**.
Equipment 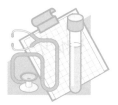	1. Watch with a second hand.
Guidelines and rationale for this nursing practice 	▪ this is the one assessment that is best carried out without the patient's knowledge **because if the patient becomes aware that the respiration rate is being assessed, this can cause the rate to change** ▪ ensure that the patient is in a comfortable position and is as relaxed as possible **as this will help to ensure an accurate assessment** ▪ observe the patient throughout for any signs of discomfort or distress **in order to monitor any adverse effects** ▪ this practice is usually carried out immediately after the assessment of the patient's pulse while the nurse still has his or her finger in position to palpate the radial pulse (Fig. 36.1). **This helps to reduce the risk of the patient becoming aware that the respiration rate is being assessed**

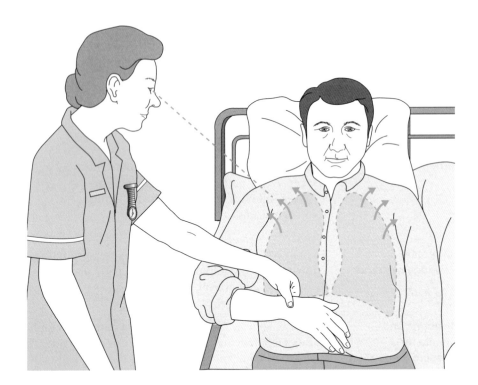

FIGURE 36.1
Monitoring the respiration rate while apparently counting the pulse
From Nicol et al 2003, with permission

- count the respirations for 60 seconds by observing the rise and fall of the patient's chest. One respiration consists of an inspiration and an expiration. The normal respiratory rate is between 12 and 18 respirations per minute
- observe the rhythm, depth and noise of respiration. Respirations should be quiet, have a regular rhythm with the depth neither shallow nor very deep
- assessment for 60 seconds *enables the nurse to become aware of any irregularities or abnormalities in the patient's breathing pattern*
- document the findings appropriately, comparing them against past recordings. Report any abnormal findings immediately and be aware of any possible complications *so that remedial action can immediately be taken* (Nursing and Midwifery Council 2005)
- in undertaking this practice, nurses are accountable for their actions, the quality of care delivered and record-keeping according to the Code of Professional Conduct: Standards for Conduct, Performance and Ethics (Nursing and Midwifery Council 2004) and Guidelines for Records and Record Keeping (Nursing and Midwifery Council 2005).

Patient/carer education
Key points

In partnership with the patient and/or carer, ensure that they are competent to carry out any practices required. Information should be given on an appropriate point of contact for any concerns that may arise.

Explain techniques that may help to ease breathing difficulties to patients who have respiratory problems. Such advice may include the avoidance of restrictive clothing, resting positions and breathing techniques. The effects of exercise on breathing rates and patterns should also be explained.

References

Nicol M, Bavin C, Bedford-Turner S et al 2003 Essential nursing skills, 2nd edn. Mosby, London

Nursing and Midwifery Council 2004 Code of professional conduct: standards for conduct, performance and ethics. NMC, London

Nursing and Midwifery Council 2005 Guidelines for records and record keeping. NMC, London

Websites

Asthma UK: http://www.asthma.org.uk/

Living with Chronic Obstructive Pulmonary Disease: http://www.livingwithcopd.co.uk

Workwithus: http:// www.workwithus.org/charities-scotland/health/ asthma-support-group

Self assessment

1. You are asked to measure and record your patient's respirations. What other indicators of respiratory function can be assessed at the same time as counting the respiratory rate?
2. What is the normal respiratory rate and why is it necessary to count respirations with the patient unaware?

Practice 37
Skin Care

Learning outcomes	**By the end of this section, you should know how to:** ▪ prepare the patient for this nursing practice ▪ collect the equipment ▪ carry out skin care.
Background knowledge required	Revision of the anatomy and physiology of the skin Revision of the predisposing factors for the development of a pressure ulcer The health authority policy regarding risk assessment, pressure ulcer classification, care implementation and criteria for the use of aids to prevent pressure ulcers should be reviewed Revision of 'Moving and handling' a patient (*see* p. 213) and 'Exercises: active and passive' (*see* p. 135).
Indications and rationale for skin care	This care involves the maintenance of a patient's skin viability by ensuring skin cleanliness, relieving skin capillary pressure, ensuring adequate nutritional status and monitoring potential problems. Skin care is indicated for every patient, but specific circumstances increase the need for care when: ▪ ***the patient is incontinent*** ▪ ***the patient's mobility is temporarily or permanently impaired***, e.g. a bedfast, paralysed or unconscious patient ▪ ***the patient has a poor nutritional status*** ▪ ***the patient has impaired peripheral circulation***.
Equipment 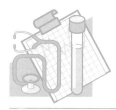	1. Appropriate risk assessment scale, e.g. the Norton (Fig. 37.1), Waterlow (Fig. 37.2) or Braden (Bergstrom et al 1987) Scale 2. Pressure-relieving devices (Bale 2006).
Guidelines and rationale for this nursing practice 	▪ explain the nursing practice to the patient ***to gain consent and co-operation*** ▪ ensure the patient's privacy ***to reduce anxiety*** ▪ wash the hands ***to reduce the risk of cross-infection*** (Jeanes 2005) ▪ observe the patient throughout this activity ***to note any signs of distress or discomfort*** ▪ assess the risk factor of the patient developing a pressure ulcer, utilising one of the assessment scales, such as the Norton (Fig. 37.1) or Waterlow (Fig. 37.2)

		A		B		C		D		E		Total Score
		Physical Condition		Mental Condition		Activity		Mobility		Incontinent		
		Good	4	Alert	4	Ambulant	4	Full	4	Not	4	
		Fair	3	Apathetic	3	Walk/help	3	Sl. limited	3	Occasionally	3	
		Poor	2	Confused	2	Chairbound	2	V. limited	2	Usually/ur.	2	
Name	Date	V.bad	1	Stuporous	1	Bedfast	1	Immobile	1	Doubly	1	

FIGURE 37.1
Norton Scale
From Roper et al 1985, with permission

Build/weight for height		Visual skin type		Continence		Mobility		Sex Age		Appettite	
Average	0	Healthy	0	Complete	0	Fully mobile	0	Male	1	Average	0
Above average	2	Tissues paper	1	Occasionally	1	Restricted/	1	Female	2	Poor	1
Below average	3	Dry	1	incontinent		difficult/		14-49	1	Anorectic	2
		Oedematous	1	Catheter/	2	Restless/	2	50-64	2		
		Clammy	1	incontinent		figety		65-75	3		
		Discolour	2	of faeces		Apathetic	3	75-80	4		
		Broken/spot	3	Doubly incontinent	3	Inert/traction	4	81+	5		

Special risk factors:
(1) Poor nutrition, e.g. terminal cachexia — 8
(2) Sensory deprivation, e.g. diabetes, paraplegia, cerebrovasular accident — 5
(3) High dose anti-inflammatory or steroids in use — 3
(4) Smoking 10+ per day — 1
(5) Orthopaedic surgery/fracture below waist — 3

Assessment value
At risk   = 10
High risk   = 15
Very high risk = 20

Directions for use:
1 Assess the patient, circling the number in each category in which the patient fits
2 Add up all the numbers, including 'special risk factors'
3 If the total places the patient within the 'at risk' high risk or 'very high risk' areas, turn the card over and read suggested preventive aids listed on the back
4 Record the circled numbers in the patient's documentation, giving the total and the date
5 Assess each patient every third day, unless the need to reassess the patient earlier becomes evident

FIGURE 37.2
Waterlow Scale

Scale *to permit preventive care to be implemented*. This should be performed as part of the initial assessment process and at regular intervals throughout care when the patient's condition alters (Waterlow 1992, Bale 2006)

■ assess the patient using a nutritional risk assessment tool such as the Burton Score (Russell 2000) *to assess the patient's nutritional status as malnutrition increases the risk of skin breakdown*

■ identify individual patient problem areas, such as a patient with peripheral vascular disease whose affected limb may be at greater risk than the rest of his or her body *as there will be increased risk of the development of a pressure ulcer* (Royal College of Nursing 2001)

■ when a risk factor is noted, institute preventive skin care (Royal College of Nursing 2001), *which will reduce the risk of development of a pressure ulcer*

- relieve the pressure exerted on the skin surface by regularly changing the patient's body position (Lowthian 1987) and using pressure-relieving devices (Bale 2006) **to prevent or reduce devitalisation of the healthy tissue**
- support the patient's body and limbs in natural positions **to promote comfort and prevent damage, and maintain joint and muscle movement** with passive and active exercises (*see* p. 135)
- a patient who is assessed as having a high risk factor will require frequent, for example 2 hourly, changes of position **to relieve the pressure of the soft tissues against bone** (Bale 2006). A turning chart may be used to record the time, position of the patient and signature of the nurse or carer
- reduce the pressure, friction and shearing forces on the skin by the use of any of the recommended aids available, such as static load distribution, posture changing or dynamic load distribution beds or mattresses (Lowthian 1995, Morison 2001), which **reduce the factors contributing to pressure sore development**
- cleanse the skin of an incontinent patient or a patient who is perspiring profusely **as the number of micro-organisms will be greatly increased**. Use soap with caution **as the alkaline content tends to dry the skin and deplete it of its natural oils**
- thoroughly dry the skin by patting gently. These measures will **decrease the number of skin micro-organisms and lessen the development of infected skin tissue**
- examine and classify (Box 37.1) the patient's skin during the nursing practice for signs of hyperaemia or loss of integrity, **which signifies the development of a pressure ulcer** (Reid & Morison 1994)
- **reduce the shearing and friction forces exerted on a patient's skin** by using a skilled moving and handling technique when repositioning him or her, and proper positioning of the patient to prevent sliding down in the bed or chair
- maintain, or improve when appropriate, the patient's nutritional status, using the services of a dietician if necessary, **as poor nutritional and hydration status greatly increases the risk of pressure sore development** (Bale 2006, Russell 2000)
- educate the patient about preventive care for pressure ulcer development when his or her condition permits; a patient nursed in traction can, for example, assist in pressure relief measures. Co-operation on the part of and care by the patient are vital in the overall prevention of pressure ulcers
- after giving any of the forms of care above, ensure that the patient is left feeling as comfortable as possible **to ensure quality of patient care**
- dispose of used equipment safely **to reduce any health hazard**
- document the nursing practice appropriately, monitor the after-effects and report any abnormal findings immediately, **providing a written record and assisting in the implementation of any action should an abnormality or adverse reaction to the practice be noted**
- in undertaking this practice, nurses are accountable for their actions, the quality of care delivered and record-keeping according to the Code of Professional Conduct: Standards for Conduct, Performance and Ethics (Nursing and Midwifery Council 2004) and Guidelines for Records and Record Keeping (Nursing and Midwifery Council 2005).

The UK consensus classification of pressure sore severity

Stage 0
No clinical evidence of a pressure sore
0.0 Normal appearance intact skin
0.1 Healed with scarring
0.2 Tissue damage, but not assessed as a pressure sore

Stage 1
Discoloration of intact skin (light finger pressure applied to the site does not alter the discoloration)
1.1 Non-blanchable erythema with increased local heat
1.2 Blue/purple/black discoloration. The sore is at least stage 1

Stage 2
Partial-thickness skin loss or damage involving epidermis and/or dermis
2.1 Blister
2.2 Abrasion
2.3 Shallow ulcer, without undermining of adjacent tissue
2.4 Any of these with underlying blue/purple/black discoloration or induration. The sore is at least stage 2

Stage 3
Full-thickness skin loss involving damage or necrosis of subcutaneous tissue but not extending to underlying bone, tendon or joint capsule
3.1 Crater, without undermining of adjacent tissue
3.2 Crater, with undermining of adjacent tissue
3.3 Sinus, the full extent of which is not certain
3.4 Full-thickness skin loss but wound bed covered with necrotic tissue (hard or leathery black/brown tissue or softer yellow/cream/grey slough), which masks the true extent of tissue damage. The sore is at least stage 3. Until debrided it is not possible to observe whether damage extends into muscle or involves damage to bone or supporting structures

Stage 4
Full-thickness skin loss with extensive destruction and tissue necrosis extending to underlying bone, tendon or joint capsule
4.1 Visible exposure of bone, tendon or capsule
4.2 Sinus assessed as extending to bone, tendon or capsule

Third digit classification
For the nature of the wound bed
x.x0 Not applicable: intact skin
x.x1 Clean, with partial epithelialisation
x.x2 Clean, with or without granulation, but no obvious epithelialisation
x.x3 Soft slough, cream/yellow/green in colour
x.x4 Hard or leathery black/brown necrotic (dead/avascular) tissue

Fourth digit classification
For infective complications
x.xx0 No inflammation surrounding the wound bed
x.xx1 Inflammation surrounding the wound bed
x.xx2 Cellulitis bacteriologically confirmed

From Reid & Morison 1994, with permission

Patient/carer
education
Key points

In partnership with the patient and/or carer, ensure that they are competent to carry out any practices required. Information should be given on an appropriate point of contact for any concerns that may arise. The patient and carers should also be given information on the care implemented to reduce the risk of pressure ulcer development.

A patient who is permanently at risk of pressure ulcer development must take an active role in the preventive care. This may involve the nurse in teaching the patient how to inspect the skin tissue regularly, for example using a mirror to assess skin areas that are difficult to access.

When a prolonged or permanent use of pressure-relieving aids by a patient is implemented, the patient and carers should be given information on the safe, continued care of the equipment and on appropriate action should a fault occur.

References

Bale S 2006 Wound healing. In: Alexander M, Fawcett J, Runciman P (eds) Nursing practice – hospital and home: the adult, 3rd edn. Churchill Livingstone, Edinburgh

Bergstrom N, Braden B, Laguzza A 1987 The Braden Scale for predicting pressure sore risk. Nursing Research 36(4): 205–210

Jeanes A 2005 Infection control. A practical guide to the use of hand decontaminants. Nursing Times 101(20): 46–48

Lowthian P 1987 The practical assessment of pressure sore risk. Care, Science and Practice 5(4): 3–7

Lowthian P 1995 Pegasus Airwave and Bi-Wave Plus. British Journal of Nursing 4(17): 1020–1024

Morison M (ed) 2001 The prevention and treatment of pressure ulcers. Mosby, Edinburgh

Nursing and Midwifery Council 2004 Code of professional conduct: standards for conduct, performance and ethics. NMC, London

Nursing and Midwifery Council 2005 Guidelines for records and record keeping. NMC, London

Reid J, Morison M 1994 Towards a consensus: classification of pressure sores. Journal of Wound Care 3(3): 157–160

Roper N, Logan W, Tierney A 1985 The elements of nursing, 2nd edn. Churchill Livingstone, Edinburgh

Royal College of Nursing 2001 Clinical practice guidelines. Pressure ulcer risk assessment and prevention. RCN, London

Russell L 2000 Malnutrition and pressure ulcers: nutritional assessment tools. British Journal of Nursing 9(4): 194–204

Waterlow J 1992 A policy that protects: the Waterlow pressure sore prevention/treatment policy. In: Horne E, Cowan T (eds) Staff nurse's survival guide, 2nd edn. Wolfe, London

Websites

Nursing and Midwifery Council: http://www.nmc-uk.org

Royal College of Nursing: http://www.rcn.org.uk

Self assessment

1. Under what circumstances would a nurse be required to provide increased levels of skin care?
2. What are the risk factors associated with pressure ulcer development?
3. What assessment tools are available for nurses to use to assess patients?
4. What actions can be taken by the nurse to minimise risk of pressure ulcer development?
5. What role can the patient play in pressure ulcer prevention?

Practice 38
Specimen Collection

Learning outcomes

By the end of this section, you should know how to:

- identify the need for laboratory investigations
- facilitate the obtaining of the necessary specimens
- be aware of the different containers used for each type of specimen
- arrange the correct storage and delivery of the specimens to the laboratory.

Background knowledge required

Revision of appropriate microbiology and pathology
Review the chapter on 'Infection prevention and control' (*see* p. 151)
Review of local policies referring to principles of infection control
Review of local policies referring to the collection and transportation of specimens.

Indications and rationale for collecting specimens

A specimen may be required:
- **as an aid to the diagnosis of disease**
- **for the purposes of screening in health to facilitate cancer diagnosis, staging and typing**
- **to monitor the effect of treatment**
- to permit laboratory culture **to identify pathogenic micro-organisms and determine drug sensitivity**.

Equipment

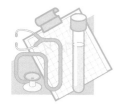

1. Appropriate container clearly labelled with the patient's details
2. Equipment to enable the collection of the specimen
3. Laboratory form
4. Plastic specimen bag for transportation.

General guidelines and rationale for this nursing practice

- explain the nursing practice to the patient **to gain consent and co-operation. Patients should be encouraged to be active partners in care**
- ensure the patient's privacy **to help to maintain dignity and a sense of self**
- the nurse and the patient (if he or she is involved in the collection of the specimen) should wash their hands **to reduce the risk of cross-infection** (Jeanes 2005, NHS Education for Scotland 2005)
- ensure that the appropriate precautions are observed **to reduce the risk of contact with body fluids during the collection and transportation of the specimen** (Roberts 2000, Clark et al 2002)

- collect the specimen at the most appropriate time **to facilitate obtaining accurate results**. This time will vary depending on the specimen; the optimum time for the collection of a specimen of urine for culture is, for example, from the first voiding of the bladder in the morning
- **to avoid interference with accurate results**, ensure that no substance that might cause an inaccurate result has been used prior to collection (Wilson 1996). A specimen of sputum could, for example, be adversely affected by the patient using an antiseptic mouthwash before giving the specimen
- ensure that sufficient quantities of the specimen have been collected **to assist the laboratory staff in preparing the specimen for analysis, which will lead to accurate results**
- avoid contamination of the specimen by the hands of the nurse or patient **as this could invalidate the results of the culture and be a hazard to the individual's health**
- avoid contamination of the outside of the container with the specimen substance **as this could pose a health risk to anyone handling the specimen** (Wilson 1996)
- ensure that the patient is left feeling as comfortable as possible after collecting the specimen
- immediately dispatch the labelled specimen container to the laboratory with the completed form; **any delay may alter the reliability of any results obtained**. If a delay is unavoidable, the specimen can usually be stored in a specimen refrigerator until it can be sent for analysis
- document this nursing practice appropriately, monitor the after-effects and report any abnormal findings immediately **so that appropriate measures can be instigated to relieve the problem**
- in undertaking this practice, nurses are accountable for their actions, the quality of care delivered and record-keeping according to the Code of Professional Conduct: Standards for Conduct, Performance and Ethics (Nursing and Midwifery Council 2004) and Guidelines for Records and Record Keeping (Nursing and Midwifery Council 2005).

Swab collection

Specific equipment

- Sterile swab
- Disposable gloves
- Sterile water for a nose swab
- Sterile vaginal speculum for a vaginal swab
- Sterile lubricating jelly for a vaginal swab
- Spatula for a throat swab.

Specific guidelines and rationale for these nursing practices

Wound swabs
- obtain a specimen before the wound is washed **so that the specimen material is not contaminated by the washing agent**
- rotate the swab in the wound **to obtain a sufficient quantity for examination**.

Throat swabs

- help the patient to sit in an appropriate position **to facilitate a good view of the faucial tonsils**
- depress the patient's tongue with a spatula **to facilitate access to the site**
- speedily and gently rub the swab over the faucial area
- avoid touching any other area of the mouth as the swab is being removed **so that the specimen will not be contaminated.**

Ear swabs

- help the patient to sit in a comfortable position with the head slightly tilted to the unaffected side
- gently pull the adult's pinna upwards and backwards to straighten the external canal. **This facilitates the insertion of the swab to obtain a specimen of the discharge**
- insert the swab into the external canal and rotate gently **to ensure that the swab is well coated with the discharge.**

Nasal swabs

- help the patient to sit in a comfortable position **to allow access to the nasal cavity**
- moisten the swab in sterile water before insertion into the nose **to make the procedure more comfortable for the patient** as the nasal cavity can be dry
- insert the swab into the nose, rotating it as it moves upwards towards the tip of the nose.

Vaginal swabs

- help the patient into an appropriate position **to allow access to the vagina** (*see* 'Vaginal examination', p. 363)
- gently insert a lubricated speculum into the vagina to separate the vaginal walls. **This allows the area to be swabbed to be visualised**
- introduce the swab into the high vaginal area and gently rotate it. Charcoal-impregnated swabs should be used if a *Trichomonas* infection is suspected **as the organism survives for longer in this medium.**

Penile swabs

- help the patient into a comfortable position **to allow access to the penis**
- retract the prepuce to allow the area to be swabbed to be visualised
- rotate the swab gently in the urethral meatus **to collect a sample of the secretions.**

Faeces

Specific equipment

- Disposable gloves
- Bedpan
- Sterile spatula
- Sterile container
- Receptacle for soiled disposable items.

Specific guidelines and rationale for this nursing practice

- ask the patient to defecate into a clean bedpan, ensuring that the faecal matter does not become contaminated with urine **as this could affect the analysis results**

- use a spatula or implement provided to fill about one-third of the specimen container with faecal material
- if the faeces are being tested for occult blood, follow the instructions on the packaging in which the occult blood testing equipment is supplied.

Urine

Specific equipment

- Sterile container
- Disposable gloves
- Bedpan or urinal may be necessary
- Sterile receiver may be necessary to receive the specimen
- Washing equipment to wash the surrounding tissue
- Midstream specimens of urine: a sterile tinfoil bowl
- Catheter specimens of urine: a sterile needle, syringe and alcohol-impregnated swab (Fig. 38.1)
- 24-hour urine collection: a large plastic/glass sterile container with a lid.

Specific guidelines and rationale for this nursing practice

- to facilitate the collection of a midstream specimen of urine, ask the patient to start passing urine to flush out the urethra *so that urethral organisms will not interfere with the analysis*
- collect the middle section of the stream directly into the container or, for a female, into a sterile bowl, then pour this into the container

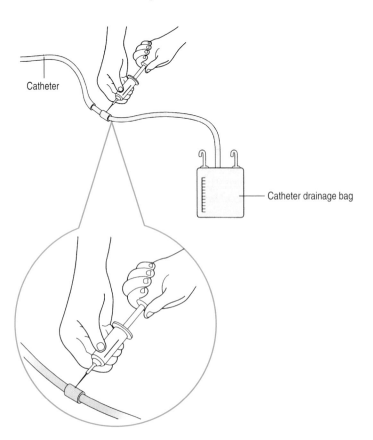

Catheter

Catheter drainage bag

FIGURE 38.1
Collecting a specimen of urine when a catheter is in position

- to facilitate the collection of a catheter specimen of urine, wipe the catheter with an alcohol-impregnated swab (Skinner 2002)
- connect the needle to the syringe and insert it into the specially marked section of the collecting bag tube. This section is made of a self-sealing material **so that the needle will not damage it**. Some collecting tubes now have a special port to which the syringe connects directly
- withdraw the required amount of urine into the syringe and then transfer it to the sterile container
- to commence a 24-hour collection, ask the patient to void his or her bladder and discard the urine **so that the patient and staff know the exact time the collection commences**
- collect all the urine passed in the next 24 hours.

Cervical smear

This should only be undertaken by a nurse following specific education and training in this practice (McQueen 2006).

Specific equipment

- Disposable gloves
- Lubricating gel
- Vaginal speculum
- Container with appropriate fixative
- Glass slide
- Cervical spatula or brush
- Medical wipes/tissues.

Specific guidelines and rationale for this nursing practice

- help the patient into the most appropriate position **to facilitate the collection of the specimen** (*see* 'Vaginal examination', p. 363)
- put on the disposable gloves
- lubricate the spatula
- gently insert it into the vagina and open it slowly until the cervix can be visualised
- insert the brush or spatula and rotate it twice round the cervix, ensuring that it is at the entrance (Fig. 38.2)
- immediately transfer the cells to the glass slide and insert this into the container holding the fixative
- close the speculum and withdraw it gently
- offer tissues to the patient for her to clean the outside of her vagina and then provide privacy for dressing
- allow the patient time to recover from this procedure before sitting her upright, as handling the cervix can cause a feeling of faintness as the result of a vasovagal response.

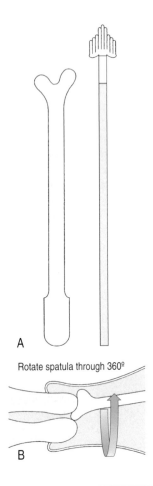

FIGURE 38.2
Cervical smear
A Cervical spatula and brush
B Correct use of cervical spatula

Patient/carer education **Key points** 	In partnership with the patient and/or carer, ensure that they are competent to carry out any practices required. Information should be given on an appropriate point of contact for any concerns that may arise. The actions associated with this practice may challenge the cultural norms of the patients and their carers. The nurse should be sensitive to these issues when discussing this practice with the patient and carers. An explanation of the method and reasons for collecting the specimen will help the patient to understand how and why the practice is necessary. This is particularly important if the patient is in the community and the specimen is being collected in his or her home. If the specimen is collected at home, the patient will need clear instructions on the storing of the specimen and where and when to deliver it so that it arrives at the laboratory in optimum condition.

References

Clark L, Smith W, Young L 2002 Protective clothing – principles and guidance. Infection Control Nurse Association of the UK, Harrogate, UK

Jeanes A 2005 Infection control. A practical guide to the use of hand decontaminants. Nursing Times 101(20): 46–48

McQueen A 2006 The reproductive systems. In: Alexander M, Fawcett J, Runciman P (eds) Nursing practice – hospital and home: the adult, 3rd edn. Churchill Livingstone, Edinburgh

NHS Education for Scotland 2005 Promoting hand hygiene in healthcare: a short self-directed web-based learning package for healthcare workers. NES, Edinburgh

Nursing and Midwifery Council 2004 Code of professional conduct: standards of conduct, performance and ethics. NMC, London

Nursing and Midwifery Council 2005 Guidelines for records and record keeping. NMC, London

Roberts C 2000 Universal precautions: improving the knowledge of trained nurses. British Journal of Nursing 9(1): 43–47

Skinner S 2002 Clinical investigations. In: Walsh M (ed) Watson's clinical nursing and related sciences, 6th edn. Baillière Tindall, London

Wilson J 1996 General principles of specimen collection. Clinical Infectious Diseases 22(5): 766–777

Websites

Department of Health: http://www.dh.gov.uk (advice and national publications)

Infection Control Nurses Association: http://www.icna.co.uk (publications)

NHS Education for Scotland: http:// www.nes.scot.nhs.uk (publications and web-based materials)

Nursing and Midwifery Council: http://www.nmc.org.uk (publications)

Royal College of Nursing: http://www.rcn.org.uk (publications)

Self assessment

1. List and discuss three reasons for specimen collection.
2. What measures can the nurse employ to ensure that accurate results from the collected specimen are achieved?
3. Discuss how you would explain to a patient the collection of a clean urine specimen while they are at home.

Practice 39
Stoma Care

Learning outcomes

By the end of this section, you should know how to:
- prepare the patient for this nursing practice
- collect and prepare the equipment
- carry out stoma care for the patient
- help patients to accept and care for their stoma themselves, both at home and in an institutional setting.

Background knowledge required

Revision of the anatomy and physiology of the digestive system, with special reference to the small and large intestines

Review of local policy regarding the role of the stoma care nurse and the literature available for patient education in an institutional and a community setting

Knowledge of the information and level of counselling given to the patient before the operation to create a stoma.

Indications and rationale for stoma care

A stoma is an artificial opening from the small or large intestine or bladder onto the surface of the abdomen through which the bowel contents or urine is diverted for excretion (Fig. 39.1). The stoma is formed after surgical intervention for the treatment of intestinal or bladder disease. Different names are used according to the site of the stoma.

Stoma care involves cleansing the stoma and surrounding skin, and providing a suitable appliance for the safe collection and disposal of excreta. Nurses either perform this on the patient's behalf or educate and support patients until they or a carer are able to competently care for the stoma.

A **colostomy** is an opening from the colon, usually the transverse or descending colon, and may be required:
- *for patients who have malignant disease of the rectum or colon*
- *for patients who have diverticular disease of the colon*
- *for patients who have inflammatory disease of the intestine, e.g. Crohn's disease or ulcerative colitis*
- *for patients who have suffered trauma to the abdomen or rectum*
- *for patients who suffer faecal incontinence*.

An **ileostomy** is an opening from the ileum and may be formed for the same reasons as a colostomy, although it is more often seen in patients who have inflammatory disease of the intestine, for example Crohn's disease or ulcerative colitis. In some cases, a temporary stoma may be formed so that once the disease has resolved, the stoma may be closed and the intestine anastomosed to function as before.

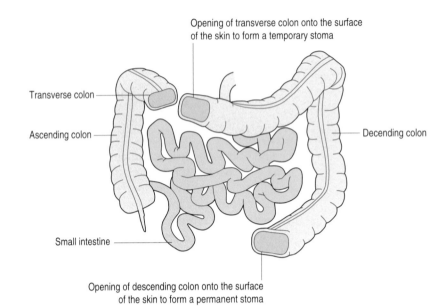

Opening of transverse colon onto the surface of the skin to form a temporary stoma

Transverse colon

Ascending colon

Decending colon

Small intestine

FIGURE 39.1
Sites that may be chosen for colostomy

Opening of descending colon onto the surface of the skin to form a permanent stoma

A **jejunostomy** is an opening from the jejunum.

A **urostomy** is an opening from the bladder or ureter into a segment of the ileum, this being used as a channel for the urine to be diverted through an abdominal stoma. This is also known as an ileal conduit, and it may be required for the treatment of malignant disease of the bladder or in the management of the neuropathic bladder or urinary incontinence (Black 2000).

A stoma may be temporary or permanent. A temporary stoma is often created to divert faeces away from an operation site (anastomosis) to allow healing to occur. The stoma is then reversed by the surgeon with minimal or no loss of intestinal function. A permanent stoma implies that the bowel cannot be reconnected (Porrett & McGrath 2005).

Equipment

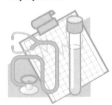

1. Trolley or tray
2. Bowl of warm water (or warm water in sink if patient mobile to toilet)
3. Soft wipes
4. Suitable appliance (stoma pouch)
5. Scissors
6. Measuring guide
7. Measuring jug (if appropriate)
8. Gloves (non-sterile) and apron
9. Deodorant as required
10. Receptacle for soiled disposable items.

Stoma appliances

There is a wide range of appliances available, and, with the guidance of a stoma care nurse, the patient will choose the one most suitable for his or her needs. Stoma pouches may have pre-cut apertures or may have to be cut to fit individually. They may be closed pouches or open ended to allow emptying (Fig. 39.2).

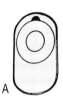

A

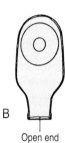

B

Open end

FIGURE 39.2
Examples of disposable stoma bags
A Closed pouch
B Open lower end to permit emptying of the contents

The pouches may be one-piece or two-piece appliances. A one-piece appliance is one in which the adhesive flange and pouch are sealed together. The backing paper is removed from the adhesive ring prior to application and the whole pouch is removed and discarded when appropriate. A two-piece appliance consists of a baseplate which is placed around the stoma and is secured onto the abdomen. The pouch is then clipped or secured onto the baseplate. The pouch can be renewed without changing the baseplate.

Postoperatively, the surgeon will place a clear plastic appliance over the stoma. This allows the observation of the stoma and its function. It may be 2–5 days before the appliance needs to be changed for the first time.

Guidelines and rationale for this nursing practice

- explain the nursing practice to the patient *to gain consent and co-operation, and encourage participation in care*
- ensure the patient's privacy *to maintain self-esteem and prevent embarrassment* (Royal College of Nursing 2002)
- wash hands *to reduce the risk of cross-infection* (Nicol et al 2001)
- collect and prepare the equipment *so that everything is ready*
- help the patient into a comfortable position *to reduce any distress and to help him or her see the area of the stoma*
- help to adjust the clothing *to expose the patient's abdomen in the area of the stoma for easy access and so that the patient can observe the practice*
- put on gloves and apron *to prevent any contamination from body fluids*
- place soft wipes appropriately *to protect the surrounding area from spills or leakage*
- observe the patient throughout this activity *to monitor any adverse effects*
- empty the appliance and, if required, measure its contents *for an evaluation of the elimination fluid balance*
- gently remove the appliance *to expose the stoma area*

- wash the skin around the stoma with soft wipes and warm water only, *soap may cause skin irritation*
- encourage the patient to look at the stoma and explain what you are doing *so that he or she gradually accepts the change of body image and to encourage early independence*
- observe the colour and condition of the stoma and the surrounding skin *to evaluate the wound healing process*
- dry the skin around the stoma thoroughly *to maintain healthy intact skin and prevent excoriation*
- prepare the appliance as required by measuring the size and shape of the stoma, cutting the aperture of the pouch *so that it is tailored to fit the individual stoma*
- apply any prescribed barrier wipes or spray if required *to heal any excoriation of the peristomal skin area*
- place the new appliance in position *so that it fits comfortably and permits no leakage round the stoma* (Fig. 39.3)
- seal an open-ended bag with an appropriate closure *to prevent leakage*
- ensure that the patient is left feeling as comfortable as possible *to limit distress and promote the healing process*
- dispose of any waste products and soiled appliances according to health authority policy *to prevent the transmission of infection*
- wash the hands *to reduce the risk of cross-infection* (Nicol et al 2001)
- document the nursing practice appropriately, monitor the after-effects and report any abnormal findings immediately. *This will ensure safe practice and enable prompt, appropriate medical and nursing intervention to be initiated*
- in undertaking this practice, nurses are accountable for their actions, the quality of care delivered and record-keeping according to the Code of Professional Conduct: Standards for Conduct, Performance and Ethics (Nursing and Midwifery Council 2004) and Guidelines for Records and Record Keeping (Nursing and Midwifery Council 2005).

FIGURE 39.3
Positioning an appliance over a stoma
A Removing the protective covering from the adhesive ring before placing the appliance over the stoma
B Applying a stoma pouch. The open-ended pouch is sealed with a clip ready for use; when the clip is removed, the stoma pouch can be emptied without removing the appliance from the skin

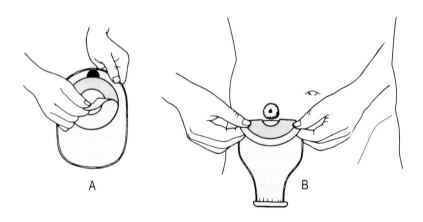

A   B

**Patient/carer
education**

Key points

Patient support and education begins prior to surgery. As the presence of a stoma completely changes the way in which bodily waste is eliminated from the body, patients need education and support to adjust to this change. Ideally the stoma nurse should meet with the patient and a relative before surgery to discuss the forthcoming procedure, the likelihood of a stoma, the implications that this will have on his or her lifestyle and some potential postoperative complications. The patient should be shown an appropriate appliance and be given written literature relative to the surgery. By offering preoperative support and education, patients are less likely to develop psychological problems following surgery.

Stoma siting is also a vital preoperative role of the stoma nurse as the site where the stoma is placed on the abdomen can have an effect on the recovery process. Attention must also be paid to the patient's employment status, leisure activities, religious and cultural influences and these must be taken into consideration when siting (Black 2000, 2004, Porrett & McGrath 2005).

Before, during and after admission stoma support and education is shared with stoma nurses and nurses from both the acute and community setting. The main aim of stoma education is to provide patients with the right skills and support to enable them to be independent in the care of their own stoma. Where this is unlikely, a relative or carer may be taught the skill to carry this out on the patient's behalf.

The presence of a stoma has a major impact on the patient's sexuality and body image. Body image has been described as the way in which we see ourselves in the world (Porrett & McGrath 2005) and the presence of a stoma can place challenges on an individual's physical, emotional and psychological wellbeing. Sexuality involves much more than the physical act of sexual expression. For some it is a measure of self worth, acceptance, security, comfort, human contact as well as cohesion in a relationship. Nurses involved in the care of a patient with a stoma should demonstrate knowledge of actual and potential problems with sexuality and body image (Junkin & Beitz 2005). Nurses should create an environment that encourages patients to talk about the stoma and any worries or concerns that they may have with regard to the threat on their body image and sexuality. Effective listening skills can be used to ensure that both the physical and psychological needs of the patient are met (Porrett & McGrath 2005). The patient may wish to discuss with the stoma care nurse any concerns he or she may have about emotional and psychological adjustment to life with a stoma.

The practical aspect of stoma education encourages patients to be fully prepared prior to starting to change the pouch. To gather all necessary equipment and to carry out the step-by-step process of removing the old pouch, washing and drying the peristomal skin area and then reapplying and securing the new pouch. Pouches should be emptied or changed as often as necessary to prevent overfilling and leakage onto the surrounding skin area. This is usually when they are one third to one half full, to prevent them becoming heavy. In hospital the contents of the pouch should be emptied into the toilet or Clinimatic. The soiled pouch should be treated as clinical waste. The faecal output from the stoma should initially be measured and observed for any abnormality.

Following discharge home, the patient will be instructed to place the soiled pouch in a disposal bag and then to double bag it in a plastic bag and place it in the waste bin outside their house. Stoma care should be regarded as a form of toileting and appropriate handwashing performed to reduce the incidence of cross-infection (Nicol et al 2001).

Nutritional advice

During the first few days following surgery, the patient will have nothing orally and will receive nutrition via intravenous infusion (Porrett & McGrath 2005). Oral fluids will be gradually introduced and increased to light diet when the stoma becomes active. Once the patient is allowed a normal diet, the stoma will discharge faecal material more frequently. By a process of observation, the patient should be encouraged to introduce new foods slowly into their diet and notice the effect that these different foods have on faecal elimination. Some foods may produce more undesired flatus, others may make the effluent looser or more bulky. This may help the patient to manage their own output from their stoma. This process may take a few weeks and the stoma nurse can provide some written information and advice regarding diet following surgery. Patients with ileostomies should be aware that foods like mushrooms, nuts, sweetcorn, coconut and some tough fruit skins may not be digested properly and may block the stoma. Ileostomy patients are also advised to drink about one litre to one and a half litres of fluid per day and to add extra salt to their diet to maintain fluid and electrolyte balance. Urostomy patients are advised to drink one and a half to two litres of fluid per day to keep the urine as dilute as possible to prevent urinary tract infections. Cranberry juice or capsules may also be taken to prevent growth of bacteria in the urinary tract.

Potential postoperative complications

Patients and carers should be aware that there are some potential complications that may occur following stoma formation (Porrett & McGrath 2005).

Oedema

All stomas are swollen immediately after surgery due to handling of the bowel, but this oedema should reduce gradually over the following weeks and the stoma size should be established at six weeks (Collett 2002). During this time the stoma should be observed. The size of the stoma has to be measured regularly so that the aperture of the flange is cut correctly. If cut too big any leakage of effluent onto the peristomal skin area may cause irritation and if cut too small ischemia may occur.

Necrosis

This is most common in the first 48 hours following surgery and is caused by inadequate blood supply to part of the bowel that is used to form the stoma (Porrett & McGrath 2005). Initially the stoma will become a dusky purple colour due to the impaired blood supply. Ischaemia may develop into necrosis, which results in a black odorous bowel. The necrosis may be superficial, which will result in sloughing off of the tissue, or it may be deep, which will require surgical excision (Lee 2001, Collett 2002).

Mucocutaneous separation

This occurs when there is a breakdown of the suture line securing the stoma to the abdominal surface, leaving a wound cavity (Collett 2002). Management is by use of stoma pastes and an adhesive washer.

Dermatitis

This is defined by inflammation or excoriation of the peristomal skin. Contact dermatitis occurs when there is a sensitivity or allergy to the appliance. It can occur at any time. It is easily identified as the outline of the pouch remains visible on the skin after the pouch has been removed. Effluent dermatitis occurs when the patient has suffered from leakages from the pouch or when the pouch has been cut too big. Barrier wipes or sprays or hydrocolloid dressings can be used to protect the area. Topical steroids may be prescribed in extreme circumstances.

Retraction

This is when the stoma lies on or recedes below the surface of the abdominal wall and is caused by the bowel being under tension. Retraction can cause leakages of effluent and contact dermatitis. Management is through the use of convexity appliances. A convexity appliance is one where the outward curving of the adhesive on the flange begins at the stoma. This helps to secure a seal around the stoma providing security and promoting physical and psychological wellbeing (Boyd et al 2004). Washers and pastes may also be used to fill in any dips or creases on the abdominal wall.

Prolapse

This is when a length of the bowel protrudes from the abdomen. This can be very alarming for the patients, it can cause leakages of effluent and odour from the appliance and it can cause body-image problems. Some patients may require a larger pouch and the aperture resized. The prolapsed stoma can sometimes be manually reduced when the patient is supine, but always prolapses again when the patient mobilises (Collett 2002). A support belt or garment can then be worn to prevent future prolapse in the short term. However, the stoma may have to be surgically refashioned for long-term management if the prolapse proves a major problem for the patient.

Stenosis

Stenosis occurs when the opening of the stoma narrows. It can be caused by non-elastic scar tissue forming around the stoma following retraction, mucocutaneous separation and necrosis. It is characterised by abdominal pain and difficulty of the stoma expelling the stool. Management of stenosis is to educate patients to maintain soft stools through diet and stool-softening agents (such as lactulose) and also by introducing a dilator into the lumen of the stoma to keep it patent. The long-term management may be that the patient will require surgical refashioning of the stoma.

Hernia

When a stoma is formed a potential site of weakness in the abdominal muscle is created. A hernia occurs when the peritoneum bulges through the weakened muscle wall (Collett 2002, Kane et al 2004). A parastomal hernia occurs when a hernia develops around the stoma. Patients can present with anything from a slight swelling around the stoma to a large uncomfortable mass causing pain and discomfort. Patients with parastomal hernias have problems with body image as the swelling may be obvious and some may have to wear a hernia support. Patients should be informed that the presence of a hernia may cause bowel obstruction. Signs and symptoms may include non-function of the stoma and abdominal pain and discomfort. These should therefore be explained to the patient as well as giving information on who to contact should they experience them. Some patients with larger hernias may have them surgically repaired.

All stoma patients should have contact details of their nearest stoma care nurse who can review them in the hospital or at home if necessary should they experience any problems.

Patients should also be encouraged to contact local and national support groups by attending meetings or via the Internet.

References

Black P 2000 Practical stoma care. Nursing Standard 14(41): 47–55

Black P 2004 Psychological, sexual and cultural issues for patients with a stoma. British Journal of Nursing 13: 692–697

Boyd K, Thomson MJ, Boyd-Carson W et al 2004 Management of convexity. Nursing Standard 18(20): 34–38

Collett K 2002 Practical aspects of stoma management. Nursing Standard 17(8): 45–52, 54–55

Junkin J, Beitz J 2005 Sexuality and the person with a stoma: implications for comprehensive WOC nursing practice. Journal of Wound, Ostomy and Continence Nursing Practice 32(2): 121–128

Kane M, McErlean D, McGrogan M et al 2004 Management of parastomal hernia. Nursing Standard 18(19): 43–44

Lee J 2001 Common stoma problems: a brief guide for community nurses. British Journal of Community Nursing 6: 407–413

Nicol M, Bavin C, Bedford Turner S et al 2001 Essential nursing skills. Nursing Standard 15(21): 56–57

Nursing and Midwifery Council 2004 Code of professional conduct: standards for conduct, performance and ethics. NMC, London

Nursing and Midwifery Council 2005 Guidelines for records and record keeping. NMC, London

Porrett T, McGrath A 2005 Stoma care. Blackwell Publishing, Oxford

Royal College of Nursing 2002 Standards of care – colorectal and stoma care nursing. RCN, London

Websites

British Colostomy Association: http://www.bcass.org.uk

Gay Ostomists Association: http://www.welcome.to/gay.ostomates

Ileostomy and Internal Pouch Association: http://www.ileostomypouch.demon.co.uk

Urostomy Association: http://www.uagbi.org

Self assessment

1. Name the different types of stomas that can be created and name two predisposing factors for each one.
2. What equipment is necessary to renew a stoma pouch?
3. What dietary advice would you give an ileostomy patient?
4. What advice would you give a patient with a parastomal hernia?
5. What can happen if the aperture of the flange is cut wrongly after surgery?

Practice 40
Suppositories

Learning outcomes	**By the end of this section, you should know how to:**
	▪ prepare the patient for this nursing practice
	▪ collect and prepare the equipment
	▪ administer rectal suppositories
	▪ describe some of the types of suppository and their function.

Background knowledge required

Revision of the anatomy and physiology of the colon, rectum and anus

Revision of 'Administration of medicines', particularly checking the medication against the prescription (*see* p. 13)

Common causes of constipation

Appropriate health education in relation to the prevention of constipation.

Indications and rationale for administering suppositories

A suppository is a cone or cylinder of a medicinal substance that can be introduced into the rectum, will eventually dissolve and may be absorbed through the rectal mucosa. It is used:

▪ *to relieve constipation*

▪ *to evacuate the bowel prior to surgery or certain investigations*

▪ *to treat haemorrhoids or anal pruritus*

▪ *to administer medication*, e.g. antibiotics, bronchodilators or analgesics.

An appropriately trained nurse prescriber has the ability to assess, diagnose and prescribe an appropriate suppository to rectify severe constipation. This is a specialised extended role, recognised by a registerable qualification with the Nursing and Midwifery Council. An awareness of the Rome II criteria for constipation (*see* p. 130) offers guidance to the practitioner when diagnosing constipation, as will a digital rectal examination (DRE; *see* p. 289).

Equipment

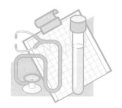

1. Tray/flat surface
2. Disposable gloves
3. Apron
4. Medical wipes/tissues
5. Water-soluble lubricant
6. Protective covering
7. Receptacle for soiled disposable items
8. Prescribed suppository
9. Access to toilet facilities.

Suppositories are of value in evacuating the rectum. Glycerine suppositories lubricate dry, hard stools and have a mild stimulant effect on the rectum. Other suppositories with a stimulant effect are Beogex® and bisacodyl.

Medication is well absorbed through the rectal mucosa and is of benefit for patients who may be unable to swallow medication, e.g. during an epileptic seizure; severe nausea and vomiting; low level of consciousness.

Guidelines and rationale for this nursing practice	Moppett (2000) discusses the latest guidance on the insertion of suppositories, suggesting that, for physiological reasons, the suppository should be inserted blunt end first into the anus. It is proposed that this will aid the retention of the suppository, as the anal sphincter muscles will close tightly round the apex of the suppository, propelling it inwards. If it is inserted apex first, as is traditional, the sphincter closes incompletely over the blunt end, and the muscles are stimulated to expel the suppository. The introduction of the blunt end of the suppository also reduces the need to insert the full length of a finger.

It is important to note that this is an invasive and embarrassing procedure for the patient. Care and consideration should be taken by the practitioner at all stages of this procedure, remaining alert to potential issues that could arise, e.g. previous radiotherapy to this area, detection of a previously undiagnosed rectal carcinoma or a past history of abuse.

- explain the nursing practice to the patient **to gain consent and co-operation**
- ensure the patient's privacy and assist him or her into the left lateral position with the buttocks near the edge of the bed **to allow ease of access to the rectal sphincter**
- observe the patient throughout this activity **for any signs of distress or discomfort**
- place the protective covering under the patient's buttocks **in case of soiling by faecal matter**
- check with the prescription sheet and with a qualified member of staff that the suppository is the correct one and is being administered to the correct patient, **in order to avoid mistakes**
- squeeze some lubricating gel onto a medical wipe or tissue and lubricate the blunt end of the suppository **for ease of insertion**
- put on disposable gloves and apron **for your protection**
- part the patient's buttocks with the non-dominant hand **to allow easier access to the anal sphincter**
- with the dominant hand, insert the blunt end of the suppository into the rectum in an upwards and slightly backwards direction **to follow the natural line of the rectum** (Fig. 40.1)
- push the suppository in gently as far as possible with the middle finger **to optimise the effect**
- withdraw the gloved finger
- wipe the patient's anal area with a medical wipe or tissue **to clean any soiling**
- remove the protective covering
- remove the gloves and apron
- provide toilet facilities when this is required. **To reduce embarrassment** for the patient, try to provide as much privacy as possible, remembering that curtains do not act as sound or smell filters
- ensure that the patient is left feeling as comfortable as possible, **maintaining the quality of this practice**

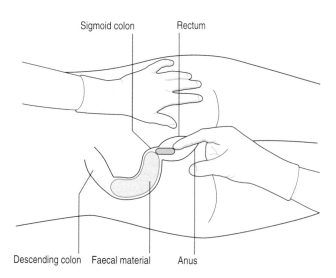

FIGURE 40.1
Insertion of a rectal suppository

- dispose of the equipment safely **_to prevent the transmission of infection_**
- document this nursing practice appropriately, monitor the after-effects and report any abnormal findings, **_ensuring safe practice and enabling prompt, appropriate medical and nursing intervention to be initiated_**
- in undertaking this practice, nurses are accountable for their actions, the quality of care delivered and record-keeping according to the Code of Professional Conduct: Standards for Conduct, Performance and Ethics (Nursing and Midwifery Council 2004) and Guidelines for Records and Record Keeping (Nursing and Midwifery Council 2005).

Patient/carer education

Key points

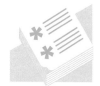

In partnership with the patient and/or carer, ensure that they are competent to carry out any practices required. Information should be given on an appropriate point of contact for any concerns that may arise.

The patient should be told the reasons for administering his or her medication via the rectal route as this route of administration may be unknown to the patient. The patient may also require education in the self-administration of suppositories.

If suppositories are being prescribed to relieve constipation, it may be appropriate to discuss ways in which increased exercise, fluid and diet may relieve this problem. The development of a habit that encourages the bowel to empty at the same time each day and allows adequate time for this to happen is also worth discussing. A self-completion bowel chart may be useful for helping to resolve the problem of constipation.

References

Moppett S 2000 Which way is up for a suppository? Nursing Times Plus 96(19): 12–13

Nursing and Midwifery Council 2004 Code of professional conduct: standards for conduct, performance and ethics. NMC, London

Nursing and Midwifery Council 2005 Guidelines for records and record keeping. NMC, London

Clinical Nursing Practices

Self assessment

1. List four indications why a suppository may be prescribed.
2. List some common types of suppository and their action.
3. What position should a patient be in before you administer a suppository?
4. Which way should a suppository be inserted?
5. What health education should you give a patient who has received a suppository to relieve constipation?

Practice 41
Toileting

Learning outcomes	**By the end of this section, you should know how to:** ▪ prepare the patient for this nursing practice ▪ collect and prepare the equipment ▪ provide facilities for the patient to empty his or her bladder or bowel, at home or in an institutional setting.
Background knowledge required	Revision of the anatomy and physiology of the urinary system, with special reference to micturition Revision of the anatomy and physiology of the rectum and anus, with special reference to defaecation Review of health authority policy regarding the disposal of excreta and the control of infection in both community and institutional care Revision of continence management.
Indications and rationale for toileting	Toileting aims ***to provide the appropriate facilities for the patient to micturate or defecate***. This may be a toilet, a commode, a bedpan or a urinal. A bedpan, urinal or commode should be provided for patients who are confined to bed or allowed up only for short periods. Assistance to the toilet should be provided for those who are too frail or immobile to be self-caring in relation to toileting.
Equipment	1. Bedpan, urinal, commode or toilet, as appropriate 2. Toilet paper 3. Disposable cover for the bedpan or urinal 4. Gloves 5. Measuring jug 6. Bedpan disposer, e.g. Clinamatic 7. Bedpan washer for non-disposable equipment 8. Facilities for handwashing 9. Facilities for communicating the patient's need for toileting to the nurse, e.g. a bell 10. Appropriate aids for moving and handling 11. Receptacle for soiled disposable items.
Bedpan	For female patients, a bedpan may be used for micturition and defaecation. For male patients, it may be used for defaecation, but a urinal should be offered at the same time for micturition. Toilet ware may be disposable or non-disposable; non-disposable equipment usually being made of plastic. Disposable equipment is, however, increasingly being used. A traditional or a slipper bedpan may be used, the latter having the advantage of being easier to insert and more comfortable to use.

Disposable bedpan

This should be placed in a rigid bedpan holder and taken to the bedside under a disposable cover. The used bedpan should be flushed in the bedpan disposer according to the manufacturer's instructions. The holder should be washed and dried before storage.

Plastic bedpan

This should be covered with a disposable cover and the used bedpan placed in the bedpan washer according to the manufacturer's instructions. The bedpan should be washed and dried before storing, and regular sterilisation should be performed according to health authority policy. In the community, waste should be disposed of in the toilet and the equipment cleaned according to local infection control policy.

Urinal

This is used for male patients for micturition and should be covered with a disposable cover when taken to and from the patient. Like a bedpan, it may be disposable or non-disposable; after use, it is processed in the same way. A female urinal is available and may be suitable for some patients (Fader et al 1999).

Commode

This is a mobile chair constructed to hold a bedpan, which can be taken to the bedside for the patient's use (Fig. 41.1 and 41.2). It may also be built to transport the patient to the toilet so that the commode seat fits over the toilet seat. Many mechanical lifting aids incorporate a commode seat so that the patient may be taken safely to the ward toilet or use it as a conventional commode (see the

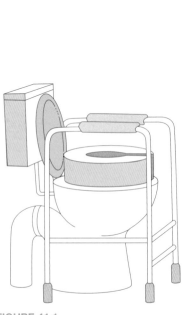
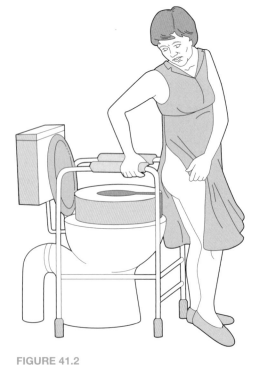

FIGURE 41.1
Use of hand rails and a raised seat to promote independence at home

FIGURE 41.2
Adaptation of clothing for ease of access when toileting

manufacturer's instructions). A commode can be made available for patients at home to maintain their independence, or as a temporary help for toileting if access to the bathroom is difficult.

Guidelines and rationale for this nursing practice	Guidelines are given for the provision of a bedpan to a female patient and a urinal to a male patient.

The provision of a bedpan for a female patient

- explain this nursing practice to the patient **to gain consent and co-operation, and encourage participation in care**
- ensure that the patient knows how to request a bedpan when needed, **to reduce anxiety about this activity of living**
- respond immediately to the patient's request for a bedpan **to prevent incontinence and patient distress**
- don a plastic apron after washing the hands **to prevent contamination** (Jeanes 2005)
- don plastic gloves **to prevent contamination from body fluids**
- collect and prepare the bedpan, carrying it to the bedside under a disposable cover **to maintain self-esteem and reduce embarrassment**
- ensure the patient's privacy **to respect her individuality**
- observe the patient's condition throughout this activity **to monitor any adverse effects**
- help the patient into a comfortable sitting position, supporting her back with pillows **so that she will be in the best position for micturition**
- help the patient to adjust her clothing **to expose the buttocks and perineum**
- if the patient's condition allows, ask her to lift her buttocks. A monkey pole or similar equipment may be used to facilitate this procedure, and two nurses may be required depending on the patient's condition. A hoist with a toileting sling may be used. The patient's moving and handling plan should be followed **to ensure safe technique** (Royal College of Nursing 1999)
- slide the bedpan into position with the shaped rim under the patient's buttocks **so that it is safely in place**
- adjust the patient's pillows **to ensure that she is sitting comfortably**
- leave the patient to use the bedpan, ensuring privacy **to maintain her self-esteem**
- remain in the vicinity **to be available when the patient is ready**
- assist with wiping the perineum and/or anus if necessary **to maintain healthy skin in the area**
- remove the bedpan **once toileting is complete**
- give the patient a bowl to wash her hands **for her own personal hygiene and to prevent cross-infection**, or help her to the washbasin if it is more appropriate

- ensure that the patient is left feeling as comfortable as possible *to minimise any distress*
- observe the contents of the bedpan *for any abnormalities*; these should be reported and the bedpan saved for inspection
- measure the urine and retain a labelled specimen *for ward testing if required* (*see* 'Urine testing', p. 357)
- dispose of the equipment safely *to prevent the transmission of infection*
- wash the hands using a good handwashing technique *to maintain a safe environment*
- document the nursing practice appropriately and report any abnormal findings immediately. *This will ensure safe practice and enable prompt, appropriate medical and nursing intervention to be initiated*
- in undertaking this practice, nurses are accountable for their actions, the quality of care delivered and record-keeping according to the Code of Professional Conduct: Standards for Conduct, Performance and Ethics (Nursing and Midwifery Council 2004) and Guidelines for Records and Record Keeping (Nursing and Midwifery Council 2005).

Guidelines for providing a commode

In principle these are the same as those for using a bedpan. Once the prepared and covered commode has been taken to the bedside, the patient should be helped out of bed *to sit on the commode in privacy*, and the guidelines as for a bedpan followed. Help from one or two nurses may be needed *to assist the patient in and out of bed*, depending on the patient's condition and the mechanical aids being used for safe moving and handling (Royal College of Nursing 2002, National Back Pain Association & Royal College of Nursing 2005).

The provision of a urinal for a male patient

- explain this nursing practice and *gain the patient's consent and co-operation*
- ensure that the patient knows how to request a urinal when needed *to reduce anxiety about this activity of living*
- collect and prepare the urinal and take it to the bedside under a disposable cover *to maintain self-esteem and reduce embarrassment*
- ensure the patient's privacy *to respect his individuality*
- help the patient to place the urinal in position if required *so that no urine is spilled*
- remain in the vicinity *to be available when the patient is ready*
- remove the urinal and proceed as for the guidelines for providing a bedpan.

Principles of continence assessment

The key principles of continence assessment are outlined in this section. Problems of continence can apply to both urine and faeces, and the majority of people with a continence problem can be cured, or have their condition improved, if they are assessed and managed appropriately (Bradley & Moran 1998). Evidence shows, however, that nursing intervention could be improved in this area of care (Bayliss et al 2000). It is also important to remember that continence is not just a problem for the older patient.

There are five main types of incontinence – stress, urge, overflow, neurogenic/reflex and functional – a detailed structured assessment being the key to the development of a management and treatment plan for the patient. The Department of Health (2000) recommends that all patients with a continence problem receive an initial assessment undertaken by a suitably qualified person that includes the following areas:

- a detailed description of the symptoms with regard to continence
- the effect on lifestyle and motivation for treatment
- a physical examination of the abdomen for a palpable mass or bladder distension; of the perineum to identify prolapse and excoriation, and to assess pelvic floor contraction; and of the rectum to check for faecal impaction
- urinalysis to exclude infection or identify potential underlying disease such as renal disease or diabetes
- an assessment of manual dexterity
- an assessment of the physical and social environment, for example the toilet and laundry facilities
- the use of an activities of living diary (including diet, exercise and bowel and urinary habits)
- an identification of the underlying conditions or medication that may exacerbate the problem.

A frequency–volume chart may be used to identify the patient's usual voiding pattern. This records the number and types of drink taken, the volume of urine passed at each voiding and the number of incontinent episodes. This is recorded over 24 hours for 3–5 days (Bardsley 2000). A variety of continence assessment forms are available, and health authorities will have developed one as part of their continence management protocol.

Following the initial assessment, it will be possible to determine the possible causes for the incontinence and from this establish a treatment plan – using locally developed protocols – that is acceptable to the patient. The role of the continence advisor is important in educating staff and auditing continence services.

Patient/carer education

Key points

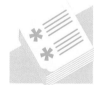

In partnership with the patient and/or carer, ensure that they are competent to carry out any practices required. Information should be given on an appropriate point of contact for any concerns that may arise.

The importance of regular toileting should be explained and, if necessary, reinforced with simple aids such as adapted clothing and the help of carers.

The reason for the use of mechanical aids for help with toileting should be explained.

Maintaining a healthy perineal area, and the efficient, safe cleaning of the area, should be emphasised. This may be achieved using something as simple as wet wipes or as specialised as a bidet.

The availability of special equipment to aid continence should be discussed with the patient according to his or her individual needs, as part of continuing care in an institutional setting or included in the goals for discharge to community care. This may include adaptations to the toilet area in the patient's home.

When a patient has had a full continence assessment, a plan of care should be discussed with the patient and mutually agreed with the community team.

References

Bardsley A 2000 Assessment of incontinence. Elderly Care 11(9): 36–39

Bayliss V, Cherry M, Lock R et al 2000 Pathways for continence care: background and audit. British Journal of Nursing 9(9): 590–596

Bradley S, Moran R 1998 Better continence care through the use of research in clinical practice. Nursing Times 94(34): 52–53

Department of Health 2000 Good practice in continence services. HMSO, London

Fader M, Petterson L, Dean G et al 1999 The selection of female urinals: results of a multicentre evaluation. British Journal of Nursing 8(14): 918–925

Jeanes A 2005 Infection control. A practical guide to the use of hand decontaminants. Nursing Times 101(20): 46–48

National Back Pain Association and Royal College of Nursing 2005 Guide to the handling of patients, 5th edn. NBPA, Middlesex, UK

Nursing and Midwifery Council 2004 Code of professional conduct: standards for conduct, performance and ethics. NMC, London

Nursing and Midwifery Council 2005 Guidelines for records and record keeping. NMC, London

Royal College of Nursing 1999 Manual handling assessments in hospitals and the community. RCN, London

Royal College of Nursing 2002 Code of practice for patient handling. RCN, London

Self assessment

1. What is the aim of toileting?
2. Where/how should toileting take place?
3. What equipment may be required for toileting?
4. What observations may you be required to carry out during/after toileting?
5. What are the principles of continence assessment?

Practice 42
Tracheostomy Care

There are three parts to this section:

1 Principles of tracheostomy care

2 Removal of respiratory tract secretions via a tracheostomy tube

3 Changing a tracheostomy tube/tube management

Learning outcomes	**By the end of this section, you will be able to:**
	▪ Understand the rationale for tracheostomy
	▪ Identify the equipment used in this nursing practice
	▪ Discuss the care of a patient with a tracheostomy in situ
	▪ Identify the potential problems a patient with a tracheostomy may experience.

Background knowledge required	Revision of the anatomy and physiology of the upper respiratory tract, and the anatomy of the upper gastrointestinal tract
	Revision of local policy or guidelines on the care of a patient with a tracheostomy
	Revision of your knowledge in relation to wound care.

Indications and rationale for the creation of a tracheostomy	A tracheostomy is an artificial opening, which is surgically created by an incision made into the anterior wall of the trachea (Docherty & Bench 2002). The incision is usually made at a level between the 2nd and 4th cartilaginous rings of the trachea.
	A tracheostomy can be **temporary**, e.g. left in situ for a number of days, weeks or months before removal, or **permanent**, i.e. for the remainder of the patient's life. Most tracheostomies are temporary (Docherty & Bench 2002).

Temporary tracheostomy

This involves the opening of the surgical incision and the insertion of a tracheostomy tube. The tube is then held in place by tapes secured around the patient's neck (Fig. 42.1).

Permanent tracheostomy (or tracheostoma)

This involves the incision of the circumference of the trachea so that it forms a permanent stoma or opening on the surface of the skin, i.e. the trachea is incised and sutured to the skin surface. In these cases a tracheostomy tube may remain in situ until the stoma has healed or if there are any complications with healing or stoma formation.

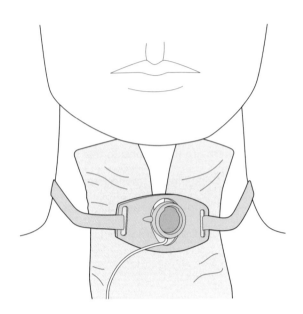

FIGURE 42.1
**Tracheostomy dressing
and securing device
in situ**

1. PRINCIPLES OF TRACHEOSTOMY CARE

Tracheostomy is becoming more common in both acute and community settings (Serra 2000). As a nurse, you therefore need to understand the rationale for this surgical procedure and utilise evidence-based knowledge in caring for your patient who has a tracheostomy in place. In doing this you will promote clinical effectiveness and prevent potential complications, as well as reassure your patient and their family.

**Indications for
tracheostomy**

These can be listed (Serra 2000) as:

- *the need to bypass potential or actual airway obstructions*, e.g. tumour, inflammation, trauma, foreign body
- *to support prolonged and assisted ventilation* in certain neuromuscular disorders, e.g. motorneurone disease, certain chronic respiratory disorders, e.g. chronic obstructive pulmonary disease, and in patients who are sedated or comatose
- *to aid in the expectoration and/or removal of bronchial secretions*, thus reducing the risk of respiratory infection or to prevent other respiratory complications such as atelectasis
- *in laryngectomy, where a permanent tracheostoma is formed*.

Equipment

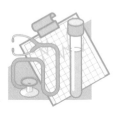

1. Plastic disposable or single-patient tracheostomy tubes are usually used in the management of both temporary and long-term tracheostomies. Tubes can either have a single cannula or consist of two parts – an outer and inner cannula. Each healthcare provider will have guidelines on the type of tube they prefer to use. A tube without an inner cannula can be left in situ for a few days or removed and replaced as and when necessary. A two-part tube can be left for a longer period. In both cases the manufacturer's instructions should be read

carefully as this will give guidance as to the length of time the tube can remain in situ – this refers to the ***licensed use*** of the product.

2. Most of your patients will have a tracheostomy tube that incorporates an inner cannula that can be changed and cleaned regularly, reducing the need to perform a complete change of the outer tracheostomy tube. The inner cannula also provides essential protection against potentially life-threatening problems, such as tube obstruction, as it can be removed quickly and safely thus providing prompt relief to your patient (Oxford Radcliffe NHS Hospital Trust 2005). A patient may occasionally have a silver tube in situ that also incorporates an inner cannula, although this is now rare due to the extensive range of plastic tubes available.

3. A ***cuffed*** tube (Fig. 42.2) may be used in your patient's immediate postoperative phase of care as they assist in airway maintenance and prevent the potential aspiration of secretions from the recently formed wound around the tube. Your patient may feel the cuff pressing against their throat so you should provide meaningful explanation at this point. Once any secretions from the wound have ceased an ***uncuffed*** tube may be considered. Finally, tubes can either be ***fenestrated*** or ***unfenestrated***. Fenestrated tubes are used when weaning off the tube or to enable phonation. Therefore tubes can be (Fig. 42.3):
   — single/double cannula
   — cuffed/uncuffed
   — fenestrated/unfenestrated.

4. Tracheostomy tubes come in a variety of sizes for adult use: 7.0 mm, 7.5 mm, 8.0 mm, 8.5 mm and 9 mm. The diameter and length of the tube selected will be

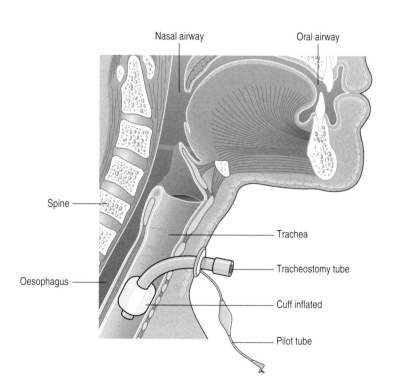

FIGURE 42.2
Anatomy of the trachea with a tracheostomy tube in place
From Woodrow 2002. Copyright RCN Publishing Company 2002. Reproduced by permission of Nursing Standard

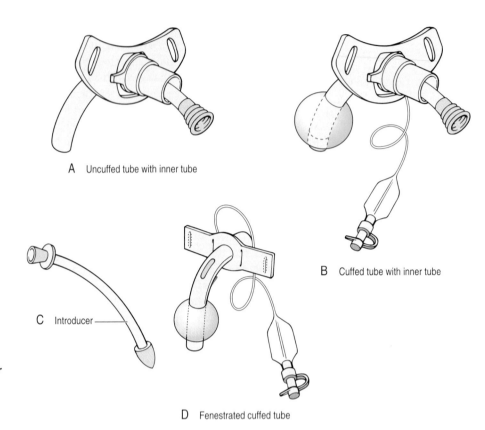

A   Uncuffed tube with inner tube

B   Cuffed tube with inner tube

C   Introducer

D   Fenestrated cuffed tube

FIGURE 42.3
**Tracheostomy tubes in
common use**
**A Uncuffed tube with
inner tube**
**B Cuffed tube with inner
tube**
C Introducer
**D Fenestrated cuffed
tube**

dependent upon your patient's needs and will always be slightly smaller than
the diameter of the trachea (Dickson & Martindale 2002).

Essential equipment

The essential equipment to be at the bedside of **all** patients with a tracheostomy
should include the following (Serra 2000; Oxford Radcliffe NHS Hospital Trust
2005):

1. Spare tracheostomy tubes – same size and type as well as a tube the next size
   down
2. Tracheal dilators
3. Stitch cutter (if the tracheostomy tube is stitched to the skin)
4. Suction equipment: suction catheters (no larger in diameter than half the
   diameter of the tracheostomy tube), connection tubing, suction container,
   gloves, aprons
5. Sterile water and normal saline
6. Humidification equipment and tracheal masks
7. Tracheostomy dressings
8. Scissors
9. Cuff manometer if cuffed tube in situ
10. Tracheostomy tapes

11. Catheter mount (so as to enable attachment to an Ambu bag should your patient require resuscitation)
12. Cuffed tube (if your patient has an uncuffed tube in situ)
13. Equipment for oral hygiene.

The Code of Professional Conduct (Nursing and Midwifery Council 2004) states that all nurses are individually accountable for their own actions. It is therefore imperative that you ensure that you are familiar not only with your local policies regarding tracheostomy care but are able to identify and use safely, all equipment related to this practice.

Guidelines and rationale

Successful tracheostomy care is dependent upon a multi-disciplinary approach to care as well as collaborative care involving healthcare professionals, patients and their families. Where possible, patients should be educated regarding their treatment and care in the preoperative phase and introduced to all members of the multi-disciplinary team who will include:

- nurses
- consultant surgeon and medical team
- specialist nurse
- speech and language therapist
- physiotherapist
- dietician
- pharmacist.

Collaborative care will not only improve communication but will assist in ensuring patient satisfaction, reduce anxiety, promote self-care, improve the patient's self-esteem and enable your patient to take an active part in the decisions made regarding their care.

Communication

Because a tracheostomy tube is inserted below the level of the vocal chords in the larynx, patients with a tracheostomy may encounter difficulties in communicating, which can have a psychological impact on both the patient and their family (NHS Quality Improvement Scotland 2003). An individualised assessment of the patient's needs must be made and referral to a speech and language specialist where appropriate. An initial assessment should be undertaken including the patient's ability to communicate using hearing, sight and writing. An individualised care plan should be devised and implemented. Your patient, for example, may be able to use a pen and paper to communicate effectively while the tube remains in situ or until a speaking valve can be fitted.

Your patient may have a fenestrated tube (Fig. 42.4) in situ, which enables speech. Some patients may find that, with uncuffed tubes, placing a finger over the tube and forcing expired air over the vocal chords restores the voice. This latter practice should be discouraged as it promotes the risk of respiratory infection (Woodrow 2002). Woodrow (2002) suggests that the use of a speaking valve should be favoured to reduce this risk.

Regular evaluation of the effectiveness of a plan of care must be made as needs may change in line with the patient's altered health status (NHS Quality

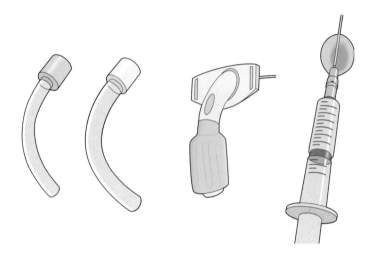

FIGURE 42.4
**Double-lumen,
fenestrated
tracheostomy tube**

Improvement Scotland 2003). A call bell should be left in reach of the patient at all times. Nurses should also continually reflect upon their own communication skills and be able to adapt to utilise alternative means of communication effectively.

Nutrition

The presence of a tracheostomy tube can lead to an impaired nutritional status (Bond et al 2003). It should be remembered that adequate nutritional intake will promote health and, in particular, provide the patient with energy, help prevent infection and promote healing. Dickson & Martindale (2002) suggest that a minimum fluid intake of 3000 ml (unless contraindicated) is achieved to help respiratory secretions remain liquefied. The presence of a cuffed tube can cause anxiety on the patient's behalf with regard to swallowing. Serra (2000) suggests that this problem can often be due to *over-inflation* of the cuff and cuff pressure must therefore be checked regularly. It has been suggested that the patient remain nil by mouth when the cuff is inflated as it places pressure upon the oesophagus and anchors the larynx thus disabling the normal swallow (Fig. 42.5). In any case an individual assessment of the patient's swallowing status *must* be made and involve multi-disciplinary decision making. Again local healthcare provider policy should be sought.

In patients who are at risk of aspiration, it will be recommended that the patient remains nil by mouth and an alternative method of feeding sought. This may involve nasogastric feeding in the short term or gastrostomy feeding in the longer term. It is therefore essential that a swallowing assessment involving the dietician, nurse specialist and speech and language therapist is performed. By doing so any swallowing difficulties can be identified early and an individualised plan of care to support the patient's nutritional needs put in place.

In patients who remain nil by mouth effective oral care should involve regular cleaning of the oral mucosa, observation of the condition of the mouth and tongue and brushing of teeth or dentures (Russell 2005).

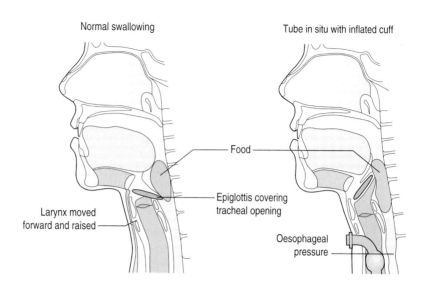

Normal swallowing

Tube in situ with inflated cuff

Food

Epiglottis covering
tracheal opening

Larynx moved
forward and raised

Oesophageal
pressure

FIGURE 42.5
Swallowing
From Russell 2005.
Copyright MA Healthcare
Ltd 2005. Reproduced
by permission of British
Journal of Nursing

2. REMOVAL OF RESPIRATORY TRACT SECRETIONS VIA A TRACHEOSTOMY TUBE

Suction must only be performed by a suitably qualified practitioner or under the direct supervision of such a person.

Equipment

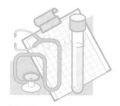

1. Tray
2. Sterile disposable gloves
3. Sterile suction catheters with a thumb control
4. Sterile container and water for flushing the catheter and tubing
5. Receptacle for soiled disposable items
6. Suction apparatus, e.g. a portable machine or centralised suction.

Guidelines and rationale for this nursing practice

- tracheal suction should be carried out only when secretions are audible in the tracheostomy tube and the patient is unable to cough up secretions or when the patient feels that the tube is blocked. ***This reduces the risk of trauma to the mucosa***
- if possible, explain the nursing practice to the patient ***to gain consent and co-operation***. Patients should be encouraged to participate actively in their care
- ensure the patient's privacy ***to maintain dignity and a sense of self***
- wash hands (Jeanes 2005) and collect the equipment ***for efficiency of practice***
- assist the patient to a suitable position such as the Fowler's position ***for ease of access to the tracheostomy tube***
- if the patient has a fenestrated tube in situ, an inner tube without a hole must be inserted prior to the procedure ***to prevent damage to the mucosal lining of the trachea***

- 100% oxygen therapy (care must be taken in patients with chronic obstructive pulmonary disease) prior to and following the procedure is recommended **to prevent hypoxia**
- observe the patient throughout this activity **for any signs of discomfort or distress**
- fill the sterile container with sterile water **to flush the suction catheter**
- open the end of the pack containing the connecting end of the suction catheter and connect it to the tubing of the suction machine. The diameter of the catheter should not exceed half the diameter of the tracheostomy tube **to ensure that hypoxia does not occur**
- put a disposable glove on the dominant hand
- slide the cover off the catheter and rinse it through with sterile water **to lubricate it**
- insert the catheter into the tracheostomy with the gloved hand but without any suction for the length of the tracheostomy tube
- withdraw the catheter, applying suction by covering the thumb control hole and rotating the catheter while this is being done. If the secretions are tenacious and difficult to remove, nebulised saline or mechanical humidification may be administered. **This loosens the secretions for easier removal**. Intermittent humidification helps the patient **to expectorate spontaneously**
- allow the patient to rest and re-oxygenate before repeating insertion of the catheter **to prevent hypoxia and reduce the risk of a vasovagal response**
- a maximum of two suctioning attempts is recommended **as repeated attempts above this place the patient at risk of cardiovascular complications**
- dispose of the catheter at the end of the practice after rinsing both the catheter and the tubing with sterile water
- ensure that the patient is left feeling as comfortable as possible
- dispose of the equipment safely and wash hands **for the protection of others**
- document the nursing practice appropriately, monitor the after-effects and report any abnormal findings immediately **to provide a written record and enable prompt intervention should an adverse reaction to the procedure be noted**
- in undertaking this practice, nurses are accountable for their actions, the quality of care delivered and record-keeping according to the Code of Professional Conduct: Standards for Conduct, Performance and Ethics (Nursing and Midwifery Council 2004) and Guidelines for Records and Record Keeping (Nursing and Midwifery Council 2005).

3. CHANGING A TRACHEOSTOMY TUBE/TUBE MANAGEMENT

Two nurses MUST be present during a tube change.

Equipment

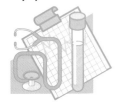

1. Tray or trolley
2. Sterile dressings pack
3. Sterile tracheostomy tube, taped and with an obturator, and a tube one size smaller in case of difficulty recannulating the stoma
4. Sterile KY jelly
5. Sterile tracheal dilators

6. Sterile scissors
7. Tracheostomy dressing, e.g. Lyofoam
8. Container of sterile normal saline with which to clean the soiled tube
9. Disposable gloves
10. Instrument brush
11. Receptacle for soiled disposable items.

Guidelines and rationale for this nursing practice

- explain the nursing practice to the patient **to gain consent and co-operation. Patients should be encouraged to be active participants in care**
- ensure the patient's privacy **to maintain dignity and a sense of self**
- collect and prepare the equipment and hands (Jeanes 2005) **for efficiency of practice**
- assist the patient to a suitable position such as the Fowler's position **to allow this practice to be carried out**
- observe the patient throughout this activity **for any signs of discomfort or distress**
- open the dressings pack and the tracheostomy tube pack
- check that the obturator fits. Check in particular that it can be easily removed **as it blocks the airway once the tube is in situ**
- lubricate the end of the tube and obturator **for ease of insertion**
- make a slit in the end of the protective pad **so that it will easily wrap round the tube**
- put on the disposable gloves **for your own and the patient's protection**
- if applicable deflate the cuff on a cuffed tube and administer suction prior to changing the tube **to prevent trauma and remove any secretions**
- remove the soiled tube with a smooth outward and downward motion, discarding it into the receptacle for disposable items if it is plastic. The tube should be soaked in normal saline and left to air dry
- remove the gloves **to allow more dextrous hand movements**
- hold the new tube by the tapes and insert it smoothly from below in an upwards, inwards and downwards movement into the trachea. **This follows the line of the stoma**
- immediately remove the obturator while holding the tube in place **to free the airway** and inflate the cuff if applicable
- tie the tapes at the side of the patient's neck. **This is a more comfortable position than the back**
- slide the protective pad into position round the stoma **to protect the skin beneath the tube flange**
- ensure that the patient is left feeling as comfortable as possible
- dispose of the equipment safely and wash hands (Jeanes 2005) **for the protection of others**
- record this nursing practice appropriately, monitor the after-effects and report any abnormal findings immediately, **providing a written record and enabling prompt intervention should an adverse reaction to the practice be noted**
- in undertaking this practice, nurses are accountable for their actions, the quality of care delivered and record-keeping according to the Code of Professional Conduct: Standards for Conduct, Performance and Ethics (Nursing and Midwifery Council 2004) and Guidelines for Records and Record Keeping (Nursing and Midwifery Council 2005).

Additional information	The presence of a tracheostomy tube means that the normal route of airflow via the nose and nasal passages is bypassed. It is therefore important that you ensure that air entering the tracheostomy tube is humidified and in some cases warmed. Dry humidification can be achieved by attaching a 'Swedish nose' to the end of the tube. By providing humidification in this way, the risk of tube blockage, crusting and damage to the lungs is reduced.

Cleaning an inner tube

The cleaning of the inner tube should take place every four hours (Docherty & Bench 2002) or as required by your patient. Using a clean technique, the inner tube can be turned anticlockwise, removed and cleansed using running tap water (Docherty & Bench 2002). The tube is then dried using sterile gauze and reinserted. Prior to cleansing the tube a spare inner tube should be inserted. The use of brushes is no longer advocated in the cleansing of tracheostomy tubes as damage can be sustained to the side of the plastic tube (Sierra 2000). While cleansing the inner tube take the opportunity to inspect the skin around the stoma site to determine whether it requires to be cleansed and a new dressing applied. This will save the need to perform this later and will reduce the amount of manipulation around the tracheostomy.

Patient/carer education

Key points

Patient/carer education depends upon the nurse having the necessary knowledge, skills and competence to provide meaningful explanations and support. In partnership with the patient and/or carer, ensure that they are competent to carry out any practices required. Information should be given on an appropriate point of contact for any concerns that may arise.

Patients require planned education to help them cope with the anxiety that most people experience when they first have a tracheostomy. If the tracheostomy tube does not have a speaking flap, they will need help and advice about alternative ways of communicating.

Patients who have permanent tracheostomies will require a structured teaching programme of self-care.

References

Bond P, Grant F, Coltart L et al 2003 Best practice in the care of patients with a tracheostomy. Nursing Times 99(30): 24–25

Dickson A, Martindale G 2002 Caring for the patient with a respiratory disorder. In: Walsh M (ed) Watson's clinical nursing and related sciences, 6th edn. Baillière Tindall, Edinburgh, pp 333–370

Docherty B, Bench S 2002 Tracheostomy management for patients in general ward settings. Professional Nurse 18(2): 100–104

Jeanes A 2005 Infection control. A practical guide to the use of hand decontaminants. Nursing Times 101(20): 46–48

NHS Quality Improvement Scotland 2003 Caring for the patient with a tracheostomy. Best practice statement. NHS QIS, Edinburgh

Nursing and Midwifery Council 2004 Code of professional conduct: standards for conduct, performance and ethics. NMC, London

Nursing and Midwifery Council 2005 Guidelines for records and record keeping. NMC, London

Oxford Radcliffe NHS Hospital Trust 2005 Adult tracheostomy management. Guidelines for best practice. Oxford Radcliffe NHS Hospital Trust, Oxford

Russell C 2005 Providing the nurse with a guide to tracheostomy care and management. British Journal of Nursing 14(8): 428–433

Serra A 2000 Tracheostomy care. Nursing Standard 14(42): 45–55

Woodrow P 2002 Managing patients with a tracheostomy in acute care. Nursing Standard 16(44): 39–48

Self assessment

1. List three indications as to why your patient may have a tracheostomy.
2. While nursing a patient who has a temporary double-lumen tracheostomy tube in place, the tube blocks. What do you do?
3. Identify the means by which you, the nurse, could ensure effective communication with a patient who has a tracheostomy tube in situ.
4. What kind of dressing should be applied around a tracheostomy tube?
5. Write brief notes on the key practices that will ensure the risk of potential complications is reduced.

Practice 43
Transfer of Patients Between Care Settings

Learning outcomes	**By the end of this section, you should know how to:**
	▪ prepare the patient and carer for transfer to another care setting
	▪ complete patient transfer documentation.
Background knowledge required	Carers and Disabled Children Act 2000
	Revision of local policy on the transfer of patients
	Achieving Timely 'Simple' Discharge from Hospital: A Toolkit for the Multidisciplinary Team (Department of Health 2004)
	Discharge from Hospital: Pathway, Process and Practice (Department of Health 2003a).
Indications and rationale for patient transfer	Healthcare reform has resulted in a much greater focus on the appropriate use of the services available for patient care. Thus, the patient may be transferred between institutional and community settings within the statutory health and social care agencies or in the voluntary or private/independent sectors, *as is judged appropriate for his or her individual needs and benefit*.
Outline of the procedure	'Patient transfer' (rather than discharge) is the term used in this section as it demonstrates a continuum rather than a cessation of care. The procedure may be simple or complex, depending on the needs of the patient and carer. The systematic approach to care – namely assessment, planning, implementation and evaluation – may, however, be used as a framework for the patient transfer process:
	▪ the assessment phase involves the collection of data pertinent to the patient and/or carer. A variety of sources may be used to build up a holistic picture of the patient and the caring environment. Some of this information will already have been collected during the patient admission assessment
	▪ the planning stage utilises the assessment data to provide a plan of transfer. Liaison with other agencies to request and discuss their input will also be carried out at this stage of the process
	▪ the implementation phase involves putting the plan into action and completing patient transfer documentation
	▪ the evaluation stage of the transfer procedure is essential in order to assess the effectiveness of the process and to identify any difficulties or problems.

Guidelines and rationale for this nursing practice

General principles will be given, followed by guidelines for planning and implementing the transfer process. Some of the guidelines may not be applicable to patients transferring from community to institutional settings.

Transfer and discharge to and from hospital can be a distressing time for individuals, their families and friends (Department of Health 2003a). As health professionals it is important that nurses develop and adapt practice and respond to the ever-changing needs of the service provided (Department of Health 2004). The multidisciplinary team can make a significant difference to the speed and quality of the patient journey (Department of Health and Royal College of Nursing 2003). A crucial factor in planning transfer and discharge is the process of communication, co-operation and collaboration between health and social care, the multidisciplinary team, patients and relatives (Hoban 2004, Lees 2004).

Principles

- the patient and carer should be involved in all stages of the transfer process, *enabling a consideration and discussion of their needs prior to the transfer plan being completed and implemented* (Department of Health 2004, Lees & Holmes 2005). Older people, in particular, often find it a major life transition, particularly when it means having to move home or establish new routines (Lishman 2003)
- patient transfer is normally a multidisciplinary procedure that may involve social, voluntary and independent care agencies as well as different healthcare professionals, *ensuring a holistic approach to patient transfer*
- good communication is an essential part of the patient-transfer process *as poor communication patterns affect continuity of care* on transfer from community to institutional settings as well as from institutional to community care (Department of Health 2004)
- it is essential that there be early involvement of and liaison with staff from the receiving care setting (which may be a hospital ward, an intermediate care facility, a nursing home or the patient's own home). Some areas have a designated liaison nurse who provides a link between institutional and community care *to promote continuity of care* (Hoban 2004, Lees 2004)
- the multidisciplinary team can speed up the transfer process and manage the care pathway to an expected or predicted date of transfer, including weekends (Department of Health 2004)
- with the development of hospital at home and supported discharge teams, patients may be transferred to where their individual needs can be appropriately met (Department of Health 2004)
- an evaluation system should be in place *to judge the effectiveness of the patient transfer process* (Rudd & Smith 2002).

Planning patient transfer

- discuss care needs with the patient and carer *to ascertain their views and requirements, and involve them in the decision-making process*
- information related to risk factors should be recorded and shared between care settings (e.g. the patient being at risk of falls or any sensory deficit that may put the patient at risk)
- plan and initiate any teaching programmes for the patient and/or carer. Examples include a self-medication programme for patients being

transferred from institutional to community care (Banning 2004) and a moving and handling teaching session for carers **to prepare the patient and carer for tasks that they will be required to undertake in the community**

▪ consult, liaise with and refer to the appropriate care agencies (health, social, voluntary or independent). If the patient has complex care needs, it may be necessary to invite all the relevant personnel, including the patient and/or carer, to a case conference **to ensure that support services are in position prior to transfer** (Department of Health 2003b)

▪ order any equipment or patient aids (e.g. moving and handling equipment or oxygen cylinder) **to ensure that the receiving care setting meets the patient's needs**

▪ if the patient has complex needs and is being transferred from institutional care, it is valuable to organise a home-assessment visit prior to transfer. This will involve the patient, carer and district nurse as well as other relevant personnel such as the liaison nurse, occupational therapist, physiotherapist and social care staff **to enable the patient's needs to be assessed within his or her own environment and to enable an assessment of the carer's ability to provide care**

▪ arrange for transport between care settings **to ensure that the transport is appropriate for the patient's needs**

▪ information related to any infection that may put the patient, carers or other healthcare personnel at risk should be recorded. If appropriate, the MRSA status of the patient should be given (*see* 'Isolation nursing', p. 187)

▪ order a small supply of continence, dressing or medicinal products **to ensure that products are available for the immediate transfer period**

▪ assess the patient's ability to administer medication. If deficits are identified, a teaching programme may have to be initiated for the patient and carer, and/or patient compliance devices can be introduced. This should be carried out in conjunction with the pharmacist **to check that the patient and carer are able to administer the medicines correctly**

▪ consult with the carers about access arrangements to the patient's home on the day of transfer **to enable access arrangements to be made in advance of the transfer**

▪ give an approximate expected time of arrival to the patient, carer and any other personnel who require this information (for example, the district nurse and home help, or the continuing care facility) **to enable the caring network to be organised**.

Implementing the transfer process	▪ complete the patient transfer documentation (Box 43.1) and retain a copy **to provide a permanent record of the transfer process**
	▪ ensure that the medical staff have completed a transfer form to give to the patient's general practitioner. This usually comprises a summary of diagnoses, treatments, medication and follow-up appointments and **provides a permanent summary of admission details**
	▪ send the documentation to the personnel in the receiving care setting. This should be carried out according to local health authority policy but may involve an internal mailing system, the postal service, delivery by the patient/

BOX 43.1

Example of a checklist of contents for transfer documentation

Social data
- Patient details – name, date of birth, address, telephone number, occupation, housing and any dependants
- Carer details – name, address, telephone number, occupation, any relevant health problems or disabilities, other dependants and ability/willingness to care

Health data
- Diagnosis (including patient/carer's knowledge and understanding of the diagnosis)
- Disability/impairment
- Prognosis (if applicable)
- Medication (including any specialised instructions or medicine aids)
- Treatment (this might include details of procedures such as wound care, catheter management or continence products)
- Investigations carried out and results if known

Current status
- Information relating to assessed needs and planned care of the patient

Patient/carer's needs
- These will be specific to the service user and should be decided in conjunction with the patient/carer. A multidisciplinary assessment of the patient's current status is essential to establish their needs

Support services
- Details of care/therapy provided by professionals from other services (such as dieticians, physiotherapists or occupational therapists) in the current care setting
- Information – name, contact number and type of input – on any support services arranged for the post-transfer period (including the date of commencement)
- Most care settings will have a directory of services in the local area. For information on national services, contact the NHS Helpline (*see* text)

Financial data
- Details of welfare benefits (either in place or applied for)

Equipment data
- Details of equipment, either in place or requested (indicating the source of the equipment)
- Equipment should be in place prior to transfer

Health promotion/patient education
- Provide a summary of:
  —health promotion activities
  —information on any education programmes
- Enclose a copy of the patient education or health promotion literature given to the patient

All documentation should be signed and dated by the named nurse responsible for the patient's care

carer, faxing or a computer network. In the future, patient-held records (which stay with the patient as he or she moves between care areas) may be the way in which information is communicated, ***thus enabling the sharing of information between care settings***

- discuss any medication with the patient. This includes reinforcing information provided by the medical staff such as the reason for the drug, its dosage, timing or frequency and route of administration, and any special instructions. The use of a personal medical record card may be of value to some patients, ***to reinforce the information given on the container label and to facilitate understanding***
- follow-up care can be offered by pharmacists, GPs or nurses as an important aspect of discharge planning to ensure that patients understand the types of medication they are taking, especially with regard to new medication (Lowe et al 2000)
- check that the patient has all his or her personal belongings ***to ensure that no property is lost during transfer***
- arrange any follow-up outpatient appointment ***so that the patient and carer are aware of follow-up care***
- provide the patient and their next of kin or carer with details of the receiving care setting (the named nurse and contact number)
- in undertaking this practice, nurses are accountable for their actions, the quality of care delivered and record-keeping according to the Code of Professional Conduct: Standards for Conduct, Performance and Ethics (Nursing and Midwifery Council 2004) and Guidelines for Records and Record Keeping (Nursing and Midwifery Council 2005).

Additional information

Information related to any risk factors should be recorded. This might include:
- moving and handling factors
- difficulties related to the self-administration of medication
- the patient being at risk of falls
- any infection that may put the patient or carers at risk
- any sensory deficit that may put the patient at risk.

Whereas patients may function effectively within their existing environment, they may be at risk (for example by becoming disorientated) in a new care setting.

The patient's ability to communicate and understand information, as well as any deficits such as of hearing, sight or speech, should be noted. Information on equipment such as hearing aids or spectacles that the patient may require to communicate effectively should be provided.

It is essential that staff communicate with the patient/carer to ensure that they are fully informed and understand all aspects of the transfer. Any anxieties or concerns should be discussed and documented.

If transfer is taking place to a continuing-care facility, the patient should, whenever possible, visit the facility prior to transfer.

Record any difficulties that the patient has with breathing, as well as treatments such as inhalers or oxygen therapy. For the patient being transferred to the community, arrangements should be made for the delivery of oxygen cylinders or a concentrator, teaching being given to the patient and carer on its use and precautions.

The nutritional status of the patient can affect the healing process so any problems should be documented. Information should be provided on any special dietary requirements and whether there has been input from a dietician. Information is also needed on patients' ability to feed themselves and on the equipment required to aid this activity.

Equipment and feeding regime details should be provided for patients with enteral feeding requirements. Carers or patients will usually be taught this procedure prior to leaving hospital.

Bladder and bowel function are essential activities. Like nutrition, they may be affected by a change in environment or illness. A record of the patient's current bladder and bowel pattern should therefore be given, together with a note of any difficulties related to function, including abnormal patterns such as diarrhoea, constipation or urinary incontinence. Any investigations should be documented, and a record of necessary continence aids or toilet equipment should be given.

The patient may be at risk of pressure sores. The risk factors and score (*see* 'Skin care', p. 297) should be documented, along with the plan of care and any special equipment required. If pressure sores are present, a full description (including tracings) should be documented as baseline data for the staff in the receiving care setting.

The condition of the patient's mouth may affect his or her health. Thus, any problems such as ulceration, oral infection or problems with dentition, plus details of treatment, should be described.

The following should be documented:
- deficits in the patient's ability to mobilise
- information on any rehabilitation programmes
- the equipment required to aid mobility
- the level and type of assistance required from another person
- any active or passive exercises that need to be followed up in the receiving care setting.

Concerns regarding a change in body image caused by the illness should be discussed and documented. Sexual issues require sensitivity and diplomacy. The patient may discuss issues of a highly confidential nature, and it may not always be appropriate to document this information.

Patients may contemplate death during an episode of illness. Such thoughts may be transitory or may be longer lasting when the patient has a life-threatening or terminal illness. It is important that the staff in the receiving care environment are aware of the information and understanding that the patient has about his or her condition and prognosis. Counselling initiated with the patient should be outlined.

**Patient/carer
education**

Key points

In partnership with the patient and/or carer, ensure that they are competent to carry out any practices required. Information should be given on an appropriate point of contact for any concerns that may arise.

Education for the patient and carer will depend on the needs identified in the planning phase of transfer. Patient education may take the form of:

- health-promotion initiatives
- the teaching, demonstration and supervision of a practical procedure such as the administration of insulin
- literature on a specific illness or disease such as myocardial infarction. This will be used in conjunction with discussion
- verbal discussion to evaluate understanding (for example of an illness or medication) as verbal advice is not always assimilated by patients.

Information on support groups is available from local health, social and voluntary agencies or at a national level from the National Health Service Telephone Helpline Scotland (0800 224488) or NHS Direct – England (0845 4647)/NHS 24 – Scotland (08454 24 24 24), or via the Internet: http://www.nhsdirect.nhs.uk and http://www.nhs24.com.

Details of patient education programmes should be recorded in the transfer documentation.

References

Banning M 2004 Enhancing older people's concordance with taking their medication. British Journal of Nursing 13(11): 669–674

Department of Health 2003a Discharge from hospital: pathway, process and practice. The Stationery Office, London

Department of Health 2003b Definitions of medical stability and 'safe to transfer' produced by Health and Social Care Change Agent/Reimbursement Implementation Team. The Stationery Office, London

Department of Health 2004 Achieving timely 'simple' discharge from hospital: a toolkit for the multidisciplinary team. The Stationery Office, London

Department of Health and Royal College of Nursing 2003 Freedom to practise: dispelling the myths. Department of Health, London

Hoban V 2004 How easy is it for nurses to take over simple discharge. Nursing Times 100(41): 20–22

Lees L 2004 Making nurse-led discharge work to improve patient care. Nursing Standard 100(37): 30–32

Lees L, Holmes C 2005 Estimating date of discharge at ward level: a pilot study. Nursing Standard 19(17): 40–43

Lishman G 2003 Delayed discharge from the perspective of older people. British Journal of Nursing 12(5): 269

Lowe CJ, Raynor DK, Purvis J et al 2000 Effects of medicine review and education programme for older people in general practice. British Journal of Clinical Pharmacology 50: 172–175

Nursing and Midwifery Council 2004 Code of professional conduct: standards for conduct, performance and ethics. NMC, London

Nursing and Midwifery Council 2005 Guidelines for records and record keeping. NMC, London

Rudd C, Smith J 2002 Discharge planning. Nursing Standard 17(5): 33–37

Websites

National Health Service: http://www.nhsdirect.nhs.uk
National Health Service 24: http://www.nhs24.com

Self assessment

1. What are the four main areas within the framework for the patient transfer process?
2. Who would be involved in the patient transfer process?
3. List the areas that may involve patient/carer education.
4. What types of information should be shared with staff in the receiving care area?

Practice 44
Unconscious Patient

Learning outcomes	**By the end of this section, you should know how to:** ▪ maintain an adequate airway for the unconscious patient ▪ assess and record the level of consciousness using the Glasgow Coma Scale ▪ care for the unconscious patient.
Background knowledge required	Revision of the anatomy and physiology of the nervous system, with special reference to the brain Review of local policy and national guidelines relating to the care of the unconscious patient.
Indications and rationale for care during a state of unconsciousness	Nursing intervention is required when a patient's level of consciousness is such that, unaided, he or she can no longer maintain a clear airway, the normal protective reflexes are so reduced that the patient can no longer maintain the safety of the environment, and the patient is unable to perform the everyday activities of living (Hickey 2003).

The unconscious state is most commonly associated with:
▪ patients who have a cerebral vascular accident, **when areas of brain tissue will be damaged and have a diminished blood supply**, e.g.:
  — cerebral haemorrhage
  — cerebral embolus or ischaemia
  — subarachnoid haemorrhage
▪ patients who have taken an overdose of analgesic drugs, **which will affect the function of the brain cells**
▪ patients who have a traumatic head injury **as brain cells may be damaged by the injury**
▪ patients who have a brain tumour **causing pressure on and damage to the brain**
▪ patients who are in a comatose state caused by:
  — severe infection **as hyperpyrexia may affect brain cell function**
  — hypothermia **because a severe temperature change reduces brain cell activity** (Hickey 2003)
  — metabolic disturbances, i.e. uncontrolled diabetes mellitus (hyperglycaemia or hypoglycaemia), **which may result in reduced brain cell function**
▪ patients who have received prescribed anaesthetic medication during and following surgery, **which affects the patient's neurological state**
▪ patients in the terminal stage of illness **when cerebral function is diminished**.

Clinical Nursing Practices

Equipment

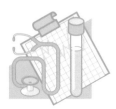

1. Bed with a detachable head
2. Padded cot sides
3. Disposable airway – either Guedel oropharyngeal or nasopharyngeal
4. Ambu bag with valve and mask
5. Equipment for oral, pharyngeal or tracheal suction
6. Equipment for oxygen therapy
7. Equipment for a nasogastric, PEG or total parenteral nutrition feeding system
8. Mouth care tray
9. Eye care tray
10. Catheter care tray
11. Equipment for endotracheal intubation if required.

Details of the equipment for specific nursing practices can be found in the relevant sections of this book.

Equipment for assessing the level of consciousness

Pen torch to assess eye pupil size and reaction
Level of consciousness assessment chart, e.g. the Glasgow Coma Scale (GCS)
Sphygmomanometer and stethoscope to measure blood pressure
Thermometer
Pulse oximeter – to measure peripheral oxygen saturation (Spo_2).

The Glasgow Coma Scale

This enables an assessment of level of consciousness to be made, using a numbered scale (Fig. 44.1). The assessment involves examining the patient's behavioural responses to the environment. Three categories are examined: eye opening, verbal response and motor responses, for example limb movements. Each level of behavioural response is recorded during the assessment and given a maximum score of 4, for a spontaneous eye-opening response, 5, for an orientated verbal response, and 6, for obeying commands in the motor response category (National Institute for Clinical Excellence 2003). A total score of 15 indicates fully conscious.

If the patient does not respond to voice or command, central painful stimuli may be applied. Pressure can be applied to the supra-orbital area for up to 30 seconds. This is contraindicated if there are any facial fractures. Painful stimuli can also be applied to the trapezius muscle, which extends from the neck across the back of the shoulders. A third method incorporates pressure to the angle of the jaw for a maximum of 30 seconds. Nail-bed pressure and sternal rubbing are methods of stimuli that can establish peripheral reflex responses to the environment. As such they provide little information about the level of consciousness (Waterhouse 2005).

Pupillary reactions to light are examined during the assessment and also recorded on the Glasgow Coma Scale chart (*see* Fig. 44.1). Pupils should be equal in size and react to light.

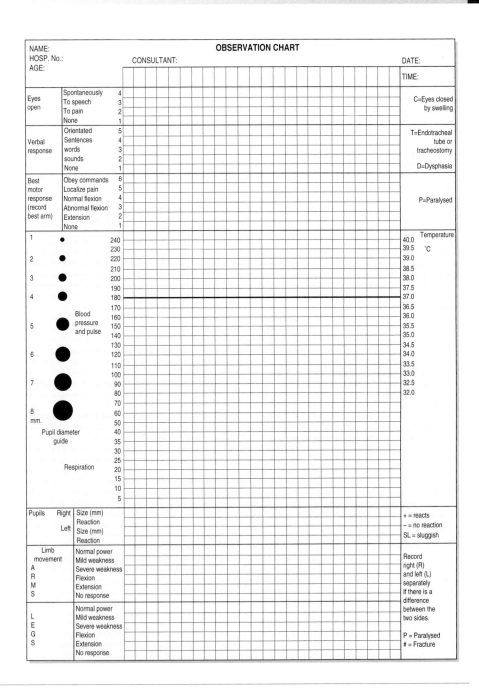

FIGURE 44.1
Glasgow Coma Scale: chart for documenting the assessment of a patient's level of consciousness

Guidelines and rationale for this nursing practice

The most important aspect of nursing is the maintenance of a clear airway and oxygenation while the reason for the patient's unconsciousness is being diagnosed and treated *so that the patient's respiratory function is as efficient as possible in the circumstances*.

- remove any dentures that may be present *to avoid obstruction of the airway*
- turn the patient into a lateral recumbent position (Figs 44.2 & 44.3) with the head of the bed elevated between 10 and 30 degrees – *to maintain the airway and prevent restricted lung ventilation* (Allan 2002)

FIGURE 44.2
Unconscious patient: the semi-prone position
From Roper et al 1985, with permission

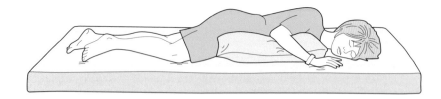

FIGURE 44.3
Unconscious patient: the lateral position

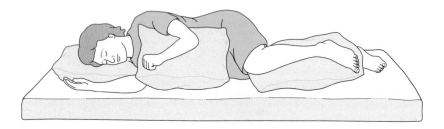

- observe the patient throughout this activity **to monitor any adverse effects**
- perform oral and pharyngeal suction, through the oral airway if necessary – endotracheal suction being carried out only by an appropriately skilled practitioner – **to prevent the aspiration of bronchial or oral secretions** (*see* 'Tracheostomy care', p. 331)
- insert an airway if required, **to help to maintain an adequate airway**
- measure peripheral oxygen saturation **to detect hypoxia**
- administer oxygen therapy as prescribed **to prevent hypoxia** (*see* 'Oxygen therapy', p. 245)
- assess and record the level of consciousness and pupillary response to light (Fig. 44.4) at every 30 minutes for the first 2 hours following deterioration of GCS. Assessment intervals can be reduced if the patient's GCS improves, to one hourly for the next 4 hours, 2 hourly for ensuing 6 hours and then 4 hourly until discharge, **to monitor and evaluate the patient's progress** (Scottish Intercollegiate Guidelines Network 2000, National Institute for Clinical Excellence 2003)

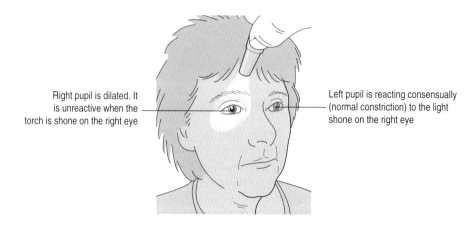

Right pupil is dilated. It is unreactive when the torch is shone on the right eye

Left pupil is reacting consensually (normal constriction) to the light shone on the right eye

FIGURE 44.4
Fixed and dilated pupils
From Brooker & Nicol 2003, with permission

- observe and record blood pressure, pulse rate, respiratory rate and temperature *to detect other physiological changes associated with a deterioration in level of consciousness* (Scottish Intercollegiate Guidelines Network 2000, National Institute for Clinical Excellence 2003)
- position the patient's limbs *to maintain his or her position comfortably and to allow an adequate flow of blood to the extremities*
- nurse the patient on a high-dependency pressure-relieving mattress system, and alternate the patient's side of lying every 2 hours *to maintain healthy tissue at the pressure areas and to aid the expansion of each lung* (*see* 'Skin care', p. 297)
- provide all nursing care as frequently as required, explaining the care to the patient despite the unconscious state and ensuring privacy before commencing care. The patient will be completely dependent for all his or her needs, and the nurse must *respect the patient's individuality and maintain his or her dignity at all times* (Hickey 2003)
- document all nursing practices appropriately and report abnormal findings immediately *to ensure safe practice and enable prompt, appropriate medical and nursing intervention to be initiated*
- in undertaking this practice, nurses are accountable for their actions, the quality of care delivered and record-keeping according to the Code of Professional Conduct: Standards for Conduct, Performance and Ethics (Nursing and Midwifery Council 2004) and Guidelines for Records and Record Keeping (Nursing and Midwifery Council 2005).

Patient/carer education Key points 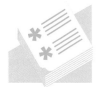	In partnership with the patient and/or carer, ensure that they are competent to carry out any practices required. Information should be given on an appropriate point of contact for any concerns that may arise. Education primarily involves the family. Explanations of the rationale for the nursing interventions and the expected outcome should therefore be shared with them. The family should be encouraged to talk to the patient about his or her interests and hobbies, this being reinforced with tapes and music if appropriate. They should understand that hearing is the first avenue of communication that returns as the patient recovers consciousness (National Institute for Clinical Excellence 2003). The family should also be encouraged to touch the patient and hold his or her hand; they may even wish to help with some of the nursing care. The family should be made to feel welcome at the bedside (National Institute for Clinical Excellence 2003).

References

Allan D 2002 Caring for the patient with a disorder of the nervous system. In: Walsh M (ed) Watson's clinical nursing and related sciences, 6th edn. Ballière Tindall, London, pp 665–745

Brooker C, Nicol M 2003 Nursing patients with neurosurgical problems. Nursing adults. The practice of caring. Mosby, London

Hickey JV 2003 Management of the unconscious patient. In: Hicey JV (ed) The clinical practice of neurological and neurosurgical nursing, 5th edn. Lippincott Williams & Wilkins, Philadelphia, PA

National Institute for Clinical Excellence 2003 Head injury: assessment, investigation and early management of head injury in infants children and adults. Clinical Guideline 4. NICE, London

Nursing and Midwifery Council 2004 Code of professional conduct: standards for conduct, performance and ethics. NMC, London

Nursing and Midwifery Council 2005 Guidelines for records and record keeping. NMC, London

Roper N, Logan W, Tierney A 1985 The elements of nursing, 2nd edn. Churchill Livingstone, Edinburgh

Scottish Intercollegiate Guidelines Network 2000 Early management of patients with a head injury. A national clinical guideline 46. SIGN, Edinburgh

Waterhouse C 2005 The Glasgow Coma Scale and other neurological observations. Nursing Standard 19(33): 56–64

Websites

National Institute for Clinical Excellence: http://www.nice.org.uk

Scottish Intercollegiate Guidelines Network: http://www.sign.ac.uk

Self assessment

1. Reflect on how you would conduct an assessment of an unconscious patient using the Glasgow Coma Scale and a pupil assessment.
2. What are main causes of the unconscious state?
3. Describe the care required to safely manage the patient's airway and maintenance of adequate oxygenation.

Practice 45
Urine Testing

Learning outcomes	**By the end of this section, you should know how to:** ▪ prepare the patient for this nursing practice ▪ collect the equipment required ▪ carry out testing of the urine.
Background knowledge required	Revision of the anatomy and physiology of the urinary system, with special reference to the formation of urine Revision of the manufacturer's instructions for the chemical reagents to be used Revision of local policy on urine testing.
Indications and rationale for testing urine	Testing urine involves assessing the constituents of the urine by observational, biochemical and mechanical means: ▪ ***to aid in the diagnosis of disease*** ▪ ***to assist in the monitoring of disease and treatment*** ▪ ***to assist in the assessment of the health of an individual*** ▪ ***to exclude pathology***.
Equipment 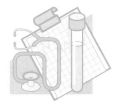	1. Clean, dry container for the urine sample 2. Bottle of reagent strips (Multistix SG8 and Multistix SG10 are the most commonly used reagent strips; Wilson 2005) 3. Jug for volume measurement 4. Bedpan or urinal 5. Watch with a second hand 6. Trolley, tray or adequate surface for equipment 7. Receptacle for soiled disposable items 8. Disposable gloves.
Guidelines and rationale for this nursing practice 	▪ explain the nursing practice to the patient and obtain consent and co-operation ***to inform the patient about the practice and ensure that he or she is aware of a person's rights as a patient*** ▪ awareness of different cultural attitudes towards handling and collecting body fluids and sensitivity to patients' individual needs is essential (Solomon 2004) ▪ wash the hands ***to reduce cross-infection and contamination by the nurse's and patient's hands*** (Swales 2003, Jeanes 2005) ▪ testing urine does not require an aseptic technique, however it is essential that all equipment should be clean or disposable, and all precautions should be taken to prevent cross-infection ▪ nurses should wash their hands before commencing and on completing this nursing practice (Swales 2003, Jeanes 2005)

- instruct or assist the patient to collect urine in the clean, dry container the next time that he or she empties the bladder *as this will ensure that the urine specimen is fresh and uncontaminated before testing*
- micturition is an activity associated with privacy *so collecting a specimen of urine is an unfamiliar and embarrassing experience for the patient* (Solomon 2002)
- provide privacy and give an adequate explanation of the practice, *this will be conducive to an uncomplicated collection of the specimen* (Bardsley 2003)
- collect and prepare the equipment *to ensure that the equipment is available and ready for use*
- apply gloves *to protect the nurse's hands from contamination by body fluids*
- measure the volume of urine if the patient has a fluid balance chart *as this will ensure accurate fluid balance monitoring*
- observe and note any sediment present in the urine *as this may indicate an abnormality of the patient's renal tract*
- observe and note the colour of the urine *as an unusual colour of the urine may indicate an abnormality*
- note any smell *as this may suggest an infection*: infected urine has a foul, fishy odour
- check the expiry date on the container of reagent strips *to prevent inaccurate results from using out-of-date reagents*
- reagent strips must be stored in their original container and kept dry using the desiccant provided *to prevent contamination* (Bayer Diagnostics Europe 2004)
- remove a reagent strip, being careful not to touch the test squares on the strip *as contamination of the reagent strip may give a false reading*
- replace the lid of the container quickly and securely following the removal of a reagent strip *as the strips are particularly sensitive to changes in temperature and humidity, which will affect the accuracy of the result recorded* (Nicol et al 2004)
- immerse the reagent strip fully in the urine. Note the time *to permit an assessment of the results after the correct interval*
- withdraw the strip, removing any excess urine by gently tapping the strip on the rim of the container (Bayer Diagnostics Europe 2004); *this will reduce the risk of contamination to the tester*
- hold the strip at an angle *to prevent cross-contamination from one reagent pad to another* (Mallett & Dougherty 2000)
- hold the strip vertically or horizontally against the results guidance chart *to ensure an accurate interpretation of the colour change* (Bayer Diagnostics Europe 2004) (Fig. 45.1)
- read the reagent strip after the recommended time has elapsed *to ensure an accurate result*
- note the result, *providing an accurate written record*
- it is important to follow the specific instructions written by the manufacturer and included with the reagent strips – refer to the label and packaging on the container (Wilson 2005) *to prevent error in interpretation*
- dispose of the equipment safely, *reducing any risk to staff and other equipment*

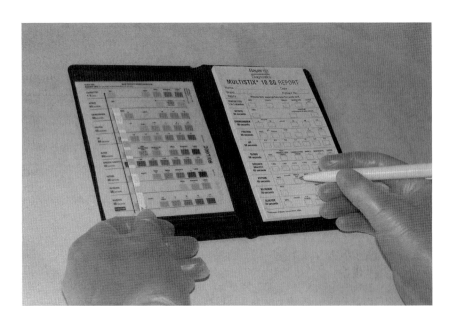

FIGURE 45.1
Result guidance chart
From Bayer Diagnostics
Europe 2004, with
permission

- document the nursing practice appropriately and report any abnormal findings immediately ***to provide a written record and assist in the implementation of any action should an abnormal result be noted***
- in undertaking this practice, nurses are accountable for their actions, the quality of care delivered and record-keeping according to the Code of Professional Conduct: Standards for Conduct, Performance and Ethics (Nursing and Midwifery Council 2004) and Guidelines for Records and Record Keeping (Nursing and Midwifery Council 2005).

Additional information

Fresh urine from a healthy individual should not have an offensive odour, but decomposing urine will smell like ammonia.

When urine is found to have a 'sweet' smell it may be necessary to investigate further for diabetes mellitus.

The normal colour of urine ranges from pale straw to dark amber and will vary according to the amount of fluid that has been taken into the body.

The type and amount of urinary constituents also affect the colour of urine; a dark-coloured urine can, for example, be an indication of dehydration or the presence of bile pigments, a manifestation of liver or biliary tract disease.

Certain foods and drugs alter the colour of a patient's urine: beetroot can cause the urine to take on an orangey-red hue.

'Haematuria' is the term used to describe blood in the urine. This can vary from microscopic haematuria, i.e. that detected only by testing, to frank haematuria, with an obvious red colouration. Blood in the urine is suggestive of disease or damage to the renal system (Selfe 2006).

Glycosuria refers to the presence of glucose in the urine. This is suggestive of diabetes mellitus.

'Proteinuria' is the term used when there is protein in the urine, which can be a manifestation of acute or chronic renal disease.

When the body metabolises fat, ketones are one of the products of this metabolism. Ketones are acidotic so if the excessive metabolism of fat persists, a state of metabolic acidosis develops, which can, if untreated, lead to coma and death. At a certain stage of acidosis, the ketones are excreted by the urinary system; when they are identified in the urine, they may be indicative of excessive fasting or uncontrolled or poorly controlled diabetes mellitus.

The specific gravity is a measure of the concentration of the substances dissolved in the urine, the normal range being 1.005–1.025. A single measurement of the specific gravity of the urine provides little information as the specific gravity varies with the state of hydration of the body. Urine that continually has a low specific gravity indicates renal damage or diabetes insipidus.

The pH of a urine sample reflects the function of the kidney in maintaining the acid–base balance within the body.

Patient/carer education

Key points

In partnership with the patient and/or carer, ensure that they are competent to carry out any practices required. Information should be given on an appropriate point of contact for any concerns that may arise.

Should the patient be collecting the urine specimen unassisted, ensure that he or she is aware of the importance of placing the urine in a clean, dry, leakproof container for transport to the doctor's practice or hospital.

Inform the patient of the results and any action required should an abnormality be detected.

A patient or carer may need to be taught this nursing practice, therefore the nurse should devise a suitable educational programme.

References

Bardsley A 2003 UTI: prevention and treatment of a common problem. Nurse Prescribing 1(3): 113–117

Bayer Diagnostics Europe 2004 Your practical guide to urine analysis. Bayer Healthcare, Newbury, Berkshire, UK

Jeanes A 2005 Infection control. A practical guide to the use of hand decontaminants. Nursing Times 101(20): 46–48

Mallett J, Dougherty L 2000 The Royal Marsden manual of clinical nursing procedures, 5th edn. Blackwell Science, Oxford

Nicol M, Bavin C, Bedford-Turner S et al 2004 Essential nursing skills, 2nd edn. Mosby, London

Nursing and Midwifery Council 2004 Code of conduct: standards for conduct, performance and ethics. NMC, London

Nursing and Midwifery Council 2005 Guidelines for records and record keeping. NMC, London

Selfe L 2006 The urinary system. In: Alexander M, Fawcett J, Runciman P (eds) Nursing practice – hospital and home: the adult, 3rd edn. Churchill Livingstone, Edinburgh

Solomon J 2004 Eliminating. In: Holland K, Jenkins J, Solomon J et al (eds) Applying the Roper–Logan–Tierney model in practice. Churchill Livingstone, Edinburgh

Swales J 2003 Why handwashing is fundamental to good practice. Nursing and Residential Care 5(9): 424–427

Wilson L 2005 Urinalysis. Nursing Standard 19(35): 51–54

Self assessment

1. List the reasons for testing urine.
2. Explain the importance of correct storage of reagent strips.
3. Outline infection control measures required during this practice.

Practice 46
Vaginal Examination

Learning outcomes	**By the end of this section, you should know how to:**
	■ prepare the patient for this procedure
	■ collect and prepare the equipment
	■ describe the various positions that enable this examination to be carried out most easily
	■ assist the examiner as necessary.

Background knowledge required	Revision of the anatomy and physiology of the female reproductive system
	Revision of 'Infection prevention and control' procedures (*see* p. 151)
	Revision of local policy on vaginal examination.

Indications and rationale for a vaginal examination	The vagina can be examined visually or digitally for the following reasons:
	■ *to assess the position, size, texture or appearance of the cervix and vagina*
	■ *to obtain a swab from the cervix or vagina*
	■ *to obtain a cervical smear for cytological examination* (*see* 'Specimen collection', p. 303)
	■ *to administer treatment to the cervix or vagina*
	■ *to determine the site of a haemorrhage*
	■ *to insert an intrauterine contraceptive device*.

Outline of the procedure	Prior to undertaking this procedure, the examiner will normally take a gynaecological history (Young 2002). The examiner puts on a pair of disposable gloves and applies some water-soluble lubricant to the dominant hand. Two or three fingers of the dominant hand are then inserted into the vagina, and the uterus is palpated through the abdominal wall with the non-dominant hand. This is known as a digital or bimanual examination.
	For a visual examination of the vagina and cervix, the examiner will insert a lubricated speculum – usually a Sims' or Cusco's speculum (Fig. 46.1) – into the vagina. The speculum should be warmed in water to body temperature and the sides lubricated with water-soluble lubricant (Rawlinson 2002). The speculum is gently opened to separate the vaginal walls and enable an inspection of the vagina and cervix; a good light is required for this. A pair of vulsellum forceps may be used to hold the cervix while it is examined. A pair of swab-holding forceps and some swabs may be necessary to wipe away any blood or vaginal discharge that might be obstructing the inspection of the mucosa. After the examination, the speculum is closed and removed gently from the vagina.

Clinical Nursing Practices

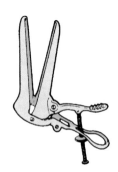

FIGURE 46.1
**Cusco's vaginal
speculum**
From Chilman & Thomas
1987, with permission

Equipment

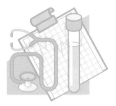

1. Tray or trolley.

For digital examination:

— disposable gloves
— water-soluble lubricant
— wipes or tissues
— receptacle for soiled disposable items.

For visual examination, in addition to the above:

— sterile vaginal speculum
— sterile vulsellum forceps
— sterile swab-holding forceps
— swabs
— light source.

Additional equipment may be required depending on the purpose of the examination.

The position of the patient

There are several suitable positions for this procedure, the position of choice usually being the one most convenient for the medical practitioner and patient.

The recumbent position

The patient lies on her back with her knees drawn up and separated and the sides of her feet resting on the bed (Fig. 46.2).

The lithotomy position

The patient lies on her back on a specially designed gynaecology couch with her legs elevated and supported on leg rests. To avoid injury to the patient, both legs must be lifted gently into position at the same time.

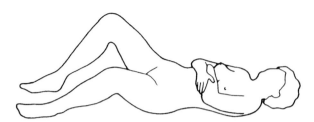

FIGURE 46.2
Recumbent position used for vaginal examination

Guidelines and rationale for this nursing practice

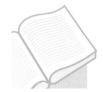

- help to explain the procedure to the patient **to gain her consent and co-operation**. Ensure that the woman is aware of her pelvic anatomy and physiology
- prior to the procedure give the patient the opportunity to empty her bladder **as discomfort may be experienced with a full bladder** (Young 2002)
- ensure as much privacy as possible for the patient and provide a blanket to cover the patient's lower body during examination **as the majority of patients are very embarrassed about having this examination**
- collect and prepare the equipment **for efficiency of practice**
- assist the patient into the agreed position with a pillow to support her head **for ease of examination**
- fold back the blanket **to enable the examiner to carried out the procedure**
- observe the patient throughout this activity **to detect any signs of discomfort or distress**
- assist the examiner and the patient as necessary
- ensure that the patient is left feeling as comfortable as possible afterwards, with protection for her underwear if there is any risk of discharge from her vagina
- ensure that the patient is aware of the location of toilet or washroom facilities **so that she can freshen up and remove traces of water-soluble gel**
- dispose of the equipment safely **for the protection of others**
- dispatch any specimens to the laboratory with the completed form and in a plastic specimen bag
- document this procedure, monitor the after-effects and report any abnormal findings immediately **to provide a written record and assist in the implementation of any action should an abnormal result be noted**
- in undertaking this practice, nurses are accountable for their actions, the quality of care delivered and record-keeping according to the Code of Professional Conduct: Standards for Conduct, Performance and Ethics (Nursing and Midwifery Council 2004) and Guidelines for Records and Record Keeping (Nursing and Midwifery Council 2005).

Additional information

Examiners are advised to use a disposable vaginal speculum to prevent cross-infection

Elderly patients may have problems adopting a position appropriate to the examination; help may be required and support necessary to promote comfort, ease of examination and safety. Care must be taken when handling joint areas such as hips and knees so that injury is not inflicted.

If the patient can co-operate by relaxing as much as possible, it is easier for the examiner to carry out the examination and also reduces the patient's discomfort. A clear explanation of why the examination is needed is necessary.

Slow, regular, concentrated deep breathing will help the patient to relax the abdominal and perineal muscles.

The patient should be given the opportunity to empty her bladder before the examination. This makes it easier for the examiner to palpate the uterus and is also more comfortable for the patient, who is usually feeling apprehensive.

If treatment that may result in vaginal discharge is to be given during the examination, the patient should have prior information so that appropriate underwear can be worn. The provision of washroom facilities after the procedure or examination has been completed is important to help patients maintain their self-esteem. Assistance with dressing and undressing should be offered.

Many patients find this examination stressful and embarrassing so the best privacy possible should be provided and the patient covered up as much as is feasible. The surroundings need to be as calm and relaxed as possible.

Women who have had no heterosexual experiences and women who have suffered from abuse should be offered extra time, support, information and counselling before and after this examination. Nurses should also demonstrate an awareness of the significance and implications of vaginal examination for women from a variety of cultural and lifestyle backgrounds and following pelvic surgery (Marquiegui & Huish 1999) and plan for this when caring for these patients.

Patient/carer education
Key points

In partnership with the patient and/or carer, ensure that they are competent to carry out any practices required. Information should be given on an appropriate point of contact for any concerns that may arise.

Encourage an open discussion with the patient about her vaginal anatomy and the details of the practice. Appropriate written information given to patients prior to attendance at the examination may help to reduce their anxiety and embarrassment.

References

Chilman A, Thomas M (eds) 1987 Understanding nursing care, 3rd edn. Churchill Livingstone, Edinburgh

Marquiegui A, Huish M 1999 A woman's sexual life after an operation. British Medical Journal 318: 178–181

Nursing and Midwifery Council 2004 Code of professional conduct: standards for conduct, performance and ethics. NMC, London

Nursing and Midwifery Council 2005 Guidelines for records and record keeping. NMC, London

Rawlinson M 2002 The gynaecological system. In: Cross S, Rimmer M (eds) Nurse practitioner manual of clinical skills. Ballière Tindall, Edinburgh

Young F 2002 Vaginal health. Nursing Standard 16(23): 47–55

Self assessment

1. Which body positions are suitable for conducting a vaginal examination?
2. What are the indications for undertaking a vaginal examination?
3. How can the nurse help the patient to relax during the procedure?

Practice 47
Vaginal Ring Pessary Insertion

Learning outcomes	**By the end of this section, you should know how to:** ▪ prepare the patient for this practice ▪ collect and prepare the equipment ▪ assist the qualified practitioner in the insertion of a ring.
Background knowledge required	Revision of the anatomy and physiology of vagina, cervix and uterus Revision of 'Infection prevention and control' procedures (*see* p. 151) Revision of local policy on vaginal ring pessary insertion.
Indications and rationale for the insertion of vaginal ring pessaries	Ring pessaries are made of a PVC type of material that is flexible and compressible by hand but springs back into shape when in situ (Fig. 47.1). The pessaries are supplied individually wrapped and sterile. There is a range of sizes; the patient should be measured and the most appropriate size fitted (Colpman & Welford 2004). Ring pessaries are used to relieve the symptoms caused by 1st, 2nd and 3rd degree uterine prolapse (James & Jenner 2002) when the patient: ▪ is unfit for a surgical repair of her prolapse ▪ does not wish to undergo surgery ▪ requires a temporary treatment to alleviate problems while awaiting surgery.
Equipment 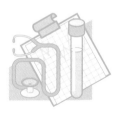	1. Selected pessary 2. Disposable gloves 3. Water-soluble lubricant 4. Protective pad 5. Receptacle for soiled disposable items 6. Warm water.
Guidelines and rationale for this nursing practice 	▪ explain the nursing practice to the patient ***to gain her consent and co-operation*** ▪ collect, check and prepare the equipment ***for efficiency of practice*** ▪ ensure maximum privacy for the patient and assist her into the position selected after she has agreed consent with the person inserting the pessary (*see* 'Vaginal examination', p. 363, for a list of appropriate positions) ▪ observe the patient throughout this activity ***to detect any signs of discomfort or distress*** ▪ put on the disposable gloves ***for protection***

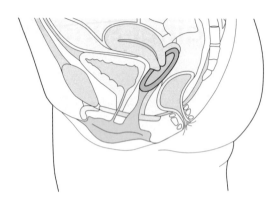

FIGURE 47.1
Vaginal ring pessary in position

- soften the pessary in warm water **to ease fitting** (James & Jenner 2002)
- lubricate the pessary and, using the thumb and forefinger of the dominant hand, squeeze the pessary into a figure of eight shape (James & Jenner 2002) **for ease of insertion**
- with the non-dominant hand, part the labia **to expose the entrance to the vagina**
- slide the pessary into the posterior part of the vagina and gently push it downwards and backwards until it settles in the posterior fornix
- once it is in this position, it will spring into its normal shape. The person inserting the pessary then needs to hook the front portion of the pessary into the anterior fornix behind the symphysis pubis **to enable protrusion of cervix through the pessary ring**
- following insertion the patient should stand and bear down and any discomfort or displacement should be noted to **check correct positioning and sizing** (James & Jenner 2002)
- dispose of the equipment safely **for the safety of others**
- document this nursing practice appropriately including details of ring pessary, monitor the after-effects and report any abnormal findings immediately **to provide a written record and assist in the implementation of any action should an abnormal result be noted**
- in undertaking this practice, nurses are accountable for their actions, the quality of care delivered and record-keeping according to the Code of Professional Conduct: Standards for Conduct, Performance and Ethics (Nursing and Midwifery Council 2004) and Guidelines for Records and Record Keeping (Nursing and Midwifery Council 2005).

The patient should attend for a clinical check 1 week following initial fitting and thereafter every 3 to 6 months (James & Jenner 2002, McIntosh 2005).

Additional information

Although this practice does not require an aseptic technique, the equipment used should be sterile and nurses should wash their hands before commencing and on completing the nursing practice (Jeanes 2005). Gloves should be worn for protection.

The importance of good personal hygiene practices to avoid the risk of infection should be explained to the patient: the pessary is a foreign body in the vagina and therefore a possible focus for infection.

If a clear explanation is given, and the woman understands the reasons for the insertion of the pessary and has sufficient knowledge of her anatomy to know exactly where it will be positioned, the insertion should be made easier.

The patient should be given the opportunity to empty her bladder prior to the insertion of the vaginal ring pessary. Micturition and bowel movements should not be hindered by the presence of the pessary; it may in fact improve any micturition and bowel problems that the patient has been experiencing.

It should be suggested to the patient that she move around as much as possible after the pessary has been inserted to ensure that it is correctly fitted. The patient should be unaware of its presence.

Personal hygiene is important to prevent infection. In older women, the lining of the vagina may be dry so an oestrogen cream may be prescribed to help avoid any irritation of the mucosal lining.

A slight watery discharge from the vagina is common, but patients should be advised to seek help if the discharge becomes purulent or bloodstained, or develops an offensive smell.

Patient/carer education
Key points

In partnership with the patient and/or carer, ensure that they are competent to carry out any practices required. Information should be given on an appropriate point of contact for any concerns that may arise.

An explanation of the reasons for the insertion of the pessary will help to gain the patient's co-operation. Assurance about the normal functions of micturition, bowel movement and sexual activity should be given.

It is essential to teach the patient the importance of good personal hygiene habits to reduce the risk of infection. Advice, and a contact name and telephone number, should be given in case the patient experiences problems related to the pessary.

Patients should be advised to seek medical advice if the pessary falls out, vaginal bleeding or unusual discharge occurs, pelvic or abdominal pain is experienced, or there is urinary retention or altered bowel habits (McIntosh 2005). Ensure that full details of any follow-up care are given to the patient, and encourage attendance at check-up appointments for an assessment of vaginal health.

References

Colpman D, Welford K 2004 Conservative management of urological problems. In: Fillingham S, Douglas J (eds) Urological nursing, 3rd edn. Baillière Tindall, Edinburgh

James R, Jenner C 2002 Uterovaginal prolapse and ring pessaries. Practice Nursing 13(5): 196–203

Jeanes A 2005 Infection control. A practical guide to the use of hand decontaminants. Nursing Times 101(20): 46–48

McIntosh L 2005 The role of the nurse in the use of vaginal pessaries to treat organ prolapse and/or urinary incontinence: a review of literature. Urology Nursing 25(1): 41–48

Nursing and Midwifery Council 2004 Code of professional conduct: standards for conduct, performance and ethics. NMC, London

Nursing and Midwifery Council 2005 Guidelines for records and record keeping. NMC, London

Self assessment

1. What are the indications for insertion of a ring pessary?
2. How would the nurse ensure the pessary was correctly positioned?
3. Following insertion what adverse symptoms should the women report to medical staff?

Practice 48
Venepuncture

Learning outcomes

By the end of this section, you should know how to:

- prepare the patient for this procedure
- collect and prepare the equipment
- obtain a sample of blood from the patient
- educate the patient on self-care following this procedure.

Background knowledge required

Anatomy and physiology of the venous blood system and upper limb

Principles of 'Infection prevention and control' (*see* p. 151) with respect to blood-borne infection

Different devices used in venepuncture

Available local guidelines for venepuncture

Understanding of routine blood investigations and their results.

Indications and rationale for venpuncture

Venepuncture is carried out in order:

- ***to obtain a specimen of blood for clinical analysis***. This may include measuring electrolyte, haemoglobin or antibody levels within the blood
- ***to cross-match blood for transfusion***.

Outline of the procedure

Venepuncture is performed by a medical practitioner or phlebotomist, or by a qualified nurse who has undertaken specialised education and is competent in this practice. The non-specialist nurse may be asked to assist with this procedure.

Blood can be withdrawn from the vein using a closed venepuncture system, a needle and syringe, or alternatively a butterfly infusion set, which may be more appropriate for some elderly patients. The closed system for venepuncture may utilise a vacuum effect to facilitate ease of blood withdrawal or may still require the practitioner to pull back a plunger to receive blood flow. The condition of the patient's veins will help determine the appropriate device for the collection of blood (Lavery & Ingram 2005). The practitioner may experience difficulty in gaining venous access in patients for whom venepuncture is a frequent occurrence, e.g. blood monitoring in relation to drug therapy (chemotherapy; warfarin; anti-rheumatics). Veins in the obese patient or the frail elderly may either be difficult to palpate or may collapse on introduction of the needle.

The value of the closed system is that several different samples may be taken as only the tube (rather than the syringe, as may be necessary in the traditional method) needs to be changed, thus protecting the nurse from blood spillage. There is also a reduced risk of needlestick injury because blood flows directly from the vein to the specimen bottle and does not have to be transferred to individual containers.

The general principles of venepuncture apply regardless of the system utilised, however the technique may vary slightly. For this reason the nurse should ensure a familiarity with the available systems, following both local policy and manufacturer's instructions.

Prior to discussing the equipment required it is pertinent to present the differing opinions in relation to infection control guidelines and skin cleansing prior to venepuncture. There is a lack of recent research to guide practitioners, however for skin cleansing to be effective the skin must be rubbed with an alcohol-impregnated swab for at least 30 seconds prior to insertion of a needle then left to dry for 30 seconds (Black & Hughes 1997). This rubbing and use of alcohol may cause localised skin irritation and some practitioners suggest that infection rates are unchanged if the skin is not cleansed, although again this remains anecdotal due to the dearth of evidence-based practice. The practitioner must therefore decide if this procedure is necessary within each situation where venepuncture occurs, while respecting local infection control policies.

Equipment

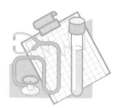

1. Clean tray/a flat surface
2. Disposable gloves/apron
3. Alcohol-impregnated cleansing swab (if required)
4. Sterile needle(s) or infusion device (20–21G)
5. Sterile syringe(s) or appropriate blood bottles for the system used and tests required
6. Disposable drape
7. Sterile adhesive plaster
8. Sterile gauze swabs
9. Tourniquet
10. Sharps box
11. Receptacle for soiled material
12. Completed laboratory form(s)
13. Plastic envelope for transferring the specimen.

Guidelines and rationale for this nursing practice

- discuss the procedure with the patient and ascertain whether he or she has an allergy to adhesive plaster, informing the patient about the procedure, discussing any concerns or queries and identifying any previous difficulties experienced with venepuncture, e.g. syncope (Lavery & Ingram 2005)
- obtain consent from the patient to undertake the procedure *to ensure that the patient is aware of a person's rights as a patient*
- select a suitable clean surface and lay out the equipment. If the procedure is being undertaken in the patient's own home, cover the surface with a waterproof cover *to provide a suitable, protected work surface*
- check that the laboratory forms have been completed and select the appropriate specimen containers *to ensure that the documentation is correct and that the samples are put into the correct specimen containers*
- cleanse the hands using soap and water *to reduce the risk of cross-infection* (Jeanes 2005)
- assemble the appropriate equipment *ensuring that equipment is ready for use*

- ensure the patient is seated (or supine if there is a history of syncope) with their arm supported and comfortable *to ensure patient comfort and prevent injury should the patient feel faint during the procedure*
- observe and palpate the veins on both arms. The vessels most commonly used are the cephalic, basilic and median cubital veins (in the forearm; Fig. 48.1), followed by the superficial veins on the dorsal aspect of the hand (Fig. 48.2). The nurse should be aware of the location of the brachial artery and median nerve (*see* Fig. 48.1) *as injury to either will cause pain and may lead to temporary or permanent damage*
- select a vein that is visible and firm to the touch. If there is lymphatic impairment or the patient has had an illness, disease or surgery affecting the limb, an alternative site should be selected. Take into account the patient's own past experience of venepuncture *to identify the vein most likely to provide the best venous access*
- place the tourniquet or sphygmomanometer cuff approximately 5–12 cm above the proposed puncture site *to promote vasodilatation*. This should not remain in situ for any longer than 2 minutes
- ask the patient to clench the fist *to promote vasodilatation*
- put on gloves *to protect both patient and nurse from potential blood-borne infection*

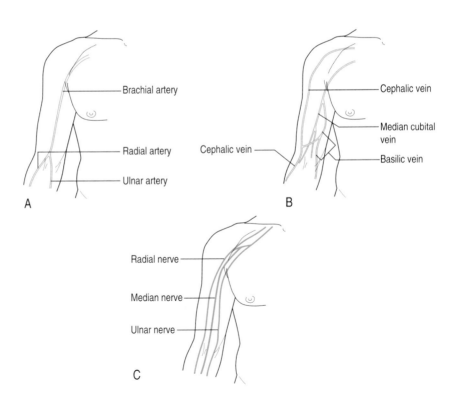

FIGURE 48.1
Anatomical features of the forearm
A Arteries
B Veins
C Nerves

A
Brachial artery
Radial artery
Ulnar artery

B
Cephalic vein
Cephalic vein
Median cubital vein
Basilic vein

C
Radial nerve
Median nerve
Ulnar nerve

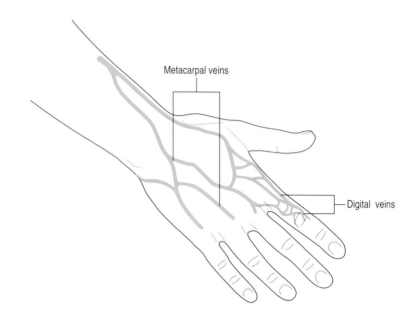

FIGURE 48.2
Superficial veins on the dorsal aspect of the hand

- select a firm visible vein and cleanse the skin if appropriate. If an alcohol-impregnated swab is used, rub area for 30 seconds then leave to dry for 30 seconds *to ensure effective removal of skin flora and prevent any stinging when inserting the needle*
- place the thumb or index finger below the proposed puncture site and pull the skin in a downward direction *to stabilise the vein*
- with its bevel facing upwards, gently and slowly insert the needle at an angle of 15° *to ensure the correct angle of entry into the vein*
- when the vessel wall has been punctured and blood appears in the barrel of the syringe, level off the needle and advance it slightly further into the vein (some systems do not allow a flash back to be seen, the needle being felt to enter the vein by a slight change in resistance) *to ensure that the opposite side of the vessel is not punctured*
- gently pull back the plunger of the syringe and collect the required amount of blood *to prevent collapse of the vein and to obtain a specimen of blood*. The vacuum system allows blood to flow directly from the vein into the specimen container
- if blood does not appear, the needle should be removed and, adhering to health authority policy, the nurse should either undertake the procedure using another vessel or seek assistance from another practitioner *to prevent undue distress to the patient and excessive trauma to the vein*
- while inserting the needle, care should be taken not to damage local nerves or other blood vessels. Bright red blood pulsating into the bottle would suggest that an artery has been pierced. If this occurs, remove the needle, apply pressure for 10 minutes and seek medical advice (Lavery & Ingram 2005).*The patient must be observed for reports of tingling in the arm, pain or any other unexpected responses*

- obtain the appropriate volume of blood, in the appropriate bottles if a closed system is used. ***Do not remove more than 20 ml of blood at a time*** (Lavery & Ingram 2005), ***do not overfill blood bottles, and fill bottles in the correct order*** (Ernst 2001)

- release the tourniquet ***to prevent further compression of the blood supply and excessive bleeding at the puncture site on removal of the needle***

- remove the needle (keeping it straight) and cover the puncture site with a gauze swab ***to prevent leakage of blood from the puncture site***

- apply pressure directly over the puncture site for 2–3 minutes (3–5 minutes if the patient has a clotting defect) after the needle has been removed. The patient may be able to undertake this activity. The patient should not bend the arm as this may enlarge the puncture wound, causing more bleeding. This pressure will ***reduce trauma to the vein and discomfort for the patient, and stop the bleeding from the vein, thus reducing the risk of formation of a haematoma***

- as soon as possible after collection, transfer the blood to the appropriate specimen container(s). This is not required for closed systems. If additives are present in the container, rotate it gently several times ***to prevent clotting of the blood***

- complete the label on the specimen container(s). Remember to apply 'high-risk specimen' labels if appropriate ***to ensure that correct investigations are carried out and that laboratory staff are aware of potential infection control issues***

- place the specimen container and laboratory form in the plastic bag (or follow health authority policy) ***to ensure that the laboratory receives the correct specimen for the correct patient***

- inspect the puncture site for bleeding and/or haematoma formation and apply adhesive plaster over the site ***to ensure that clotting has occurred and that the puncture site is protected from infection and trauma***. If the patient has an allergy to sticking plaster, apply a gauze swab and secure it firmly with hypoallergenic tape

- dispose of contaminated equipment according to health authority policy ***to prevent the transmission of infection***

- remove the gloves and dispose of as above. Wash the hands or cleanse them with bactericidal solution ***to prevent cross-infection***

- ascertain the wellbeing of the patient ***to ensure that the patient does not feel unwell as a result of the procedure***. This is especially important if the procedure is being carried out in the patient's own home

- discuss the points raised under 'Patient/carer education: key points' below. If the patient is unable to participate in this stage of the procedure, monitoring should be undertaken by the nurse or by an appropriate adult carer ***to ensure that the patient, carer or nurse is aware of, and understands, the follow-up self-care***

- in undertaking this practice, nurses are accountable for their actions, the quality of care delivered and record-keeping according to the Code of Professional Conduct: Standards for Conduct, Performance and Ethics (Nursing and Midwifery Council 2004) and Guidelines for Records and Record Keeping (Nursing and Midwifery Council 2005).

Patient/carer education

Key points

Information should be given on an appropriate point of contact for any concerns that may arise.

When preparing the patient for the procedure:
- advise the patient of any dietary restrictions that may be required for blood glucose or cholesterol investigations
- check with the medical practitioner whether there is any information that you require from the patient for more specialist investigations, for example drug doses and times or menstrual cycle dates.

With aftercare of the puncture site:
- report any bleeding oozing from under the adhesive plaster
- if itching or a rash occurs at the plaster site, remove the plaster and apply a gauze swab secured with hypoallergenic tape
- remove the adhesive plaster 24–48 hours after venepuncture.

There are potential complications following venepuncture:
- the patient should report excessive bruising radiating from the puncture site as this could relate to haematoma formation
- the patient should report any tingling, pain or swelling in the arm as this may indicate pressure on a nerve.

Inform the patient when the test results will be available and how to obtain them.

The patient may be anxious about the potential implications of the results of the laboratory investigations required. The nurse must therefore be sensitive to these issues and have an understanding both of the requested blood tests and the interpretation of these results. Health education may be appropriate for certain tests, e.g. random blood glucose or lipids. It may be beneficial for the nurse to have an awareness of local counselling services to enable them to offer support to patients receiving potentially life-changing results, e.g. HIV status, genetic profiles.

References

Black F, Hughes J 1997 Venepuncture. Nursing Standard 11(41): 49–55

Ernst DG 2001 The right way to do blood cultures. Registered Nurse 64(3): 28–31

Jeanes A 2005 Infection control. A practical guide to the use of hand decontaminants. Nursing Times 101(20): 46–48

Lavery I, Ingram P 2005 Venepuncture: best practice. Nursing Standard 19(49): 55–65

Nursing and Midwifery Council 2004 Code of professional conduct: standards for conduct, performance and ethics. NMC, London

Nursing and Midwifery Council 2005 Guidelines for records and record keeping. NMC, London

Websites

Infection Control Nurses Association: http://www.icna.co.uk

NHS Education for Scotland: http://www.nes.scot.nhs.uk

Nursing and Midwifery Council: http://www.nmc.co.uk

Self assessment

1. Describe the reasons for skin cleansing prior to venepuncture.
2. Describe the procedure for skin cleansing prior to venepuncture.
3. Describe potential complications of venepuncture.
4. List some tests that could provide opportunities for health education within venepuncture.

Practice 49
Wound Care

There are three parts to this section:

1 **Wound bed preparation**

2 **Wound drain care**

3 **Removal of stitches, clips and staples**

The concluding subsection 'Patient/carer education: key points' and the 'Self-assessment questions' refer to the chapter collectively.

Learning outcomes

By the end of this section, you should know how to:
- assess the patient for these three nursing practices
- collect and prepare appropriate equipment
- carry out these nursing practices.

The concept of wound care is vast, with an ever-evolving knowledge base offering direction for best practice. This chapter therefore presents the basic knowledge required for these practices and encourages you to reflect on your own learning needs to develop a relevant knowledge base. References and useful web addresses are provided at the end of this chapter as a starting point for this process.

Background knowledge required

Revision of the physiology of wound healing and the factors that affect wound healing

Revision of the principles of wound assessment

Review of existing local policy and national guidelines regarding all three components of this chapter

Review of common wound dressings available and their individual properties (note: in hospitals, available dressings may vary depending on the stock held by pharmacy. In the community setting a wider selection is usually accessible).

1. WOUND BED PREPARATION

Indications and rationale for wound bed preparation

Wound bed preparation is a process that assists in optimising conditions at the wound bed to encourage healing (Shultz et al 2005). This process requires the nurse to have a basic knowledge of the physiology of the stages of wound healing as this will help to understand the reasons why some wounds fail to heal effectively and/or quickly.

The main aims of wound bed preparation are:

- *to provide a method for continual assessment of the wound bed for tissue type*
- *to monitor and treat any signs/symptoms of critical colonisation/ clinical infection appropriately*
- *to address any moisture imbalance evident in the wound bed by either rehydrating sloughy/necrotic tissue or removing excess volumes of exudate*
- *to monitor the edges of the wound for signs/symptoms of effective healing.*

Assessment

The first step of wound bed preparation should involve a holistic assessment of the patient. Wound assessment tools are of value within this process as they provide prompting and direction for appropriate care (Hess & Kirsner 2003). The tool chosen should address both local and systemic factors that may impact on the ability of the patient to heal effectively (Hess & Kirsner 2003). Examples of local factors that may need to be addressed include pressure area assessments; continence assessments; and evidence of trauma. Examples of systemic factors include peripheral vascular disease; immunosuppression; and nutritional status. Once identified, action must be taken to rectify any unmet need that may delay effective wound healing, e.g.:

- use of specialist pressure reducing or continence equipment
- referral onto relevant members of the multi-disciplinary team.

Assessment tools also collect basic information such as the position and depth of the wound; the cause of the wound, e.g. trauma, surgical incision; how long the wound has been there; and any allergies the patient may have to previously tried dressings. The use of clinically assessed, research-based assessment tools not only offers direction for care but also a means of objective monitoring that can be used within clinical audit. Pressure ulcers can be graded by means of recognised classification scales, a process that will help in the accurate description of these wounds (DeFloor & Shoonhoven 2004).

A grid map can be used to assess the original size of a wound and consequent changes to size and tissue type on the wound bed. Care should be taken, however, that consensus is agreed within the clinical area in relation to the counting of the squares within the wound-bed area (Keast et al 2004). A camera may be used to record effectively both the size and tissue type of the wound bed, however this should be used in conjunction with local protocols to adhere to legal requirements including the Data Protection Act (Department of Health 1998). Again, knowledge of local guidelines and protocols should guide practice.

A Doppler ultrasound can also be used by skilled personnel in the assessment of leg ulcers to determine if they are vascular or arterial in nature. This is important as treatment will vary significantly depending on the result of this test. Vascular wounds will require referral to a vascular clinic for further assessment while venous leg ulcers are appropriate for compression bandaging. Compression bandaging must only be applied by staff who have received training in this practice as badly applied bandaging can cause damage to the lower limb.

Tissue type

There are five main types of tissue found in wounds, and a popular way to describe these types objectively is by colour (Hess & Kirsner 2003, Keast et al 2004, Shultz et al 2005):

- Black – necrotic
- Yellow – sloughy
- Green – infected
- Red – granulating
- Pink – epithelialising.

Infection

Wounds that are taking longer to heal than expected but do not appear clinically infected should be assessed for 'critical colonisation'. This means that bacteria in the wound are of a great enough number to compete for existing nutrients and oxygen against healthy cells, but are not of a great enough number to cause a clinically infected wound (Warriner & Burrell 2005). Signs of critical colonisation include delayed healing, wound breakdown and discoloration of the granulation tissue from red to dusky red/purple.

Clinically infected wounds will require further assessment by medical staff to assess if an antibiotic is required. Critically colonised wounds will benefit from the use of dressings that contain broad-spectrum antimicrobial properties such as silver or iodine. It is important to note that these dressings are expensive and require frequent reassessment to ensure their effectiveness. Once healthy tissue is observed in the wound bed these dressings can be stopped and other dressings can be applied.

Moisture

Included should be an assessment of the volume, colour and viscosity of any exudate present. Too little exudate and a scab (eschar) will form, contraindicating the moist, warm environment required for effective wound healing. High volumes of exudate will impact on surrounding tissue, causing maceration and prevent the wound from progressing further. Dressings for necrotic (black)/sloughy (yellow) tissue with low volumes of exudates should be chosen to rehydrate the eschar/slough, e.g. hydrogels or hydrocolloids. Wounds with high volumes of exudate require dressings that will absorb the exudates effectively, e.g. foams or hydrofibres.

Wound edges

As stated above, excess volumes of exudates will have a detrimental effect on surrounding tissue. Assessment should also involve gentle probing of the wound margins to rule out undermining of tissue. In a healing wound the margins of the wound advance across the wound bed thereby leading to an epithelialised (pink) wound. If this process fails then reassessment is required to identify the failure of the process.

Wound cleansing

Once a routine procedure, it is important that the nurse questions the need for wound cleansing prior to each individual dressing change. Research shows (Barber 2002) that wound cleansing is only necessary under certain circumstances:

- when specifically indicated by the dressing manufacturer, e.g. hydrogels, alginates
- in traumatic wounds to assist in visualising the wound bed.

If cleansing is indicated, again informed decision making should direct the choice of fluid used. Tap water can be used to irrigate wounds with no greater incidence of wound infection when compared to normal saline (Fernandez et al 2002). However, risk assessment guidelines should be followed to ensure the quality of the water used (Barber 2002, Fernandez et al 2002). No other fluid, e.g. chlorhexidine/betadine should be used to cleanse a wound unless within a specific aseptic technique or if requested by a clinical specialist with research to support the request.

Reference should be made to the use of an aseptic technique within this discussion. Once a routine procedure, a risk assessment will direct the nurse in the appropriate decision as to whether this practice is necessary. For certain procedures, e.g. care of a Hickman line, an aseptic technique is vital to protect the patient from infection. However, in general, wounds will not require an aseptic technique, e.g. leg ulcers, pressure sores (Barber 2002).

Choosing a wound dressing

Nurses are accountable for administering topical preparations, as they are for the administration of all other medicines, so they must be familiar with the properties and side effects of any wound-care products they are using. Up-to-date information on these preparations is available from the British National Formulary (2005). Dressings should provide a moist, warm environment for optimum wound healing to occur. They should also:
- be impermeable to bacteria
- be non-toxic and non-allergenic
- be comfortable and conformable for the patient to wear
- protect the wound from further trauma
- require infrequent dressing changes
- be cost-effective
- have a long shelf life
- be available in both hospital and community settings.

In addition to the above, it is also important for the dressing to have the necessary physiological and biochemical properties to facilitate wound healing at a cellular level. Tissue Viability Nurse specialists offer a wealth of knowledge in wound healing and treatment options and are available in both acute and community settings to provide support for 'difficult' wounds.

Larval therapy also provides an option for the debridement of necrotic/sloughy wounds (MacDougall & Rodgers 2004). Available on prescription, the larvae ingest dead tissue without affecting healthy tissue and can also be used when a wound is infected, indeed research shows that they may be effective in eradicating MRSA from infected wounds (Thomas & Jones 2000).

Due to budgetary constraints, ward-based nurses may have a limited number of dressings available via pharmacy. Within the community most district nurses have undertaken a nationally accredited course to enable them to prescribe from a wide range of wound-care products. A nurse prescriber must maintain an awareness of recent research, ensuring that decision making is grounded in a balance of both cost effectiveness and the proven effectiveness of the dressing.

Equipment required for a wound assessment and non-aseptic dressing change

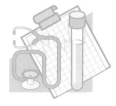

1. Wound assessment tool
2. Grid/camera
3. Dressing pack/swabs (only if required)
4. Flat surface
5. Gloves/apron
6. Disposal bag
7. Water/normal saline (only if required)
8. Alcohol-based hand rub
9. Clean scissors (to cut tape or the dressing to fit the wound)
10. Appropriate dressings/securing bandage (if required).

For many dressings a dressing pack will not be required. Simple dressings will require removal of the old dressing and application of a new dressing. Since all dressings are packaged within a sterile field, careful removal of these dressings negates the need for any further sterile field to lay them on. In an institutional environment, the number of air-borne pathogenic micro-organisms can be reduced by working in a well-ventilated room used solely for procedures involving aseptic technique, or by performing procedures at least 30 minutes after the completion of ward cleaning and bed making. This may not always be possible in the home setting, where the community nurse has little control over the environment.

There is no need for the nurse to wear a disposable cap or face mask, but verbal communication should be kept to a minimum during the aseptic technique in order to reduce droplet contamination. When a number of aseptic wound dressings are to be performed, a known contaminated and/or infected wound should be treated last to reduce environmental contamination.

Guidelines and rationale for a wound assessment and non-aseptic dressing change

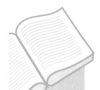

- explain the nursing practice to the patient **to gain consent and co-operation**
- collect and prepare the equipment required **to ensure that it is available and ready for use**
- ensure the patient's privacy **to reduce anxiety**
- help the patient into a comfortable position **to create a sense of wellbeing**
- place a drape/towel under the wound if possible **to protect the bed/chair/floor from potential leakage of exudates and/or to protect from irrigation fluid (if used)**
- wash hands and apply gloves/apron **to reduce cross-infection** (National Institute for Clinical Excellence 2003)
- remove any existing dressing **to allow a clear assessment of the wound**
- use an appropriate wound assessment tool to assess the patient and the wound bed **thereby ensuring a holistic assessment of the patient**
- assess and record the shape of the wound using a measured grid tracing or grid camera **to permit changes to the wound shape to be noted**. If a camera is used the appropriate paperwork must be completed to ensure both consent and legal ownership of the photos; knowledge of local guidelines and protocols should be used to guide best practice
- assess wound bed tissue; any evidence of infection; volume of exudates and wound edges exudate **as this will assist with the decision-making process to determine the choice of dressing**

- assess and document the wound bed tissue type *to provide information regarding the stage of healing*
- carry out a pain assessment *to determine the analgesic requirement and the timing of any medication required*
- discuss with the patient previous treatments and their effect, allergies and dressing preferences *to increase concordance with the treatment regime*
- decide on the most appropriate dressing for the presenting wound (if this has changed from the existing dressing, remove and dispose of gloves; collect new dressing; wash hands again and apply new gloves) *to ensure effective treatment for the patient*
- irrigate wound with either warm saline or tap water only if indicated *to ensure that research-based practice is followed*
- apply appropriate dressing
- following the initial assessment, evaluate the wound at regular intervals *to monitor the overall progress of the wound*
- ensure that the patient is left feeling as comfortable as possible, *maintaining the quality of this nursing practice*
- dispose of the equipment safely *to reduce any health hazard*
- document the nursing practice appropriately, monitor the after-effects and report any abnormal findings. *This provides a written record and assists in the implementation of any action should an abnormality or adverse reaction to the practice be noted*
- in undertaking this practice, nurses are accountable for their actions, the quality of care delivered and record-keeping according to the Code of Professional Conduct: Standards for Conduct, Performance and Ethics (Nursing and Midwifery Council 2004) and Guidelines for Records and Record Keeping (Nursing and Midwifery Council 2005).

Thorough handwashing *prior* to the dressing must be performed, further hand preparation being performed *during* the aseptic technique as stated in the guidelines above and whenever the nurse accidentally contaminates his or her hands. An alcohol-based hand rub is used for the subsequent hand preparation; it has the benefit that the nurse does not have to leave the patient during the practice (Jeanes 2005).

It is preferable for the skin-cleansing lotion to be supplied as an individual single-use sterile sachet or bottle. Once a bottle has been opened, environmental contamination can occur, so any residual lotion should be discarded. If an aerosol can of irrigating fluid is used, the nurse should ensure that the dispensing nozzle does not become contaminated and therefore act as a source of infection.

Equipment for an aseptic dressing change

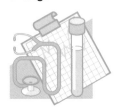

1. Dressings trolley, or an appropriate clean surface if in the patient's home
2. Sterile dressing pack containing a gallipot or similar container, low-linting swabs, disposable forceps, a drape and a disposal bag
3. Normal saline (if wound irrigation is indicated)
4. Sterile 10 ml syringe for irrigating the wound. This may not be required as some solutions are packaged to allow irrigation
5. Additional sterile dressing material, usually packed separately
6. Sterile disposable gloves
7. Hypoallergenic tape

8. Clean pair of scissors for cutting the tape
9. Clean disposable plastic apron
10. Alcohol-based hand preparation lotion
11. Appropriate dressings/securing bandage if required
12. Receptacle for soiled disposable items.

Guidelines and rationale for aseptic dressing change

The guidelines for this procedure are similar whether within a hospital setting or within a patient's home. The obvious difference is that within the hospital a dressing trolley will be available; within a patient's home there will be vastly differing levels of cleanliness. An experienced community nurse will adhere as closely to an aseptic technique as the environment allows.

- explain the nursing practice to the patient **to gain consent and co-operation**
- use a treatment room for wound dressing **as this reduces the incidence of cross-infection**. If one is not available, prepare the environment around the patient's bed appropriately. If in the community, identify an adequate surface
- wash the hands **to reduce the risk of cross-infection**
- if using a dressing trolley, wash thoroughly with detergent and water, and then dry it **to provide a socially clean surface**
- disinfect the dressings trolley with 70% ethyl alcohol immediately prior to every dressing undertaken **to reduce the number of micro-organisms on the trolley surface**
- collect and prepare the equipment, check the packaging for damage such as tears or leakage, and check the expiry dates of all the materials to be used, **ensuring that the equipment has not been contaminated**
- in the hospital – place all the equipment on the bottom shelf of the trolley, preferably in order of use, **to leave the top shelf free and clean during the practice and to permit easy access to the equipment**
- ensure the patient's privacy **to reduce anxiety**
- observe the patient throughout this activity, **noting any signs of distress**
- in the hospital – adjust the position of the bed **to ensure safe working practice and the most comfortable position to carry out this procedure** (Nicol et al 2003)
- help the patient into a comfortable position **to allow the position to be maintained during the practice**
- adjust the patient's clothing to expose the wound area **in order to give the nurse easy access to the wound**
- wash the hands **to reduce the risk of cross-infection**
- apply the plastic disposable apron **to prevent micro-organisms adhering to the nurse's uniform**, which could be a source of cross-infection
- open the outer packaging of the dressing pack and slip the contents on to the top shelf of the dressings trolley or flat surface, **allowing the inner cover of the dressing pack to come into contact with a clean surface**
- loosen the outer dressing covering the patient's wound **to ease removal after the nurse has commenced the dressing**
- wash the hands using bactericidal soap or an alcohol-based hand lotion **to reduce the risk of cross-infection** (Storr & Clayton-Kent 2004)
- open the dressing pack, touching the sterile covering as little as possible **in order to reduce contamination from the dresser's hands**

- open any additional equipment and drop it on to the sterile field. If using a sachet of saline, pour the contents into the gallipot, ***thereby preparing the equipment for use***
- wash the hands with alcohol-based lotion
- place one hand inside the disposal bag and arrange the contents of the dressing pack, ***thus reducing the risk of contamination***
- with the hand still in the bag, remove the soiled dressing from the wound, ***removing contaminated material from the wound site***
- turn the bag inside out with soiled dressing inside and, if using a dressing trolley, attach it to the side of the trolley, below the level of the top shelf ***to reduce the risk of contamination***
- apply gloves ***to prevent contact with body fluids***
- drape the wound with the sterile drape
- note the condition of the wound and the surrounding skin ***to assess and evaluate the healing rate and identify potential problems***
- if required, irrigate the wound, ensuring that the tip of the syringe or container does not come into contact with the skin surface, ***to remove debris without localised trauma***
- use the gauze swab to dry the surrounding skin, ***aiding dressing adherence and preventing maceration of the skin***
- apply the appropriate dressing ***to create the optimum wound-healing environment***
- discard the gloves or forceps, ***thus removing contaminated material***
- ***to maintain the position of the dressing***, secure it by the chosen method
- ensure that the patient is left feeling as comfortable as possible, ***thus maintaining the quality of this nursing practice***
- dispose of all equipment safely ***to reduce any health hazard***
- document this nursing practice appropriately, monitor the after-effects and report any abnormal findings immediately, ***providing a written record and assisting in the implementation of any action should an abnormality or adverse reaction to the practice be noted***
- in undertaking this practice, nurses are accountable for their actions, the quality of care delivered and record-keeping according to the Code of Professional Conduct: Standards for Conduct, Performance and Ethics (Nursing and Midwifery Council 2004) and Guidelines for Records and Record Keeping (Nursing and Midwifery Council 2005).

2. WOUND DRAIN CARE

Indications and rationale for wound drain care

Wound drains are inserted at the time of surgical intervention by the medical practitioner ***to prevent fluid collecting at the operation or wound site***, which may retard tissue healing. The extent and site of the surgery will influence the types and number of drains used. Drains may be inserted away from the original incision, to be dressed and to heal independently. ***This will help to prevent the transmission of infection between the incision/operation site and the exit site for the wound drain***. Research studies discuss the need for wound drains following certain types of surgery, e.g. total hip arthroplasty, total knee replacement, abdominal surgery. The suggestion is that drains may not decrease the risk of postoperative wound infection or the development of haematomas, indeed the presence of a wound drain may instead increase the risk of infection (Minnena et al 2004, Aldameh et al 2005, Walmsey et al 2005). Despite this emerging research, it remains important that you have an understanding of the types of wound drains that you may come into contact with and the appropriate nursing practice to manage them.

Types of wound drain

Hollow plastic tube

This is a deep drain with drainage holes at the proximal (drainage site) end, which is usually stitched in position and attached to a closed-circuit drainage bag. Such a drain may be used following major abdominal surgery to drain fluid collections.

Corrugated rubber drain

This is a superficial drain that usually drains directly into the dressing. It may be used to drain an incision site.

T-tube

A T-tube is a specialised tube inserted into the common bile duct following a cholecystectomy. It allows bile to drain into a closed-circuit bag for 6–10 days postoperatively until normal drainage is re-established.

Portable vacuum suction drain

This is a perforated plastic catheter attached to a specialised sterile vacuum suction bag (Fig. 49.1). Two or more may be attached to the same vacuum bag with a Y-connection. This system is used **to prevent the formation of a haematoma, by maintaining gentle suction**. It may be used following joint replacement surgery or surgery to the face or neck area, where fluid may collect rapidly because of the efficient local blood supply.

Soft fluted silicone drain

These may be less painful that rigid drains, especially if a large-calibre drain is required (Rayatt et al 2005).

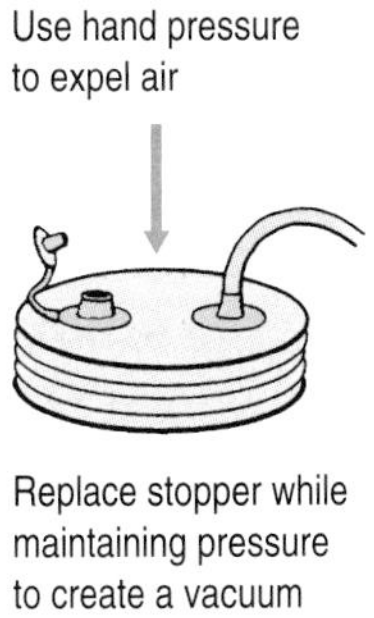

Use hand pressure to expel air

Replace stopper while maintaining pressure to create a vacuum

FIGURE 49.1
Wound care: a portable vacuum drain

Practice 49
Clinical Nursing Practices

Equipment	As for 'Aseptic technique' above.

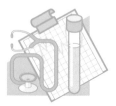

Additional equipment as required	1. Sterile gloves
	2. Sterile scissors
	3. Sterile stitch-cutters
	4. Sterile drainage bag
	5. Portable wound suction equipment
	6. Sterile specialised keyhole dressing
	7. Extra sterile dressings material
	8. Sterile safety pin
	9. Sterile wound pads
	10. Measuring jug
	11. Sterile specimen container.

Sterile gloves should be used when dressing wound drains to help to maintain asepsis.

Guidelines and rationale for this nursing practice 	▪ explain the nursing practice to the patient *to gain consent and co-operation, and encourage participation in care*
	▪ ensure the patient's privacy *to respect his or her individuality*
	▪ help the patient into a comfortable position depending on the area of the wound drain *so that the area for dressing is easily accessible and the patient is able to maintain the position with minimum distress*. In some instances, carefully timed prescribed analgesia may be given *to ensure its maximum effect during the wound care*
	▪ observe the patient throughout this activity *to monitor any adverse effects*. This continual evaluation ensures that nursing or medical intervention can be altered as necessary
	▪ collect and prepare the equipment *to ensure an efficient use of time and resources*
	▪ remove clothes and covers from the area of the wound, ensuring that, with the exception of that area, the patient remains covered, *to expose only the site for wound care and respect the patient's dignity*
	▪ perform the dressing for the surgical incision line first if necessary, maintaining asepsis. Dressings will usually be removed from the incision line after 24 hours and the wound may be covered by a plastic spray dressing *to encourage healing by first intention*. After this, only the drainage tube sites need to be dressed *to promote healing and prevent infection*
	▪ prepare the sterile field for dressing the drainage tube site *as an essential component of the aseptic technique*

- don sterile gloves after efficient handwashing *to prevent any contamination with body fluids*
- proceed as for 'Aseptic technique' above until the drainage tube has been exposed
- cleanse the skin round the wound drain with normal saline if required then dry surrounding skin *to allow any subsequent dressings to adhere properly* (Fig. 49.2)
- prepare a 'keyhole' dressing. *This allows the dressing to fit snugly round the drain*
- shorten the drain as ordered by the medical practitioner. This will depend on the healing process of the individual wound
- apply the keyhole or other dressing as required *to maintain asepsis and promote healing* (Fig. 49.3)
- secure the dressing *to prevent its slipping*
- change the drainage bag and secure it in such a position that *gravity will help the fluid to drain away from the wound efficiently*

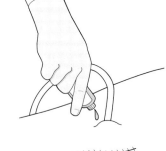

FIGURE 49.2
Cleansing the skin round the wound drain

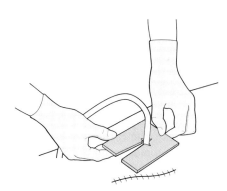

FIGURE 49.3
Applying a keyhole dressing

- measure the drainage fluid and note its colour, consistency and smell *so that the process of healing can be monitored and any adverse condition reported*
- ensure that the patient is left as comfortable as possible *to create an environment that will promote healing*
- dispose of the equipment safely *to maintain a safe environment*
- document this nursing practice appropriately, monitor the after-effects and report any abnormal findings immediately *so that any nursing or medical intervention can be evaluated and altered as required*
- in undertaking this practice, nurses are accountable for their actions, the quality of care delivered and record-keeping according to the Code of Professional Conduct: Standards for Conduct, Performance and Ethics (Nursing and Midwifery Council 2004) and Guidelines for Records and Record Keeping (Nursing and Midwifery Council 2005).

Shortening wound drains

Deep wound drains may be shortened, as ordered by the medical practitioner, once or twice during the postoperative period as healing proceeds.

- expose the drain site, maintaining asepsis and cleansing the skin as above. Sterile gloves should be worn after effective handwashing *to prevent contamination with body fluids*
- remove any stitches holding the drain in position (*see* 'Removal of stitches, clips and staples', p. 394) *to release the drain*
- support the skin round the drain site with one hand using a sterile swab and gently withdraw the drain as far as ordered by the medical practitioner, e.g. 3–5 cm. Supporting the surrounding area *reduces discomfort and prevents damage to healthy tissue*
- insert a sterile safety pin through the drain near the entry site. *This prevents the drain falling back into the wound*
- cut off the extra length of drain if necessary *so that it lies neatly at the drain site and causes no discomfort*. Drains attached to drainage bags will not need to be cut
- apply one sterile keyhole dressing under the safety pin and another over it. *This helps to maintain the drain in position and prevents the safety pin damaging the skin*
- secure the dressing in position *to prevent any drag on the drain or contamination of the wound*
- proceed as for the guidelines above.

Removing wound drains

This will be ordered by the medical practitioner when there is no longer any significant drainage from the wound.

- expose the drain site
- the skin should be cleansed only if this is needed *to ensure that the suture is visible*
- gloves should be worn *to prevent contamination with body fluids*
- release the vacuum or clamp the tubing *to prevent suction during removal*, which may cause tissue damage or pain (Nicol et al 2003)
- remove any stitches holding the drain in position

- support the skin round the drain site with one hand, using a sterile swab, and gently withdraw the drain using either a sterile gloved hand or sterile forceps held in the other hand. *This prevents damage to the surrounding tissues and helps to reduce discomfort as well as maintaining asepsis*
- maintain pressure over the wound after the drain has been removed (Smith et al 1999)
- the tip of the drain should be cut off with sterile scissors and placed in a sterile specimen container, maintaining asepsis, *if it is required for microbiological investigation*
- cleanse and dry the wound site again if necessary
- apply and secure an appropriate sterile dressing *to maintain asepsis and promote healing*
- proceed as for the guidelines above
- immediately dispatch the labelled specimen to the laboratory along with the completed form *so that investigative procedures may be completed as soon as possible*.

Emptying the portable wound suction container

The containers should be emptied as soon as they are no longer maintaining a vacuum suction, or every 12 hours as required *to measure drainage and prevent ascending infection*.

- clamp the drainage tubing above the level of the wound drainage container *to prevent backflow*
- remove the stopper or bung from the container, maintaining asepsis, *to release the vacuum*
- obtain a specimen of drainage fluid *for microbiological investigation if required*
- pour the remaining contents into a measuring jug, *avoiding contamination*
- wipe the outside of the entry channel with an alcohol solution, e.g. Mediswab, *to remove any drainage fluid that might cause infection*
- press the two rigid surfaces of the container together and maintain the pressure until the stopper is firmly in position. Once the pressure is removed, a gentle vacuum suction is created
- secure the drainage bag in position as before
- document the amount and details of the drainage fluid in the patient's records *so that accurate monitoring of the healing process and an evaluation of treatment can continue*
- in undertaking this practice, nurses are accountable for their actions, the quality of care delivered and record-keeping according to the Code of Professional Conduct: Standards for Conduct, Performance and Ethics (Nursing and Midwifery Council 2004) and Guidelines for Records and Record Keeping (Nursing and Midwifery Council 2005).

As a wound drain is in direct contact with the underlying tissues, pathogenic micro-organisms could gain entry to a wound through the drain site.
The maintenance of a closed drainage system and aseptic technique may help to reduce the chance of wound infection.

3. REMOVAL OF STITCHES, CLIPS AND STAPLES

Indications and rationale for the removal of stitches, clips and staples

Following surgery, stitches, clips, staples or tissue glue/super glue are used **to place the skin edges in apposition and promote rapid healing**. Unless absorbable, these are removed when there is:

- evidence of the wound having healed
- infection in part of the wound.

If the wound is greater than 15 cm in length, or if healing is slow, alternate sutures or clips may be removed (Nicol et al 2003). The remaining sutures should be removed when clinically indicated.

Absorbable sutures/glue are usually used for wounds that will heal quickly, requiring temporary support. Non-absorbable material (staples, non-absorbable sutures) offer longer mechanical support.

Adhesive sutures are sometimes applied to the wound edges when healing is not complete. Some wounds are sutured using a subcuticular method or tissue glue, e.g. Dermabond, and since biodegradable material is used these do not require manual removal. Research studies demonstrate ongoing discussion surrounding the various methods for surgical wound closure (Tritle et al 2001, Khan et al 2005) and the associated benefits and risks of each technique. Local preference will also influence the techniques used within different areas.

During suture, clip or staple removal, care must be taken to prevent the sharp equipment causing accidental injury to the patient.

Equipment

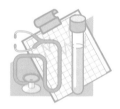

1. Dressing trolley/flat surface
2. Sterile dressing pack
3. Sterile normal saline (only if required to visualise the incision line)
4. Sterile stitch-cutter or scissors, clip or staple remover
5. Receptacle for soiled disposable items.

Guidelines and rationale for this nursing practice

- explain the procedure to the patient **to gain consent and co-operation**
- ensure the patient's privacy **to maintain dignity and a sense of self**
- collect the equipment **to help the efficiency of the practice**
- observe the patient throughout this activity **to detect any signs of discomfort or distress**
- clean the wound with normal saline only if it is necessary to gain access to the stitches, clips or staples
- examine the wound to ensure that it is appropriate to remove the sutures or clips.

Removing sutures

There are two main types of suture, continuous and individual (Fig. 49.4) – their method of removal being similar.

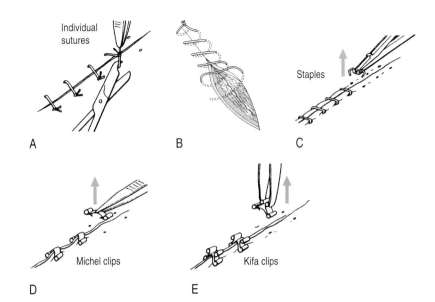

FIGURE 49.4
Removal of sutures, clips and staples
A Individual suture
B Continuous suture
C Staples
D Michel clips
E Kifa clips

For individual stitches:

- hold the stitch-cutter or scissors in the dominant hand and the dissecting forceps in the other hand **to lift the knot of the stitch gently** (*see* Fig. 49.4A)
- cut between the knot and the skin so that no part of the stitch above the skin surface is pulled under the tissues; then gently pull out the cut stitch. This helps **to reduce the risk of introducing infection**
- ensure that no piece of the stitch is left in the wound **as this could eventually form a wound sinus**.

For continuous stitches:

- hold the stitch-cutter or scissors in the dominant hand and the dissecting forceps in the other hand to lift gently the knot at one end of the suture line (*see* Fig. 49.4B)
- cut between the knot and the skin, so that no part of the stitch above the skin surface is pulled under the tissues. This helps **to reduce the risk of introducing infection**
- grasp the knot at the other end of the suture line and pull gently away from the wound **to remove the total suture intact**.

Removing clips or staples

- hold the remover in the dominant hand and the dissecting forceps in the other hand when removing clips or staples (*see* Fig. 49.4C–E)
- steady the clips or staples with the dissecting forceps. Depending on the type of clip or staple, either insert one blade of the remover under the centre of the clip or staple and the other blade over it, then gently squeeze the blades together, or place one blade of the remover on the outside of each wing on top of the clip and squeeze the blades together. Depending on the clip or staple type, one or other of these actions should lift the clip from the skin on either side of the wound

- follow local policy for the aftercare of a wound. The wound may be cleaned if necessary and then left exposed or covered with a dressing if discharge is present
- ensure that the patient is left as comfortable as possible
- dispose of all equipment safely *for the protection of others*
- document the nursing practice appropriately, monitor the after-effects and report any abnormal findings immediately
- in undertaking this practice, nurses are accountable for their actions, the quality of care delivered and record-keeping according to the Code of Professional Conduct: Standards for Conduct, Performance and Ethics (Nursing and Midwifery Council 2004) and Guidelines for Records and Record Keeping (Nursing and Midwifery Council 2005).

Patient/carer education

Key points

In partnership with the patient and/or carer, ensure that they are competent to carry out any practices required. Information should be given on an appropriate point of contact for any concerns that may arise.

The nurse should discuss the identified factors that may interfere with wound healing for each patient and, where possible, agree realistic goals for these factors with the patient. The nurse should provide information and education for the patient and/or carer relating to the care of the wound between each dressing change. The community nurse should agree and confirm the place, date and time of the next dressing change with the patient.

At home, the patient or carer may assume some or all of the responsibility for wound care; therefore the nurse has an important role in the education of all concerned.

Some education and guidance may have to be given to allay patients' fears that the wound will open up once the clips or sutures have been removed. Advice and guidance should be given on any lifestyle restrictions. Smoking in particular should be discouraged as it delays wound healing by causing vasoconstriction and reduced prostaglandin and fibrinogen production.

References

Aldameh A, McCall JL, Koea JB 2005 Is routine placement of surgical drains necessary after elective hepatecectomy? Results from a single institution. Journal of Gastrointestinal Surgery 9(5): 667–671

Barber LA 2002 Clean technique or sterile technique: let's take a moment to think. Journal of Wound, Ostomy and Continence Nursing 29(4): 29–32

British National Formulary 2005 British Medical Association/Royal Pharmaceutical Society of Great Britain, London

DeFloor T, Schoonhoven L 2004 Interrater reliability of the European Pressure Ulcer Advisory Classification System using photographs. Journal of Clinical Nursing 13(8): 952–954

Department of Health 1998 Data protection act. The Stationery Office, London

Fernandez R, Griffiths R, Ussia C 2002 Water for wound cleansing. Cochrane database of systematic reviews CD003861. Wiley, New York (Available at: http://www.cochrane.org/reviews/en/ab003861.html)

Hess C, Kirsner RS 2003 Uncover the latest techniques in wound bed preparation. Nursing Management 34(12): 54–56

Jeanes A 2005 Infection control. A practical guide to the use of hand decontaminants. Nursing Times 101(20): 46–48

Keast DH, Bowering CK, Evans AW et al 2004 A proposed assessment framework for developing best practice recommendations for wound assessment. Wound Repair and Regeneration 12(3): 51–57

Khan R, Nivbrant B, Wood D et al 2005 Different techniques of wound closure in arthroplasty surgery: a prospective randomised trial. The Journal of Bone and Joint Surgery 87-B(Suppl III): 368

MacDougall KM, Rodgers FRT 2004 A case study using larval therapy in the community setting. British Journal of Nursing 13(5): 255–260

Minnena B, Vearncombe MMD, Augustin A et al 2004 Risk factors for surgical site infection following primary total knee arthoplasty. Infection Control and Hospital Epidemiology 25(6): 477–480

National Institute for Clinical Excellence 2003 Infection control, prevention of healthcare associated infection in primary and secondary care. NICE, London

Nicol M, Bavin C, Bedford-Turner S et al 2003 Essential nursing skills, 2nd edn. Mosby, London

Nursing and Midwifery Council 2004 Code of professional conduct: standards for conduct, performance and ethics. NMC, London

Nursing and Midwifery Council 2005 Guidelines for records and record keeping. NMC, London

Rayatt SS, Dancey AL, Jaffe W 2005 Soft-fluted silicone drains: a prospective, randomised patient controlled study. Plastic and Reconstructive Surgery 115(6): 1605–1608

Shultz G, Mozingo D, Romanelli M et al 2005 Wound healing and TIME: new concepts and scientific applications. Wound Repair and Regeneration 13(4): S1–S11

Smith L, Baker F, McDougall C et al 1999 Removal of a vacuum drain. Nursing Times 95(Suppl 11): 1–2

Storr J, Clayton-Kent S 2004 Hand hygiene. Nursing Standard 18(40): 45–52, 54

Thomas S, Jones M 2000 Maggots can benefit patients with MRSA. Practice Nurse 20(2): 101–102, 104

Tritle NM, Haller JR, Gray D 2001 Aesthetic comparison of wound closure techniques in a porcine model. Laryngoscope 111(11): 1949–1951

Walmsley PJ, Kelly MB, Hill RMF et al 2005 A prospective randomised control trial of the use of drains in total hip arthroplasty. Journal of Joint and Bone Surgery 87-B(10): 1397–1401

Warriner R, Burrell R 2005 Infection and the chronic wound: a focus on silver. Advances in Skin and Wound Care 18(Suppl 8): 2–12

Websites

ConvaTec: http://www.convatec.com
Manufacturers of wound-care products

Journal of Woundcare: http://www.journalofwoundcare.com

National Institute for Clinical Excellence: http://www.nice.org.uk

Smith & Nephew: http://www.smith-nephew.com
Manufacturers of wound-care products

Wound Care Society: http://www.woundcaresociety.com

ZooBiotic Ltd: http://www.zoobiotic.com
Information about larval therapy

Self assessment

1. What is 'wound bed preparation'?
2. List the five types of tissue to be found in wound beds.
3. What properties should you look for when choosing a dressing?
4. How do you decide whether to cleanse a wound or not?
5. Discuss the different types of ways to close a surgical wound.

Index